Palgrave Studies in the History of Experience

Series Editors
Pirjo Markkola
Faculty of Social Sciences
Tampere University
Tampere, Finland

Raisa Maria Toivo
Faculty of Social Sciences
Tampere University
Tampere, Finland

Ville Kivimäki
Faculty of Social Sciences
Tampere University
Tampere, Finland

This series, a collaboration between Palgrave Macmillan and the Academy of Finland Centre of Excellence in the History of Experience (HEX) at Tampere University, will publish works on the histories of experience across historical time and global space. History of experience means, for the series, individual, social, and collective experiences as historically conditioned phenomena. 'Experience' refers here to a theoretically and methodologically conceptualized study of human experiences in the past, not to any study of 'authentic' or 'essentialist' experiences. More precisely, the series will offer a forum for the historical study of human experiencing, i.e. of the varying preconditions, factors, and possibilities shaping past experiences. Furthermore, the series will study the human institutions, communities, and the systems of belief, knowledge, and meaning as based on accumulated (and often conflicting) experiences.

The aim of the series is to deepen the methodology and conceptualization of the history of lived experiences, going beyond essentialism. As the series editors see it, the history of experience can provide a bridge between structures, ideology, and individual agency, which has been a difficult gap to close for historians and sociologists. The approach opens doors to see, study, and explain historical experiences as a social fact, which again offers new insights on society. Subjective experiences are seen as objectified into knowledge regimes, social order and divisions, institutions, and other structures, which, in turn, shape the experiences. The principle idea is to present a new approach, the history of experiences, as a way to establish the necessary connection between big and small history.

More information about this series at
http://www.palgrave.com/gp/series/16255

Ville Kivimäki • Peter Leese
Editors

Trauma, Experience and Narrative in Europe after World War II

palgrave
macmillan

Editors
Ville Kivimäki
Faculty of Social Sciences
Tampere University
Tampere, Finland

Peter Leese
Department of English, Germanic and
Romance Studies
University of Copenhagen
Copenhagen, Denmark

The book is an outcome of a workshop project "Historical Trauma Studies," funded by the Joint Committee for the Nordic Research Councils in the Humanities and Social Sciences (NOS-HS) in 2018–20.

ISSN 2524-8960   ISSN 2524-8979   (electronic)
Palgrave Studies in the History of Experience
ISBN 978-3-030-84662-6   ISBN 978-3-030-84663-3   (eBook)
https://doi.org/10.1007/978-3-030-84663-3

This Palgrave Macmillan imprint is published by the registered company Springer Nature Switzerland AG.
The registered company address is: Gewerbestrasse 11, 6330 Cham, Switzerland

Preface: Expanding the Field of Historical Trauma Studies

This book has its origins in a workshop project, "Historical Trauma Studies," funded by the Joint Committee for the Nordic Research Councils in the Humanities and Social Sciences (NOS-HS) in 2018–20. When planning the project in the mid-2010s, trauma had firmly established itself as a commonplace notion in public debate about past experiences of collective violence. Histories of both world wars, as well as many other violent aspects of the twentieth century, were increasingly being discussed from the perspective of trauma, thus emphasizing the mental shocks caused by modern industrialized warfare and genocide—and long, traumatic traces of these experiences in individual and collective memories. This development in the public discourse went hand in hand with academic research, where trauma studies have become a multifaceted research field extending across disciplines over the past 25 years. From the turn of the millennium onwards, historians too have been active in studying traumatic war experiences and their various psychiatric treatments and cultural and societal contexts, especially during and after World War I in Western Europe. Yet, as an analytical concept, trauma has been less popular in historical scholarship than in many other disciplines. Wary of the pitfalls of anachronism, historians have, for the most part, been reluctant to apply the psychological and cultural theories of trauma to past human experiences.

Consequently, in the "Historical Trauma Studies" project, we had four tasks in mind to permit furthering the discussions and debates on the applicability of trauma to history. The first three of them have sought to move the spatial, temporal, and thematic foci of empirical research, whereas the fourth aim is a more theoretical one. Spatially and temporally, we have wanted to examine a geographical area in history, an area that saw some of the most hideous violence of the twentieth century: the regions that lay between Nazi Germany and the Soviet Union between 1939 and 1945. How would the concept of trauma aid in analyzing these violent experiences in time and place, and how would this expansion of historical trauma studies from the "Western Front 1914–18" paradigm influence our understanding of traumatic pasts? Thematically, we have wanted to broaden the earlier emphasis on combatants' traumatic experiences at the front to incorporate the experiences of other, unarmed social groups whose sufferings—especially in the context of Central and Eastern Europe during World War II—often equaled and surpassed the experiences of violence at the frontlines. Another thematic expansion has been our intention to supplement the analysis of medical discourses and the treatment of psychological breakdowns with the study of *experiences* of trauma; and how people have expressed (and kept silent about) their traumatic experiences in different societal, political and cultural settings during and after the war. This leads to the project's fourth, theoretical aim: to think about new ways to study trauma in history and to recognize possible problems and shortcomings thereby. What are the limits and advantages of trauma as an analytical concept in historical study? What new interdisciplinary methodologies, concepts, and sources can we use to study historical trauma? What is the specific contribution of historical research to the study of trauma?

Inspired by these aims and questions, we organized the workshop "Aftershocks: War-related Trauma in Northern, Eastern, and Central Europe" at Tampere University, Finland, in October 2018. Most of the following chapters are based on the presentations given at this workshop. We hope that the current anthology will be a step forward in moving the discussions on historical traumas in the twentieth century into new, less studied territories—both geographical and methodological. It also seeks to be a contribution to the study of violence and its long-lasting traces in Europe. Looking at the histories of war-related trauma in Russia, Finland, former Yugoslavia, Ukraine, Slovakia, Poland, Hungary, and Lithuania, the book explores World War II and the histories of trauma from angles that have had less visibility in the Western European and American narratives. This approach reveals both cultural contingency and transnational parallels and patterns in the manner in which war-related trauma has manifested itself and affected people's lives. While expanding the scope of trauma studies within Europe, the book is further linked to the historical investigation of traumatic experiences and their treatments from a global and comparative perspective.

* * *

As the director of the "Historical Trauma Studies" project, it is a great pleasure to thank my colleagues Jason Crouthamel (Grand Valley State University, Michigan), Maria Fritsche (Norwegian University of Science and Technology, Trondheim), Peter Leese (University of Copenhagen), and Barbara Törnquist-Plewa (Lund University) most warmly for co-organizing the project. I am grateful to the authors of the book, who have shown great flexibility and commitment to our joint effort despite the practical problems and delays brought on by the Covid-19 pandemic. It has been a real joy to co-edit this anthology with Peter, whose expertise in trauma studies and editorial experience has been invaluable. Professor Mark Edele, from the University of Melbourne, accepted our invitation to read through the chapters and write a Coda for the anthology, something we appreciate very much. Carl Wieck did a wonderful job as always in checking and correcting the book's English, and Lauri Uusitalo has been a great help in copyediting. It has been a pleasure to work with Emily Russell and Antony Sami at Palgrave. My own work has been sponsored first by the Academy of Finland's postdoctoral research project "Trauma before Trauma" (2016–19) and then by the Academy of Finland Centre of Excellence in the History of Experiences, at Tampere University. Finally, I want to thank the Joint Committee for the Nordic Research Councils in the Humanities and Social Sciences most sincerely for financing our project.

Tampere, Finland   Ville Kivimäki
October 2021

CONTENTS

Part I   Comparative Approaches   1

1   The Limits of Trauma: Experience and Narrative in
    Europe c. 1945   3
    Peter Leese

2   Beyond the Western Front   27
    Mark S. Micale

Part II   Case Studies   53

3   Testing the Silence: Trauma and Military Psychiatry
    in Soviet Russia and Ukraine During and After
    World War II   55
    Robert Dale

4   Experiencing Trauma Before Trauma: Posttraumatic
    Memories, Nightmares and Flashbacks Among Finnish
    Soldiers   89
    Ville Kivimäki

5   Entangled Bystanders: Multidimensional Trauma of
    Ethnic Cleansing and Mass Violence in Eastern Galicia   119
    Anna Wylegała

6   Traumatized Children in Hungary After World War II   149
    Tuomas Laine-Frigren

7   "We will cry a little, but then we will forget": Narratives
    of Loss and Victory in Postwar Yugoslavia   177
    Ana Antić

8   Guilt, Responsibility and Trauma: Restoring the Moral
    Self-Image in Postwar Slovakia   207
    Hana Kubátová

9   "Perpetrator Trauma" in Memoirs of Veterans of the
    Polish Home Army   233
    Marta Kurkowska-Budzan

10 Environmental Trauma in the Narratives of Postwar
    Reconstruction: The Loss of Place and Identity in
    Northern Finland After World War II   267
    Outi Autti

11 Suicide Rates as a "Social Thermometer": Reading the
    Traumatized History of Lithuania   299
    Danutė Gailienė

Part III   Coda   319

12 Towards a History of Trauma in Central and Eastern
    Europe After World War II: A Coda   321
    Mark Edele

Index   333

Notes on Contributors

Ana Antić is a professor MSO of European History at the Department of English, Germanic and Romance Studies at the University of Copenhagen, Denmark. She specializes in the cultural and social history of psychiatry, war, and violence. She is currently leading an ERC project on the history of postcolonial and transcultural psychiatry. She is the author of *Therapeutic Fascism: Experiencing the Violence of the Nazi New Order* (2017).

Outi Autti works at the University of Oulu, Finland, at the School of Architecture in the interdisciplinary research area of Arctic Architecture and Environmental Adaptation. Autti specializes in multidisciplinary research in the fields of environmental sociology, migration studies, rural education, and human geography. She holds the Title of Docent in Cultural Sociology at the University of Lapland. Her current research interests include the human-environment relationship, health and well-being in the northern circumpolar areas, people's experiences, and the social contexts of their narratives. Power relations, inequality, and marginal positions have been of interest to her throughout her research career.

Robert Dale is Lecturer in Russian History at Newcastle University, UK. His work focuses on the impact of World War II on the Soviet Union, with a particular focus on the reconstruction of the late Stalinist state and society, and the traumatic memories and experiences of combatants. In addition to his monograph *Demobilized Veterans in Late Stalinist Leningrad: Soldiers to Civilians* (2015), he has written articles in the *Journal of Contemporary History*, the *Russian Review*, *Contemporary*

European History, and *Kritika: Explorations in Russian and European History*, as well as several essays on war trauma in edited volumes.

Mark Edele is the Hansen Professor in History at the University of Melbourne, Australia. His publications include *Soviet Veterans of the Second World War* (2008), *Stalinist Society: 1928–1953* (2011), *Stalin's Defectors* (2017), *The Soviet Union: A Short History* (2019), *Debates on Stalinism* (2020); *The Politics of Veteran Benefits in the Twentieth Century: A Comparative History* (2020), with Martin Crotty and Neil Diamant; and *Stalinism at War: The Soviet Union in World War II* (2021). He is a chief investigator on the ARC Discovery Grants "KGB Empire: State Security Archives in the former Eastern Bloc" (2020–23); and "Aftermaths of War: Violence, Trauma, Displacement, 1815–1950" (2020–24).

Danutė Gailienė is Professor of Clinical Psychology at Vilnius University, Lithuania. She has specialized in the field of clinical psychology and is the author of many scientific articles and books. She initiated the very first studies on suicidology and psychotraumatology in Lithuania, with special emphasis on the traumatizing effects of long-term political repression and intergenerational transmission of trauma and resilience. She has edited, inter alia, *The Psychology of Extreme Traumatization: The Aftermath of Political Repression* (2005) and *Lithuanian Faces after Transition: Psychological Consequences of Cultural Trauma* (2015).

Ville Kivimäki is a senior research fellow at Tampere University, Finland. He leads the Lived Nation research team at the Academy of Finland's Centre of Excellence in the History of Experiences (HEX). Kivimäki has specialized in the social and cultural history of World War II and its aftermath and in the intertwined histories of trauma, gender, nationalism, experience, and emotions. In his doctoral dissertation *Battled Nerves* (2013), he studied the history of traumatic war experiences and military psychiatry in Finland. He has co-edited, among others, *Finland in World War II: History, Memory, Interpretations* (2012) and *Lived Nation as the History of Experiences and Emotions in Finland, 1800–2000* (2021).

Hana Kubátová is an assistant professor at the Charles University in Prague, Czech Republic. Her areas of research include majority-minority relations in wartime Slovakia, the social history of the Holocaust, and the relationship between memory and robbery. Her contributions have appeared in *Contemporary European History, Holocaust Studies: A Journal of Culture and History, Nations and Nationalism*, and other scholarly publications. She has recently co-authored *The Jew in Czech and Slovak Imagination, 1938–89: Antisemitism, the Holocaust and Zionism* (2018), and co-edited *Jews and Gentiles in Central and Eastern Europe during the Holocaust: History and Memory* (2018).

Marta Kurkowska-Budzan is Associate Professor of History at Jagiellonian University in Krakow, Poland. She leads the "Homo [Lab]orans" interdisciplinary and international research and education initiative at Jagiellonian University. Her areas of expertise are the cultural history of twentieth century Poland, heritage studies, and the methodology of historical research (oral history in particular). Her published work includes the symbolization of the past in contemporary Polish public discourses (*Antykomunistyczne podziemie zbrojne na Białostocczyźnie: Analiza współczesnej symbolizacji przeszłości*, 2009), in addition to the cultural history of sports in Poland under the communist regime (together with M. Stasiak, *Stadion na peryferiach*, 2016).

Tuomas Laine-Frigren is a postdoctoral research fellow at the Academy of Finland's Centre of Excellence in the History of Experiences (HEX) at Tampere University, Finland. Laine-Frigren is specialized in the history of childhood, mental health, and psychological sciences. In his ongoing research project, he studies the readjustment of child evacuees returning to Finland after World War II. In his doctoral dissertation *Searching for the Human Factor* (University of Jyväskylä, 2016), he studied the history of psychological expertise and social planning in Cold War Hungary. Together with Markku Hokkanen and Jari Eilola, he has edited *Encountering Crises of the Mind: Madness, Culture and Society, 1200s–1900s* (2018).

Peter Leese is Associate Professor of Social and Cultural History, Department of English, Germanic and Romance Studies, at the University of Copenhagen, Denmark. His publications include *Shell Shock: Traumatic Neurosis and the British Soldiers of the First World War* (2002; revised paperback in 2014), *Britain since 1945: Aspects of Identity* (2006) and *Migrant Representations: Life-story, Investigation, Picture* (2022). He is the co-editor of various collections, including *Languages of Trauma: History, Memory, and Media* (2021), *Traumatic Memories of World War Two and After* (2016), *Psychological Trauma and the Legacies of the First World War* (2016), and *Narration, Migration and Identity: Cross-cultural Perspectives* (2012).

Mark S. Micale is Emeritus Professor of History at the University of Illinois in Urbana-Champaign, USA. His fields of specialization include modern European intellectual and cultural history; France from the Revolution to the present; the history of science and medicine, especially psychiatry; psychoanalytic studies, and masculinity studies. He is the author or editor of several books, including *Beyond the Unconscious* (1993); *Discovering the History of Psychiatry* (with Roy Porter, 1994); and *Hysterical Men: The Hidden History of Male Nervous Illness* (2008). In 2001, Paul Lerner and he published the edited collection *Traumatic Pasts: History, Psychiatry, and Trauma in the Modern Age, 1870–1930*. Micale's most recent books are *The Darker Angels of Our Nature: Refuting the Pinker Theory of History and Violence* (co-edited with Philip Dwyer, 2021) and *Traumatic Pasts in Asia: History, Psychiatry, and Trauma from the 1930s to the Present* (co-edited with Hans Pols, 2021). After 30 years of teaching, he retired in 2018 and now lives in Los Angeles.

Anna Wylegała is Assistant Professor of Sociology at the Institute of Philosophy and Sociology of the Polish Academy of Sciences. Her research focus is on the social history and memory of World War II and the postwar period in Poland and Ukraine. She is the author of *Displaced Memories: Remembering and Forgetting in Post-War Poland and Ukraine* (2019) and co-editor of *The Burden of the Past: History and Identity in Contemporary Ukraine* (2020).

LIST OF FIGURES

Fig. 10.1 The research area: the biggest municipality centers and hydro-
electric power plants in Northern Finland. (Map by Juhani
Päivärinta, Outi Autti and Anu Soikkeli)   271
Fig. 11.1 Suicide rates in Lithuania 1924–39 and 1962–2018. (Source:
Paulius Skruibis, Paper presented at the International
Association for Suicide Prevention conference in Derry, 2019)   301
Fig. 11.2 Lithuanian male and female suicide rates over two periods—
pre-war (1930–39) and postwar (1962–2018)   304

PART I

Comparative Approaches

The Limits of Trauma: Experience and Narrative in Europe c. 1945

Peter Leese

INTRODUCTION

The practices, technologies and narratives that constitute trauma adjust continually according to their time and place. One such time and place, Europe in the 1940s and in the later postwar era, was a site of particularly notable human destruction. While much went undocumented, the responses of perpetrators and those against whom actions were directed both register a strong psychological response that to this day remains difficult to effectively name, describe or process. Part of the difficulty is social. The debilitation of a mental wound may be difficult to admit of because it carries the strong possibility of stigmatization, discrimination and implied personal weakness. Part of the difficulty is cultural. Different norms of thinking, believing and behaving reveal or disguise mental suffering in line with local cultural criteria. Part of the difficulty is historical. Although

P. Leese (✉)
Department of English, Germanic and Romance Studies, University of Copenhagen, Copenhagen, Denmark
e-mail: leese@hum.ku.dk

© The Author(s), under exclusive license to Springer Nature Switzerland AG 2022
V. Kivimäki, P. Leese (eds.), *Trauma, Experience and Narrative in Europe after World War II*, Palgrave Studies in the History of Experience, https://doi.org/10.1007/978-3-030-84663-3_1

there is a significant brain physiology for traumatic memory, the past is also another country that needs ethnographic interpretation, for example, in relation to concepts of mental health or illness.

The past is also subject to intense present-day political demands in relation to the identity and conduct of communities, to states as well as to international relations. For many European nations, World War II and its aftermath represent a founding moment for political settlement and revision persisting into the twenty-first century, as the essays in *Trauma, Experience and Narrative in Europe During and After World War II* show. The cultural politics of the present, contemporary definitions of trauma included, also tends to obscure the recent past. Trauma in the twenty-first century is a failing concept because it has become so widely embraced, because it increasingly seems present at all times and in all places. Trauma has also been highly successful as a concept since the 1990s because it highlights otherwise difficult to see issues of human suffering and the related need for human rights, justice and reconciliation. Like the concept of trauma itself, our present-day notions of human rights, of truth, reconciliation and justice, have gained particular prominence in the wake of the Cold War. Applied retrospectively to the ideological and cultural divisions that grew so powerfully after 1945, it is difficult to avoid present-minded misreadings of trauma. Nor has the end of the Cold War lessened the retrospective tendency to divide nations and communities into "blocs" of victors, perpetrators and victims. Such distortions predispose us to particular ways of seeing, to historical and memory blind spots or to simplified assumptions of guilt, innocence and moral ascendancy.

This leads naturally to the question of how the postwar era might be reconceived thirty or more years after the end of the Cold War. While scholars from Central and Eastern Europe remain chronically underfunded and consequently do not often achieve the international reach of their western colleagues, anybody who has engaged directly with these scholarly communities knows its inventiveness and vibrancy. This is not a matter only of "younger" scholars—perhaps a polite euphemism for "more exposed to the West"—but also of many who were trained within a rigorous university education system that excluded a large portion of the population but nevertheless produced successive generations of skilled, insightful scholars both before and after 1989. I mention the material conditions of knowledge production to suggest that local conditions are easily misconstrued, that ideological coordinates set from a distant bearing and without the benefit of lived experience are rarely sufficient to survey a terrain fully. I suggest that we might gain new insights by rejecting the still persistent Cold War distinctions of West and East, by rejecting the notion that "bloodlands" belong more to one part of Europe than to another. At the very least, common western preconceptions can hardly do justice to the complexity and diversity of post-World War II developments in Central and Eastern Europe or the Baltic states.

This raises another critical question recently put forward by two Polish scholars, namely, how Europe remembers from its eastern quarters. For Małgorzata Pakier and Joanna Wawrzyniak, "regional" studies more often than not suggest work that is peripheral or "outside the norm." Yet the rapidly emergent canons of western memorialization, commemoration and recollection cannot adequately account for the local, and tend to distort by their emphasis on difference and exceptionality.[1] The intricacies and contradictions of competing memory cultures are well illustrated by the ways in which different nation states choose to remember or forget aspects of their pasts, identities, or give particular emphasis to certain memories. Taking these differences seriously, at once sets up very different genealogies of memory that may relate more closely to each other than to the predominantly western models. Notions of who or what constitutes witness, the affluent conditions of commemoration, the dynamics of memory transmission within families and across generations need to be understood within local settings rather than across transnational "regions."[2] In what follows, I use conceptualizations of trauma—its historical contexts and histories, its forms of narrative conceptualization and expression, its cultural variations—to consider some of these differences, parallels and similarities across time and space, and within Europe's early postwar era.

The Long 1945

The dynamics of cross-cultural understanding grow more complex when engaged with a central theme throughout this collection, namely traumatic memory. Such memories do not appear mechanically as an

---

[1] Małgorzata Pakier and Joanna Wawrzyniak, eds, *Memory and Change in Europe: Eastern Perspectives* (New York: Berghahn, 2015), 10–12.

[2] A still useful model of how memory genealogies may be constructed is Jay Winter's essay "The Great War in the Memory Boom of the Twentieth Century," in his *Remembering War* (New Haven: Yale University Press, 2006), 17–51.

automatic or universal response to particular events. Rather, the presence and persistence of traumatic memories depends on the subsequent life-story of the teller, on the material and political conditions within which a troubled recollection returns. As a result, traumatic memories are highly variable, subject to continual shifts across societies and generations, and only gain a limited degree of consensual canonization very gradually, over decades and generations.[3] In the context of Europe during and after 1945, the gradual, troubled and slow acknowledgment of trauma is part of a wider process: a recognition of human suffering in our present. In Targol Mesbah's formulation, this public reckoning is a counter-discourse of trauma "situated within the tradition of articulating, bringing into a field of sayable experiences, experiences [...] that have been otherwise excluded from official discourse."[4]

This introductory essay to *Trauma, Experience and Narrative in Europe During and After World War II* tries to contextualize in various settings the start of one particular "bringing into sayability," and to explain some of the ways in which this group of related essays promotes a new agenda for trauma and memory studies not only connected to Eastern European and Baltic states. In what follows, I first consider the relevant historical conditions—both before and after 1945—to stress continuity and development rather than any dramatic shift or rupture at the moment violent conflict ceased. Second, I consider the complex, diverse and shifting connections as well as the discontinuities between trauma, history and Europe at around the same time. Third, I deal with the relation of narrative, emotions and experiences as I understand them historically, conceptually and methodologically. Fourth, I address the issue of cultural, social and historical variations in the constitution of traumatic symptoms and memories. A final issue, cutting across various essays in this collection, relates to commemoration, memorialization and healing narratives. Borrowing Barbara Rosenwein's terminology for emotions in history, I suggest that there are both "generations of trauma" and "trauma communities." As Rosenwein puts it, "Emotional communities adapt the traditions to their own needs. Sometimes they produce new words and new sequences built

---

[3] Carolyn J. Dean, "Erasures: Writing History and Holocaust Trauma," in *Science and Emotions after 1945: A Transatlantic Perspective*, ed. by Frank Biess and Daniel M. Gross (Chicago: Chicago University Press, 2014), 388–93.

[4] Targol Mesbah, "Why Does the Other Suffer? War, Trauma and the Everyday," Ph.D. thesis (University of California, Santa Cruz, 2006), 44.

on the older ones. That is what I mean by 'generations of feeling': the constant availability and potentiality of older and coexisting emotional traditions."[5] This formulation is especially useful since it connects emotions to the particular time, place, and social setting in which they were experienced. Equally, it acknowledges the need to investigate the particular conditions—practices, technologies and narratives—that articulate any particular manifestation of traumatic memory.

While traumatic memory has much in common with emotional states—malleability, subjective conceptualization, environmental influences—it cannot be reduced to a bundle of mental responses. The psychological suffering that resulted from World War II was unprecedented in its breadth, reach and longevity. Its historical peculiarity lay in the powerful emotional states that accompanied fascism, in the scale and disruption caused by the war, in the mass population displacements and emotional extremities of suffering caused by family and community separations as well as by deaths. All of which pressurized rational behavior, non-expressive temperament and civic nationalism in the postwar years.[6] This response is not surprising given the conditions of the war and the inevitable longevity of its collective effects. Over half of the casualties were civilians; the legacy of physical, martial and emotional destruction was inevitable following the deaths of large portions of Europe's population, including around six million Jews as well as millions of Poles, Germans, Russians and Ukrainians.[7] Likewise, the destabilization of political regimes, retributions, and the imposition of newly established state regimes meant a decade or more of troubled, halting recovery punctuated by mass population shifts and political upheavals.[8] Given these ongoing deprivations, the struggles for physical survival, sustenance and the very gradual emergence of new stability within the civic societies, neighborhoods and local communities of Europe's eastern and Baltic reaches, it is no surprise that traumatic memories began to form, although their presence may not have been evenly or

[5] Barbara H. Rosenwein, *Generations of Feeling: A History of Emotions, 600–1700* (Cambridge: Cambridge University Press, 2016), 9.

[6] Frank Biess and Daniel M. Gross, "Emotional Returns," in Biess and Gross, eds (2014), 4.

[7] Timothy Snyder, "European Mass Killing and European Commemoration," in *Remembrance, History and Justice: Coming to Terms with Traumatic Pasts in Democratic Societies*, ed. by Vladimir Tismaneanu and Bogdan G. Iacob (Budapest: Central European University, 2015), 25–6.

[8] Mark Mazower, *Dark Continent: Europe's Twentieth Century* (London: Penguin, 1998), 221–2.

predictably mapped. If such a mapping had been possible, widespread public participation in procedures of recognition and acknowledgment would surely have been a very basic prerequisite, and, even then, might well have had only a marginal prophylactic effect. In reality, conditions were less than ideal: ideological and highly politicized versions of World War II were often compulsory in public ceremonies; the silencing or active disapproval of dissenting groups or troubling incidents prevented even local community recognition or family acknowledgments.[9]

It is also important to recognize that a diversity of war outcomes and postwar settlements is not the same as inherently greater suffering, trauma or backwardness. The highly variable presence or absence of traumatic memory is not necessarily more or less in any particular time or place; politicizations, erasures or delayed responses may occur in all kinds of conditions. Likewise, while the dynamics of connected traumatic memories are highly variable, there are some common generational features and processes. One sign of these common patterns is the delayed emergence of Primo Levi's writing, which only became well known in the 1970s as a part of the wider, emergent "memory boom" of that time. Such delays in public discourse—the transfer between private and family recollection and subsequent engagement via films, museums or book sales—relate in part to the Cold War and the rather more urgent political upheavals of 1956 or 1968. What matters here, too, is the gradual resettlement of displaced persons as well as the continuation of conflict in various zones after 1945, for example, nationalist resistance to the postwar settlement in Poland.[10] A later, equally decisive, shift in the dynamics of collective memory also takes place across the European continent following 1989, with certain kinds of events receiving new attention and new interpretations. It is particularly after 2001 that attention to trauma grows decisively and becomes a more widely recognized vector through which to register and acknowledge formerly overlooked, unrecognized past sufferings.

Among those most acutely and chronically affected, because of their wartime experiences and their lives during the aftermath of war, were children, refugees and women, both as participants and civilians. Many

---

[9] Peter Gattrell, "From 'Homelands' to 'Warlands': Themes, Approaches, Voices," in *Warlords: Population, Resettlement and State Reconstruction in the Soviet East-European Borderlands, 1945–50*, ed. by Peter Gattrell and Nick Baron (London: Palgrave, 2009), 13–4.

[10] Dan Stone, "Postwar Europe as History," in *The Oxford Handbook of Postwar European History*, ed. by Dan Stone (Oxford: Oxford University Press, 2012), 3–4.

children, for example, were witnesses to the atrocities of conflict but equally became witnesses to the aftereffects of conflict through engagement with the lives of family members. Likewise, family separation, displacement, loss or severe injury of parents had a lifelong impact. The Red Cross received over 300,000 queries in search of lost parents and children in 1945–1948. Of the approximately twelve million human beings displaced in Germany at the end of the war—from Poland, Czechoslovakia, Hungary, Romania, Yugoslavia and the Baltic states—around 1.4 million were minors under the age of fourteen.[11] Despite the increasing limitations of the trauma concept because of its current popularization and widespread usage, one effect has been fuller investigation into and recognition of the troubled experiences and memories of increasingly diverse groups. As the essays in this collection show, if ex-servicemen are the most obvious group to suffer adverse psychological effects, other less acknowledged groups include women participants and veterans, civilians and bystanders, perpetrators of atrocities and defeated populations from the very young to the elderly. Psychological injury also now attaches to a far greater variety of circumstances than direct exposure to atrocity. Among the most recently and urgently recognized is the extent to which physical environment, and infrastructural and environmental destruction impact the psyche.

For those whose lives are altered irrevocably by the events of war and its aftermath, and more particularly by the remembrance of those events, such acknowledgments are an essential act, and a precursor to any achievement of social justice. In this respect traumatic memory is an involuntary act of commemoration. Since the rememberer has no choice but to again bring to mind life-disrupting and painful past events, the opportunity for recognition and acknowledgment remains potential, although the effects of recognition can never actually be guaranteed. Moreover, the irreducible persistent presence of such traumatic pasts can be as disruptive as they are elegiac or therapeutic. Quality of life as well as personal family relations with children, parent or partner can all be long-term casualties of such conditions.[12] In this respect, successive generations have continued to live

---

[11] Tara Zahra, "'The Psychological Marshall Plan': Displacement, Gender and Human Rights after World War Two," *Central European History* 44:1 (2011), 41–3.

[12] Alice Förster and Birgit Beck, "Post-Traumatic Stress Disorder and World War II: Can a Psychiatric Concept Help Us Understand a Postwar Society?," in *Life after Death: Approaches to a Cultural and Social History During the 1940s*, ed. by Richard Bessel and Dirk Schumann (Washington D.C: German Historical Institute / Cambridge University Press, 2003), 32–3.

in the uncanny, unhomely psychological ruins of war. Relegating the past to a position of irrelevance, moving on to the possibilities of a present, or a particular future, is not possible. An ongoing sense of mortality, of the past, and of a marginal position in the world of events, are the side effects of traumatic memory. It makes the "long 1945" a persistent presence that may remain throughout the course of a lifetime to cast a shadow over the lives of future generations.[13]

Histories of Traumatic Stress

These longer-term effects are being increasingly acknowledged and investigated. As Mark Micale points out in his essay for this collection, trauma and traumatic memory have histories, and expanding historiographies. *Trauma, Experience and Narrative in Europe During and After World War II* provides an opportunity to develop both of these further by concentrated attention to a particular time and place.[14] Our interest as editors has been to reflect on commonalities and disjunctions within a particular, limited frame, but also to seek out connections to earlier and later medical, social and cultural conceptualizations of trauma. There is no simple, traceable line of connection here, but, rather, a complex set of variable concepts, mental conditions and medical understandings that need to be interpreted on their own terms. A second aspect of particular interest has been the construction of a cross-cultural perspective that avoids the imposition of normative Western European and North American frameworks.

While there is some merit to the notion of a "return from war" as a timeless, placeless condition, the limitations of such a framework are equally apparent. To go further into the time-based particularities of post-traumatic conditions, it is necessary to engage with specific medical and social practices, technologies and modes of narrative expression. It is also critical to move beyond institutional frameworks of diagnosis, treatment and representation: to engage with communal interest groups; the medical and social triage of psychological war damage; the specific efforts and

[13] Rebecca Bryant, "History's Remainders: On Time and Objects After Conflict in Cyprus," *American Enthnologist* 41:4 (2014) 681–2.

[14] For further studies using this approach see, for example, Mark Micale and Paul Lerner, eds, *Traumatic Pasts: History, Psychiatry, and Trauma in the Modern Age, 1870–1930* (Cambridge: Cambridge University Press, 2001); Jason Crouthamel and Peter Leese, eds, *Psychological Trauma and the Legacies of the First World War* (Cham: Palgrave Macmillan, 2016).

resources mobilized under local conditions.[15] One approach that would enable a comparative typology of traumatic responses across cultures, medical regimes and social practices would be an analysis of three widespread but variously employed concepts, namely "shock," "stress" and "trauma." All three terms have both physiological and psychological aspects; they also overlap in historical usage, though shock, for example, often retains a predominantly physical implication.

World War II is especially interesting in this respect as it was a moment when "shock," or similar notions of fatigue, suggesting a concussion-like impact and its after effect, were first rivaled by newer, emergent notions of "stress." The emphasis on physical conditions is still present in diagnostic terminology or related treatments. Closely related are views of moral and behavioral stigmatization associated with varied "mental" conditions. Understanding or acceptance of the legitimacy of psychological injury remains highly variable and generally only begins to gain wider acceptance—if at all—in the aftermath of World War II.[16] Attention to the effects of time, like close attention to terminologies and concepts, is a connected theme within histories of traumatic stress, especially when considering variation across cultural boundaries. The troubling event or set of circumstances may be momentary or prolonged, but, more importantly, it is either anticipated or regarded retrospectively.[17] We may see this, for example, in notions of "attendant expectation," as described in physician Daniel Hack Tuke in his 1884 account of the effects of a train crash. A related example is the conceptualization of "combat fatigue" as a depletion or diminution of physical and psychological resources.[18] While the high-modernist theoreticians of the psyche were not far removed in time from these developments, their practical influence on the everyday treatment of industrial or industrialized warfare mental conditions was

[15] Allan Young, *The Harmony of Illusions: Inventing Post-traumatic Stress Disorder* (Princeton, NJ: Princeton University Press, 1995), 5.

[16] Ferec Erős, "From War Neurosis to Holocaust Trauma: An Intellectual and Cultural History," *S.I.M.O.N.Shoah: Intervention, Methods, Documentation* 1 (2017), 41.

[17] Rhodri Hayward, "Sadness in Camberwell: Imagining Stress and Constructing History in Postwar Britain," in *Stress, Shock and Adaptation on the Twentieth Century*, ed. by David Cantor and Edmund Ramsden (Rochester, NY: Boydell and Brewer/University of Rochester, 2014), 320.

[18] Daniel Hack Tuke, *Illustrations of the Influence of the Mind Upon the Body in Health and Disease* (Philadelphia: Henry C. Lea, 1884), ix–x; Roy Grinker and John Spiegel, *Men Under Stress* (Philadelphia: Blakestone, 1945).

marginal. At best, popularization of the psyche as an explanatory model gradually allowed discussion, increased professionalization, and the potential conditions for de-stigmatization. Walter Cannon's "Voodoo Death" article, published in 1942, provides an explicit link between nineteenth and mid-twentieth century conceptualizations. Investigating unexplained deaths among "primitive peoples," Cannon also refers to soldiers both in World War I trenches and civilians in the Spanish Civil War whose sudden deaths could not be explained by physical injury, but, rather, by "the classic symptoms of mental shock" expressed in "malignant anxiety" and a "perturbed state deeply involving the sympathico-adrenal complex."[19] The intriguing implication that World War I soldiers in the trenches of the Western Front also experienced a kind of "Voodoo Death" was not much commented upon then or since, but in other ways Cannon's account previews emergent thinking after World War II. In particular, Cannon illustrates a newly developing sense of bodily sensitivity to the psyche and nervous system that gradually yields new insights for physiology, psychiatry and anthropology, among other disciplines. A longer-term consequence was the popularization and growing explanatory power of the stress concept as it emerges through the second half of the twentieth century.[20]

Recognition and investigation of mid-twentieth century traumatic memories have similarly been patchy and slow. Early acknowledgments are connected most often to the practical wartime requirements of discipline, human resource management and combat efficiency. Wider social, medical or physiological responses emerged for the most part retrospectively in response to the insistence on as well as the obvious needs of particular interest groups such as veterans. It is no coincidence that a relatively affluent, well-educated society was able to most effectively articulate, and to some extent alleviate, the mental suffering of ex-servicemen, or that the diagnosis of post-traumatic stress disorder (PTSD) was first framed in order to secure legitimate claims for financial compensation. The possibility or purpose of acknowledgment in other times or settings has been less clear. Notions of survival or witness develop in tandem with ideas of stress and trauma. Later on, the new, critical category of traumatic memory emerges more clearly and allows for fuller acknowledgment of effects on

---

[19] Walter B. Cannon, "Voodoo Death," *American Anthropologist* 44:2 (1942), 179–80.

[20] Otniel Dror, "From Primitive Fear to Civilized Stress: Sudden Unexpected Death," in Cantor and Ramsden, eds (2014), 99–101.

children and across generations. For many groups, during and after World War II, the difficulty of acknowledgment was related to social and political stigmatization—visible differences of behavior or speech that provoked fears of "madness." Unacceptable memories or stories of witness might also prompt political or communal hostility. Silence and invisibility were the inevitable result when any other response potentially caused greater harm. Marginal groups might also lack the means to articulate or advocate recognition. Hence the difficulties experienced by many groups, including first and second generation "Hibaksha"—survivors of the United States atomic bomb detonations at the end of World War II; genocide survivors of Armenian, Cambodian or Yugoslavian origin; indigenous peoples of Australian or North American descent and African origin. To the long list of twentieth-century survivors we might add populations persecuted under dictatorship regimes in Chile, Argentina, South Africa or Iran.[21]

As this list suggests, there is no simple way to reconcile or amalgamate these highly variable sets of social circumstances and memory contexts. What they have in common in the second half of the twentieth century and the early decades of the twenty-first century is a tendency towards non-articulation, incommunicability and repression, which may be self-imposed, but which might also result from particular local, communal or wider political conditions. In the case of Central and Eastern Europe as well as the Baltic states, the relative nearness as well as recent Cold-War-related constructions of east-west "difference" tend to obscure local specificities. Yet, in certain respects a similar set of historical developments since World War II is certainly present. For those most directly affected by World War II, there is a prolonged pause, a phase of collective recovery, during which time relatively little is said. The social effects of this near silence are expressed in difficulties of communication with the wider society and difficulties in resolving traumatic memories or coming to terms with the past. The turbulent political and economic conditions of the early postwar years, in contrast to slowly emergent affluence and political stability, both generated and reinforced traumatic memories. The emergence of a "multidimensional approach"—which incorporates biological, communal, cultural and religious aspects, as well as a gradually fuller understanding of cross-generation transmission—suggests some of the origins of such mental conditions. Work concerning Argentina similarly outlines both the

[21] Yael Danieli, ed., *International Handbook of Multigenerational Legacies of Trauma* (New York: Plenum Press, 1998), 4.

phases of development that enable effective coping and reconciliation as well as the social requirements necessary to enable retrospectively the resolution of traumatic memories.[22] In another study, a set of five conditions necessary for survival and adaptation following violence, conflict conditions or other potentially traumatizing circumstances also suggests a possible agenda that historians might follow when investigating particular local conditions. These are worth listing as a potential framework for future historical research: first, conditions of safety and security; second, attachment to families, social networks and rituals; third, engagement with justice, including truth, punishment and reconciliation; fourth, sufficient rebuilding of role identity; fifth, concern with existential meaning, including morality, belief systems and cultural expression.[23] The difficulties of achieving such conditions in early postwar Europe were of course substantial, given that traumatic memory can be aptly characterized as "shot through with holes," and the likely delay, postponement or abandonment of resolution even in ideal circumstances.[24]

Thinking further about the potential resolution of traumatic memories, the disparity between private reminiscence and public commemoration also matters. Violations of personhood and the traumatized memories that result are, by definition, filled with gaps and disruptions. In one interpretation of this process, personal narratives characteristically split off and slip out of speakability to become spectral and incomplete presences. The difficulties of achieving narrativization in the face of such emotional and cognitive fragmentation thereafter become all the more greater.[25] In the particular social and political conditions of early postwar Central, Eastern and Baltic European states this fragmentation was strengthened by a more general damping down of intense emotions. Passion, blind enthusiasm, extreme devotion to nation and charismatic national leaders: these were seen as the excesses that led to the conflict, violence and atrocities of World

---

[22] Elizabeth Jelin and Susana G. Kaufman, "Layers of Memory: Twenty Years After in Argentina," in *The Politics of War Memory and Commemoration*, ed. by T.G. Ashplant, Graham Dawson and Michael Roper (London: Routledge, 2000), 89–110.

[23] Derrick Silove, "From Trauma to Survival and Adaptation: Towards a Framework for Guiding Mental Health Initiatives in Post-conflict Societies," in *Forced Migration and Mental Health: Rethinking the Care of Refugees and Displaced Persons*, ed. by David Ingleby (New York: Springer, 2005), 42.

[24] Marilyn Charles and Michael O'Laughlin, eds, *Fragments of Trauma and the Social Production of Suffering: Trauma, History, and Memory* (Lanham: Rowman and Littlefield, 2014), 4.

[25] Charles and O'Laughlin (2014), 4.

War II. One postwar reaction was a more neutral mode of emotional response, a reluctance to articulate damage or damaging pasts in favor of a potentially better, more achievable future. The implication of slow recovery, a gradual loosening of memory around fifteen to twenty years after the war, fits into the larger framework of recognition. The public emergence of Holocaust memory, the beginnings of discussion and conceptualization leading eventually to the PTSD diagnosis also map onto this early postwar phase of emotional recuperation.[26] Yet, at the same time, political repression meant certain kinds of past traumatic memories, and memory conceptualization, only arrive in the wake of the PTSD diagnosis and develop in the 1990s and 2000s as an extension of the "post-traumatic stress" formulation.[27]

NARRATIVES, EMOTIONS, EXPERIENCES

The popularization of PTSD, especially since the 1990s, has led, though, to a tacit assumption that exposure to violent events, atrocities or extended periods of physical, emotional or mental deprivation all but guarantees the production of traumatic memories. What this assumption ignores is the greater physical difficulties of survival in past times—even as recently as the mid-twentieth century—which itself has a prophylactic effect. Communal resilience, the urgencies of everyday survival and material conditions that constitute a support system can equally lead to the diminution, eradication or non-formation of intrusive mental images or trigger responses based on past experience. While it is important not to underestimate the resilience effect, it is equally important to acknowledge that trauma is always mediated as memory, and that the forms by which it is transmitted also influence what stays in the mind, what is forgotten, and the degrees of recollection, amnesia or erasure.

Memory formations of all kinds mesh with local ways of living and are constituted in relation to peers as well as to wider collective interpretations of the social world. Memory also has a geological aspect. Recollections are built up in successive layers. Deeper, earlier memories may fragment,

[26] Frank Biess, "Feelings in the Aftermath: Towards a History of Postwar Emotions," in *Histories in the Aftermath: Towards a History of Postwar Emotions*, ed. by Frank Biess and Robert Moeller (New York: Berghahn, 2010), 32–4.

[27] Patrick J. Bracken, "Post-modernity and post-traumatic stress disorder," *Social Science & Medicine* 53:6 (2001), 32–4.

collapse or resurface to dominate the horizon. If later conditions do not allow the submergence of particular troubling images or sensations, their continuing presence can take many forms. When such recollections persist, they may come back to consciousness as isolated and repeated fragments that split off from more coherent recollections; as impossible, incomprehensible images that cannot be processed; as feelings of fear, disbelief and powerlessness.[28] These effects have a physiological source in the chemistry of the brain, but culture is also critical. Memories are a form of storytelling; narratives are constituted from the cultural heritage and resources available to the teller. Since many of the essays in this collection are centered on stories, it is useful here to give an account of the relation between narrative and experience as well as the relation of these two to the emotions.

Narrative constitutes a kind of distancing effect from events as they are remembered, and through this "epistemic distance" it becomes possible to reconsider meanings, re-evaluate experiences and think through possible avenues of response. As narrative psychologist Jens Brockmeier suggests:[29]

> I propose understanding narrative imagination as a form and practice of human agency. Telling stories is an advanced mode of communicating and negotiating meaning, but it is also an advanced mode of creating novel meanings [...] Even extreme experiences that seem to evade language often give shape to stories, as uncommon as these may be, that in their own way share the extreme nature of their experiences.

Reconciliation, processing and resilience are in this view implicit to the social meanings and consequences of storytelling. The narratives of traumatic memory, by contrast, continually stumble, hesitate and repeat themselves. The sense-making procedures to which Brockmeier refers are frustrated by the non-sense of fragmentation, isolation and incoherence. The nature of traumatic memory as a social act is its stuck-ness; the inability to create a meaningful explanation generates a repetitive loop of images and feelings that may last across the course of a lifetime and transmit across generations. The dissipation of traumatic memories is difficult to achieve,

---

[28] Graham Dawson, *Making Peace with the Past: Memory, Trauma and the Irish Troubles* (Manchester: Manchester University Press, 2007), 128.

[29] Jens Brockmeier, "Reaching for Meaning: Human Agency and the Narrative Imagination," *Theory and Psychology* 19:2 (2009), 227.

and by no means is it a likely effect of time's passage. Equally, narrative needs to be an extended category to incorporate the extreme experiences that are described throughout this collection. Narrating traumatic memories does not necessarily mean direct, vocal articulation. Degrees of self-expression may vary according to distance and conditions at the time of telling; changing degrees of articulacy, coherence, body language or behavior can also describe inner mental states, as can artistic forms. Nor are narrative events final, completed or ever fully resolved. Retellings across the course of a lifetime may take many different forms for both individuals and societies. The completion of one rendering may only serve as the prompt for a new recollection procedure to begin.[30]

The social and psychological uses of personal narrative have also become the subject of extensive investigation, especially in the early twenty-first century, and the complex, multiple uses to which such stories can be put by their tellers is increasingly well understood. What matters here is not that first-person or even collectively imagined stories match events in the world, nor is it necessary that the final resolution or definitive version of any such story should emerge. Rather, what matters for any given iteration of a story is its "cultural meaningfulness," since "[…] the meanings that individuals give to (or 'find' in) their lives can be manifold, open, and fleeting […]"[31] While social conditions or personal circumstances sanction the telling of particular stories with relative ease, this is not always the best outcome. Non-resolution or non-processing may also function as a self-protective mechanism. In either case, what matters is a manageable relation of the present self to a particular traumatic past. The site of a particular memory is subject to a complex set of variables in reworking and remaking the present self. A historical moment, communal and family histories, but also emotional vocabulary and constitution can all play a critical part in the purposes, formation and outcome of any given story iteration. Such specificities are, though, not easily catalogued or collated.[32]

---

[30] Peter Leese, "Traumatic Displacements: The Memory Films of Jonas Mekas and Robert Vas," in *Traumatic Memories of the Second World War and After*, ed. by Peter Leese and Jason Crouthamel (Cham: Palgrave Macmillan, 2016), 245–65.

[31] Nhi Vu and Jens Brockmeier, "Human Experience and Narrative Intelligibility," in *Theoretical Psychology: Critical Contributions*, ed. by N. Stephenson, H.L. Radke, R. Jorna and H.J. Stam (Concord, Ont.: Captus University Press, 2003), 282.

[32] Rob Boddice, "The Affective Turn: Historicizing the Emotions," in *History and Psychology: Interdisciplinary Explorations*, ed. by Christina Tileaga and Jovan Byford (Cambridge: Cambridge University Press, 2014), 155–6.

What the essays in this collection provide is a sequence of careful case studies, each of which examines the variable relations of narrative to the interpretation of traumatic experience and memory. Among these is Kurkowska-Budzan's engagement with the memoir of Stefan Dąmbski, which takes the publication and public presence of such a memory document as the pretext for an examination of culturally specific ways in which the past may be refigured to serve a particular present, in this case in Poland. While more usually medial, state administrative and institutional sources have provided a way to access a range of possible recollection strategies and the ways in which such sources reveal or conceal their subject. For wider social, communal and state affairs, such sources are invaluable; often they are also all that is available, so that the reconstruction of life experiences and stories becomes a patient procedure of putting fragments in meaningful proximity, overlapping institutional encounters, and social possibilities. These are the techniques used in contrasting ways by Robert Dale to reconstruct the lives of post-World War II Soviet veterans, and by Danutė Gailienė to consider the social functioning and traces of traumatic experience via suicide rates in twentieth-century Lithuania. Smaller autobiographical texts—diaries, memoirs, letters—are closer to the norm. Such sources are relatively available and can be used in relation to other sources to reconstruct past lives, as well as for purposes of comparison and contrast. Such sources can also be supplemented by pre-existing collections of oral history interviews, or with present day interviews, as in Anna Wylegała's essay on Eastern Galician bystanders and Outi Autti's research on postwar Finnish reconstruction. An ideal source base for this kind of study would be two or three successive reconstructions of a single life-story since this approach allows for a comparative examination of the storytelling form and narrative purposes. New kinds of sources emerge: in his chapter, Tuomas Laine-Frigren pays attention to poems written by traumatized Hungarian children as a part of their therapy. Image-based evidence is also an important supplement to word-based evidence as it allows another kind of narrative engagement. Ville Kivimäki examines films in his study of connections between Finnish ex-servicemen's dreams—recorded for ethnographic study in the postwar era—and narrative forms in popular culture, which might also serve as a source for narrative expression. Finally, Ana Antić finds in film a medium through which to access collective cultural trauma in postwar Yugoslavia.

A range of possible strategies might be extracted from this variety of source materials and approaches, but what is apparent across the range of these essays is their diagnostic function. The interpretive task of historical scholarship as it is expressed in the case studies that follow is a complex, imaginative and intricate reconstruction of past mentalities, which are constituted by the narrative expression of emotions and experiences recalled. The range of possibilities here is wide, and in many respects remains to be explored, as indicated by a recent discussion of "fear, sublimity, [and] transcendence" in the music of a composer whose work is closely associated with the most difficult experiences of World War II, Olivier Messiaen.[33]

Cultural and Social Variation

Describing the relation between psychological trauma and the contexts within which it is experienced and treated, Boris Drożđek, a specialist in intercultural psychology and the cultural sensitivities of traumatic response, uses the spider's web as a metaphor. There are various "intrapsychic, interpersonal, and socio-political domains" that particularly effect individuals. "When looking at it [the web] one sees the spider clearly and does not have to see the web at all. However, the spider does not exist and cannot live without the web. The web must not be overlooked."[34] Drożđek here alludes to the personal conditions within which any individual acts: social roles and relations, physical and material conditions, upbringing, education, community and social life, levels and varieties of social engagement, governing and ideological belief systems. Following Urie Bronfenbrenner's categories, these types of conditions can be described as micro-, meso-, exo-, and macro-.[35] Thinking historically, I would suggest that each of these levels is necessary in any given interpretive analysis in order to fully grasp the particularity of the traumatic experience in its time and place. Even in the present, and even with the full engagement of the subject, such an investigation would be difficult. The act of historical reconstruction—and the varied methodologies that can be used to access different levels of psychological experience in time and space—are in many respects

[33] Stephen Schloesser, "Fear, Sublimity, Transcendence: Notes for a History of Emotions in Olivier Messiaen," *History of European Ideas* 40:6 (2014), 826–58.

[34] Boris Drożđek, "The Rebirth of Contextual Thinking in Psychotrauma," in *Voices of Trauma: Treating Psychological Trauma Across Culture*, ed. by Boris Drożđek and John P. Wilson (New York: Springer, 2007), 10.

[35] See especially Part IV of Bronfenbrenner's *The Ecology of Human Development: Experiments in Design and Nature* (Cambridge, MA: Harvard University Press, 1981).

the central theme for the essays in *Trauma, Experience and Narrative in Europe During and After World War II.*

One effect of an analysis sensitized to particularities of time and place is to put the most prevalent present-day iteration of trauma, namely PTSD, into its own relativizing context. The PTSD concept originates within the English-speaking world in the 1970s and after; its purpose stressed one particular aspect of such diagnostic categories—to enable medically sanctioned compensation claims especially among United States veterans of the Vietnam War—but like any such category it is focused on a restricted spectrum of symptoms, cases and consequences. The analytic category of PTSD has little to say about the broader cultural web of conditions and sensitivities that shape traumatic responses; it fails to acknowledge the "cultural recipes" for signaling distress, interpreting symptoms, or recovering. These limitations were clear almost as soon as the category of PTSD was invented, and the diagnosis is no different than any other diagnostic conceptualization in having particular strengths, weaknesses or points of emphasis. Still, to explicitly or, more often, implicitly apply such a category beyond its cultural boundaries is to risk a form of "cultural bereavement."[36] Like earlier diagnostic categories as well as popularized notions of the psyche, other limitations quickly emerged in relation to PTSD. In any form of official assessment—successful medical diagnosis, or compensations-claim assessment for example—success depends on a sanctioned outward performance of an inner mental state. Especially where there are financial implications, the limitation of symptoms to a "correct" performance immediately matters: definition is as much a case of exclusion as of incorporation. Almost inevitably, a broader spectrum of post-traumatic damage is set "off limits," as are ethno-cultural and societal aspects.

To give one example of how restrictive the PTSD diagnosis has become, we might refer to the broader category of historical trauma. While there are varied definitions of the term, it is broadly connected to groups that have a sustained past of physical and psychological violation, for instance, indigenous peoples. More broadly, historical trauma is related to the experiences and psycho-social aftereffects suffered among Holocaust survivors, aboriginal colonial subjects, Allied survivors of Japanese internment

---

[36] Maurice Eisenbruch, "From post-traumatic stress disorder to cultural bereavement: diagnosis of Southeast Asian refugees," *Social Science and Medicine* 33:6 (1991), 673.

camps, Khmer Rouge victims as well as legacy descendants of slavery.[37] One such instance is reported by Aaron Denham in his study of the Si John—a Coeur d'Alene Indian family of North Idaho. Subjected to generations of racism, warfare, murder and forced land removal their reactions bear little relation to western notions of dysphoria or psychopathology. Although the historical experiences of the Si John parallel those of indigenous Australians or twentieth-century war casualties: witnesses to, or subjects against whom atrocity was perpetrated, their response is distinctive. Collective procedures of oral history-making and family narratives have produced strong group ties and collective forms of identification and powerful resilience strategies that enable post-adversity equilibrium. Where narratives of traumatic memory might more readily be transmitted within certain social milieux among the extended Si John family, employment of life events as clearly evolving stories, transmission among various family members and generational sharing by telling stories, listening to and learning from stories, have been especially beneficial. The cumulative effect of these strategies has been to retard potential manifestations of historical trauma, perhaps because collective rather than individual stress and identity are the focus of attention.[38] Such examples illustrate how current conceptions of trauma, more specifically of traumatic memory—its origins, symptomatic effects, and resolution—can easily be defined within a narrow spectrum that too easily and rigidly limits the possibility of cultural, social and historical variation.

This current state of affairs has been present since the later twentieth century and has become increasingly acute since the beginning of the twenty-first century, at which time John P. Wilson and Boris Drožđek first put forward their innovative sequence of hypotheses concerning connections between trauma and culture. What is certainly the case is that syndromes are culturally sanctioned; that healing is person-specific both in health-seeking and treatment pathways; that personal awareness enables mental processes of self-transcendence. Additionally, Wilson and Drožđek argue that cultural grounding particularizes forms of identity disruption, alienation, anxiety, distress or depression; that cultural specificities may be lessened in the current conditions of twenty-first century cross-cultural connection; that culturally specific healing rituals cohere and evolve

---

[37] Aaron R. Denham, "Rethinking Historical Trauma: Narratives of Resilience," *Transcultural Psychiatry* 45:3 (2008), 396.
[38] Denham (2008), 492–3.

according to needs and conditions; that western, twenty-first century therapies are specific to time and place while other procedures may be better suited to enhance resilience, personal growth and self-transcendence; and finally, that any effective pathway to diagnosis and healing must incorporate culturally specific as well as common aspects.[39]

Such insights, if taken seriously by historians, may enable a better understanding of trauma played out in the conditions of a particular historical, cultural and social milieu. I would suggest here that Central and Eastern Europe and the Baltic states are under-examined and misunderstood precisely because spectacularly different example of Asian localities are more readily distinguishable from Northern Europe or North America. When cultural specificities are less visible, they are more likely to be erased or ignored, but the essays in this collection nevertheless demonstrate decisively how much variation there can be in illness and healing scripts, and how landscape, politics and history can decisively reshape medical interpretations as well as individual and collective notions of suffering or psychological distress. Methodologies that help to understand the particular ways of writing trauma remain relatively underdeveloped in historical analysis, but a characteristic feature of several essays in this collection is combined close reading of one or more cultural artefacts, and a strong contextual reading of related clinical, social and political conditions. Ana Antić's examination of "Partisan Neurosis" is an example of this kind of close reading, where diagnostic interpretation is inevitably mixed in with an examination of historical and especially volatile political conditions. Antić's account is also valuable for its reading of popular cultural sources as a way to access contemporary conditions in relation to wider societal trauma effects. Tracing shifts of ideological opinion as well as tensions between state leadership elites and wider social constituencies also allows a more nuanced understanding of how political control could function, as well as the extent to which such political circumstances could direct cultural and diagnostic interpretations.

The varied methodologies of the essays in this collection further suggest some of the ways in which cultural specificities can be incorporated into comparative historical analysis. Hana Kubátová's essay, for example, notes how particular social groups might be treated in separate diagnostic

---

[39]Boris Drožđek, "Are We Lost in Translations? Unanswered Questions on Trauma, Culture and Posttraumatic Syndromes and Recommendations for Future Research," in Drožđek and Wilson, eds (2007), 381.

and etiological categories due to their status within a wider communal landscape. Unfavored or minority groups, of course, were especially disadvantaged in finding effective treatment or material sufficiency. Lack of social acknowledgment or recognition has additionally long-term mental health and clinical effects, as traumatic memories are far less likely to be resolved in later unsatisfactory conditions of reinterpretation. While the evidence is more fragmented and diverse—drawing on oral history, diary entries and written testimonies—Kubátová's composite methodology provides a powerful sense of how personal accounts allow insight into collective traumatizations as they evolve after many years and in processes of ongoing retrospection. Finally, Outi Autti addresses a growing field of research interest that remains to date underexplored, namely the traumatic effects of environmental destruction.[40] This is not necessarily a question of generalized degradation or global effects, but can also relate to the ways in which a local, lived landscape may be damaged—in this case Lapland following the withdrawal of German troops, the effect of damming on a local salmon fishing culture and the continuing human-made harm inflicted on local communities, which also has a profound impact on psychological well-being.

The "grass roots" specificity of the studies in *Trauma, Experience and Narrative in Europe During and After World War II* is valuable not only for the local knowledge each provides. The organization, content and analytic methodologies on display here also make a powerful argument for the pursuit of transnational and comparative histories of mentalities. Implicit in our analysis, too, is a continuation of the pioneering work by Jolande Withuis and Annet Mooji in *The Politics of War Trauma: the Aftermath of World War Two in Eleven European Countries* (2010).[41] A closely co-authored collaborative volume by twelve specialists, *The Politics of War Trauma* covered a coherent thematic and geographical subject area, mostly across Western Europe, and developed a strongly comparative and culturally based interpretation. *Trauma, Experience and Narrative in Europe During and After World War II* extends these themes to geographical districts less known among English-speaking readers. What

---

[40] See also E. Ann Kaplan, "Coda: Climate Trauma Reconsidered," in *Languages of Trauma: History, Memory, and Media*, ed. by Peter Leese, Julia Barbara Köhne, and Jason Crouthamel (Toronto: University of Toronto Press, 2021), 384–95.

[41] Jolande Withuis and Annet Mooij, eds, *The Politics of War Trauma: The Aftermath of World War Two in Eleven European Countries* (Amsterdam: Askant, 2010).

remains to be done is a more thematically based and comparative cultural history of the psychological aftermaths of World War II.

THE LIMITS OF TRAUMA

Describing the ideal conditions that allow recovery and reconciliation from remembered traumatic events, we can return to Derrick Silove's five necessary conditions. First, safety and security; second, attachment to families, social networks and rituals; third, engagement with justice (issues of truth, punishment and recognition); fourth, sufficient rebuilding of role and identity; and fifth, engagement with existential meaning (morality, belief systems and cultural expression).[42] Given the post-conflict turmoil that so dramatically destabilized and continually afflicted the central, eastern and Baltic states of Europe following World War II, it is inevitable that psychological survival and recovery across successive generations was only partially realized. Yet these were not the only consequences of wartime experience. Cultural artifacts across a range of media show, as they are documented and analyzed in the essays of this collection, ongoing procedures of reconciliation and processing. What matters is not that any final resolution could be achieved, as it is very doubtful that this could happen in many cases, especially with transgenerational trauma. Rather, the ongoing process of reworking troubled memories is itself the act of reconciliation.

While traumatic memories may not form even in obviously troubling conditions, and while recovery may be very easy or quick for some, it is also the case that for others there are no quick fixes. Children and grandchildren are often caught up actively in the circumstances of older family members whose ongoing lives are dominated by, or strongly determined by, traumatic memory. Beyond the third generation, in the realm of postmemory, different meanings and greater degrees of political manipulation become possible as the re-telling of events can no longer be directly contradicted. In both cases it is clear that strongly intrusive traumatic memories take generations to work their way out of the collective consciousness. At the same time, amnesia, misremembering and misinterpretation are also always present. Widely recalled or promoted past events are all the more likely to be repurposed to serve subsequent social and political agendas. This is not merely to say that events are cynically manipulated. Instead,

[42] Silove (2005), 42.

the deeper lifecycle of traumatic memory links personal recollection to wider societal purposes, since what is remembered and how it is recalled will always depend on the context of remembering. Social support may enable a sufficient, stable environment within which to resolve painful, contradictory or intrusive memories, but it is equally clear that this process is gradual and most usually progresses in two stages. First, a mastery of troubling events in memory is necessary so that the individual is no longer at the mercy of such recollections or overwhelmed when troubling events come back to mind uninvited. Second, recovery depends on the development of a sense-making narrative for the events remembered.[43] The development of sufficient contextualization is not only an individual process, but also depends on external conditions, not least sufficient public acknowledgment. When there is no such communal recognition, or where there is active suppression for political reasons or because a subject, rape for example, remains taboo, the chances of meaningful recovery are drastically diminished.[44]

Returning to my opening theme—that there is a profound imbalance between western memory's public presence and the less well-known events, languages and recollection of events across different parts of Europe—we might speculate on both the causes and consequences of this effect. Thinking first of causes, political history, and especially the prolonged effects of the Cold War, linger on in a troubled afterlife of ideological segregation. To these political aftereffects we may add the persistence of romantic nationalism as in influential ideology that promotes singular, heroic and sometimes martyrological narratives of the nation state to varying degrees in the central and eastern polities of Europe, and perhaps not only. Additionally, levels of relative affluence tend to allow the collection and preservation of different genres of recollection, remembrance and public past-making. In some Western European states, and with wider encouragement and financing from the European Union, for example, in its Platform of European Memory and Conscience, there is a degree of diversity in public and national commemorations.[45] The increasingly

---

[43] Nigel Hunt, "Memory and Social Meaning: The Impact of Society and Culture on Traumatic Memories," in *Hurting Memories and Beneficial Forgetting: Post-Traumatic Stress Disorder, Biographical Developments and Social Conflicts*, ed. by Michael Linden and Krzysztof Rutkowski (Amsterdam: Burlington/Elsevier Science, 2013), 49–50.

[44] See for example, Sandra Kessler, "Public and Private: Negotiating Memories of the Korean War," in Peter Leese and Jason Crouthamel, eds (2016), 173–96.

[45] Website https://www.memoryandconscience.eu, accessed 21 January 2021.

widespread use of oral history, although it tends sometimes in public recollection towards the tokenistic, has nevertheless encouraged and given some legitimacy to more diverse archival practices. Such deviation from state narratives can, however, still be tolerated or seen as subversive rather than recognized or valued. One example is the Polish KARTA Center Foundation, incorporating the journal *Karta*, which has long promoted a social, cultural and grass-roots methodological perspective with respect to the recent past, though such groups are unfortunately not the norm.[46] In place of wider procedures of public acknowledgment and recognition, which have a transnational aspect in relation to World War II, Europe's western, central and eastern quarters can be characterized as still caught up in procedures of involuntary commemoration. Individuals, families and communities continue to act as witnesses to the effects and aftereffects of conflict; memory and commemoration continue to snare those who are its subject, but there is equally the potential for release.[47]

[46] Website https://www.karta.org.pl, accessed 21 January 2021.

[47] Jo Stanley, "Involuntary Commemorations: Post-traumatic Stress Disorder and Its Relation to War Commemoration," in Ashplant, Dawson and Roper, eds (2000), 240–59.

CHAPTER 2

Beyond the Western Front

Mark S. Micale

SHELL SHOCK AS A HISTORIOGRAPHICAL SUCCESS STORY

As settings of psychological trauma, the trenches of the Western Front in World War I and the Nazi concentration camps in World War II have unquestionably attracted the greatest attention. In recent decades, these two sites have become historical archetypes. They have broken their specific geo-chronological boundaries to become paradigmatic instances of senseless, savage, state-sponsored killing. Viewed psychologically, both the Holocaust and World War I are now seen as illustrations of the devastating long-term damage that has been inflicted by massive, technologized violence in the modern era.

The story of the Western Front is as familiar as it is compelling. A meandering, roughly 700-kilometer line running northwesterly from the juncture of France, Germany, and Switzerland near the Rhine River city of Basel, through southern Germany, northeastern France, and Belgium, and ending at the North Sea around the Flemish city of Ostend, the front

M. S. Micale (✉)
Department of History, University of Illinois in Urbana-Champaign, Champaign, IL, USA

V. Kivimäki, P. Leese (eds.), *Trauma, Experience and Narrative in Europe after World War II*, Palgrave Studies in the History of Experience, https://doi.org/10.1007/978-3-030-84663-3_2

began to take shape in the autumn of 1914, only a few months after the war's outbreak.

When the Entente Powers halted German advances into northern France at the First Battle of the Marne in September 1914, the fighting stalled, and despite numerous large-scale frontal assaults and outflanking maneuvers, infantry and cavalry on both sides were repeatedly repelled. As a response to this stalemate, both sides constructed vast systems of defensive earthen formations in close proximity to one another. The labyrinth of trenches siphoned together hundreds of thousands of French, British, German, and eventually American soldiers who were periodically deployed in over-the-top attempts to break through the enemy's line. They proved little more than fodder for the industrialized weaponry that made its debut in the Great War: long-range artillery, machine guns, poison gas, and, during the final year of the conflict, armored tanks. Hence the concentrated human carnage.

Suffering on the Western Front did not end with the signing of the Armistice Agreement on 11 November 1918. In addition to the staggering death tolls and grievously disfiguring injuries, there occurred a third scene of intense and sustained human suffering, one that was underappreciated if not omitted altogether from earlier histories. Since the middle of the 1970s, scholars have been constructing a specifically psychiatric history of the war. What began as the story of individual ex-soldiers writing poems, novels, and memoirs about mental and emotional collapse has over the past two generations coalesced into a new enlarged narrative that is evermore integrated into the general history of World War I as well as into popular knowledge about the event.

The new psychiatric understanding of World War I is inseparably associated with the war's distinctive fighting conditions. Confronted with the unbearable, soldiers, many of them infantrymen on the front line, broke down physically, emotionally, and psychologically. A few months into the fighting, rank-and-file combatants on both sides began to show an array of symptoms: nervousness, anxiety, headaches, insomnia, depression, fainting spells, terrifying nightmares, and uncontrollable crying. In addition to these "non-specific psychogenic complaints," as they would be called today, bizarre physical, often quasi-neurological, behaviors surfaced: soldiers began to tremble without cause. Some developed painful facial tics or contractures of the arms or legs. Others began walking with a distorted gait, and still others lapsed into epilepsy-like convulsions, all of which were captured on early short medical films. Many lost their sight or ability to speak partially or fully. Short-term memory loss was one of the most commonly reported symptoms. The curious symptom profiles indicated some sort of bodily injury, and in particular central nervous system damage. But, in what became the greatest clinical conundrum of the war, military doctors on the Entente side and among the Central Powers were unable to locate any physical damage to the body or to ascertain organic causes.

At the time, the most common explanations for what afflicted these soldiers were cowardice, fakery, moral degeneration, or undiscovered nerve injury to the spine or brain. This last medical possibility—that these infirmities were caused by the concussive force of exploding ordnance close to the victims—gave rise to a diagnostic neologism: shell shock. A simple and attractively alliterative moniker, shell shock was a non-technical term and a noun that also became a verb and adjective. It had other attractions, too: shell shock implied a physical etiology, thereby protecting the reputation of a nation's fighting forces as well as the masculinity of the sufferer. As the number of cases swelled, shell shock raised serious manpower concerns.

As the war ground on, it became clearer and clearer to military doctors that what caused these perplexing symptoms was something altogether different: shell shock was in fact a mind-body revulsion against the horrific intensity of modern technological warfare—an existential *cri de coeur*. The harrowing conditions in the trenches, especially when combined with long periods of battlefield immobility, were wearing down the psychological strength and even sanity of soldiers. In the new psychoanalytic parlance of the day, they were unconsciously converting or somaticizing their intense fear into disabling mental and physical symptoms. By the war's end, a number of innovative physicians were exploring treatment techniques that would later be judged progressive and called psychotherapeutic; these included hypnosis and talk therapies that sought to recover the particular traumatic experience underpinning a patient's sickness.

As historians have pieced it together, the shell shock story extends beyond the war's end. Long after the cessation of hostilities, new shell shock-like cases continued to proliferate. Psychological and behavioral problems—including suicide, alcoholism, trouble concentrating or working, temper issues, and a greater susceptibility to physical illnesses—beset many veterans. The combatant nations responded in varied ways. In victorious, English-speaking countries (e.g., Britain, Australia, New Zealand, Canada, and the United States), the problem of "the neuropsychiatric ex-serviceman" became a major social welfare challenge throughout the

1920s, which governments met as best they could through new programs and practices. In defeated or impoverished nations, veterans were viewed far less sympathetically and fared much less well.

A final component of the story casts forward to our own time. Shell shock, including the phenomenon of the delayed onset of symptoms, presaged what physicians in the United States during World War II would call "war neurosis" and what, in 1980, the American Psychiatric Association christened "Post-traumatic Stress Disorder." If the Great War is often viewed today as the violent end of Enlightenment-Victorian civilization and the curtain-raiser on Europe's bloody and turbulent "short twentieth century," then shell shock is the prototype of war-induced psychological trauma and the ur-diagnosis of today's post-traumatic stress disorder (PTSD).

Especially since the 1990s, the outpouring of research on Western Front shell shock has included books, articles, dissertations, websites, symposia, exhibitions, novels, and films. Scores of historians—myself included—have produced publications exploring countless aspects of the shell shock story.[1] Thanks to an exemplary study by the British historian Peter Leese, published in 2002, knowledge of the subject has moved beyond the iconic works of a few "articulate sufferers"—the British "war poems," novels by Erich Maria Remarque and Henri Barbusse, the trench art of Otto Dix and George Grosz—to a much larger population of hospitalized shell shock victims.[2] Historians began researching not just male combatants, the original core population of historical trauma studies, but civilians—those in occupied territories and families back home, including parents and children.[3] A great range of topics has now been explored, from newspaper journalism about shell shock to postwar compensation for veterans, from the sex lives of the traumatized to interwar shell shock and psychoanalysis.

Before moving on, I want to salute the high scholarly and intellectual quality of this historical writing. Three book-length studies that I especially admire are emblematic. Written by the Berkeley-based film historian

---

[1] Mark S. Micale and Paul Lerner, eds, *Traumatic Pasts: History, Psychiatry, and Trauma in the Modern Age, 1870–1930* (New York: Cambridge University Press, 2001).

[2] Peter Leese, *Shell Shock: Traumatic Neurosis and the British Soldiers of the First World War* (Basingstoke: Palgrave Macmillan, 2002).

[3] For an excellent representative study, see Gregory M. Thomas, *Treating the Trauma of the Great War: Soldiers, Civilians, and Psychiatry in France, 1914–1940* (Baton Rouge: Louisiana State University Press, 2009).

Anton Kaes, *Shell Shock Cinema: Weimar Culture and the Wounds of War* (2009) shows how, among Germans, the traumatic memory of the lost war became a pervasive, if symbolic and unconscious, presence in many classic Expressionist films of the Weimar era.[4] A year later, my former University of Illinois colleague Jonathan Ebel published *Faith in the Fight: Religion and the American Soldier in the Great War* (2010). Ebel's book portrays the complex Christian religiosity of American soldiers in the field and after their return home through a sensitive analysis of their letters, diaries, and memoirs.[5] Christine Hallett's *Containing Trauma: Nursing Work in the First World War* (2009) is based on rich collections of nurses' personal writings housed in libraries and archives in London, Cambridge, Canberra, Wellington, and Ottawa. Hallett shows that, just by talking and listening compassionately to soldier-patients struggling to overcome their traumas in the hospital, nurses exerted a calming, healing influence.[6] The studies of Kaes, Ebel, and Hallett all broke new ground. They study little-known aspects of shell shock in several countries, and they creatively draw on fields such as film theory, colonial medicine studies, and the cultural history of religion. Among historians, there is no sign of slackening interest in the subject.[7]

Finally, shell shock studies have even reached a sizable popular audience. In 1976, *The Great War and Modern Memory*, by the American literary historian and World War II veteran Paul Fussell, won the National Book Award in the United States. In the first half of the 1990s, the British novelist Pat Barker published her prize-winning *Regeneration Trilogy*. Barker's trio of novels tells the story of war psychiatrist William Rivers and his pioneering treatments of World War I soldiers, including poets Siegfried Sassoon and Wilfred Owen, for shell shock at the Craiglockhart war

[4] Anton Kaes, *Shell Shock Cinema: Weimar Culture and the Wounds of War* (Princeton, NJ: Princeton University Press, 2009).

[5] Jonathan H. Ebel, *Faith in the Fight: Religion and the American Soldier in the Great War* (Princeton, NJ: Princeton University Press, 2010).

[6] Christine E. Hallett, *Containing Trauma: Nursing Work in the First World War* (Manchester: Manchester University Press, 2009). For a companion study, see Wendy Moore, *No Man's Land: The Trailblazing Women Who Ran Britain's Most Extraordinary Military Hospital during World War I* (New York: Basic Books, 2020).

[7] For the most recent survey of the subject, see Tracey Loughran, *Shell shock and Medical Culture in First World War Britain* (Cambridge: Cambridge University Press, 2017). And for the voluminous scholarship in the field, see the bibliography in Jason Crouthamel and Peter Leese, eds, *Psychological Trauma and the Legacies of the First World War* (Cham: Palgrave Macmillan, 2017), 311–27.

hospital outside Edinburgh. In 1997, the Scottish director Gillies MacKinnon produced a high-quality film adaptation of Barker's first novel, *Regeneration*, with Jonathan Pryce in the lead role. Ever since, British-made films about modern wars have invariably included scenes of nervous breakdown among soldiers, right up to the Oscar-nominated *Dunkirk* in 2017 and the 2019 film *1917*. In the later 1990s, historian Jay Winter, an international authority on World War I, devoted an hour-long installment of his multi-episode PBS/BBC documentary on the Great War to shell shock. Most recently, centennial memorializations of the 1914–1918 war offered still more opportunities for discussing and drama-tizing the subject.[8]

A New Present Requires a New Past

The success of shell shock as a historiographical phenomenon is striking. Viewed as a development in historical trauma studies, however, the shell shock industry has had an ironic and unfortunate, if wholly unintended, side effect. So much light has been shone on the experience of the Western Front in World War I that it has eclipsed many other important historical sites of suffering, including events in modern times.

Take the European Eastern Front during World War II. No region of Europe witnessed greater horrors during the years 1939 and 1945 than the lands between Nazi Germany and Stalin's Soviet Union. The Eastern Front comprised a thousand-mile north-to-south stack of nations includ-ing Finland, the Baltic States of Estonia, Latvia, and Lithuania, Poland, Soviet Ukraine, Soviet Belarus, the western portion of Soviet Russia, Slovakia, Hungary, Romania, and portions of Yugoslavia. Why, we might ask, did historical trauma studies emerge solely from the story of shell shock on the French-German-Belgian borders and not from the Eastern Front, which was equally deadly, involved more countries (from the Baltic to the Black Sea), and was fought under different conditions and among different combatants? Or, for that matter, from the study of all fronts in

---

[8] Paul Fussell, *The Great War and Modern Memory* (Oxford: Oxford University Press, 1975); Pat Barker, *Regeneration* (New York: Plume/Penguin, 1991); Pat Barker, *The Eye in the Door* (New York: Viking Press, 1993); Pat Barker, *The Ghost Road* (New York: Dutton, 1995); *Regeneration* (Directed by Gillies MacKinnon, 1997), which debuted in the United States in 1999 under the title *Behind the Lines*; Jay Winter, PBS/BBC documentary series, 8 episodes, *The Great War and the Shaping of the 20th Century*, 1996.

the war (including the Eastern Mediterranean) or from a comparative study of all fighting fronts in both world wars?

I think I know why this historiographical asymmetry arose. As Peter Leese notes in his introductory essay to this volume, several reinforcing developments are likely involved. During the decades of the Cold War, if Soviet-dominated states discussed the war at all, they tended to sponsor narratives of heroic resistance, super-human resilience, and eventual victory against the Nazi empire. Research that did not support patriotic national histories was discouraged or forbidden. The suppression extended even to autobiographical reminiscences of the war years. "The real war," as Vita Zelče of the University of Latvia has commented, "could not be discussed, nor could the trauma of the people who were part of it, the shock of the war, panic or depression could not be part of the discourse."[9]

The wholesale internal disintegration of the Soviet Union that began in the early 1980s, aided by growing unrest in a number of "Soviet Bloc" nations and spearheaded by the trade union Solidarity in Poland, came to a conclusion in December 1991 when the master Communist state, the USSR itself, imploded. This world-historical development meant that former Soviet republics, including the Eastern Bloc nations studied in this book, suddenly and unexpectedly became free and self-governing entities. One of the many consequences of this transformation was the opening of countless archives that had previously been closed or censored. All manner of subjects that were formerly taboo to discuss, and literally millions of documents that were unknown or inaccessible, began to become available to researchers. Across Central and Eastern Europe, scores of institutional repositories, especially government archives, including the records of many state-run hospitals, opened for scholarly inspection. For the first time, citizens of formerly occupied countries could start to learn "what really happened" during the war and ask why.

A result of these new conditions has been the publication of a multitude of first-person accounts by people still alive and now able to tell their stories. This "wave of testimony" includes memoirs by soldiers, officers, bureaucrats, civilians, families, doctors, and even perpetrators. These proliferating "late witness testimonies," as Hana Kubátová calls them below, written 50–60 years after the war's conclusion, are now being brought together, catalogued, and digitized—an emerging trauma archive for

---

[9] Vita Zelče, "War, History and People," in Vita Zelče and Uldis Neiburgs, eds, *(Two) Sides: Diaries of Latvian Soldiers in WWII* (Riga: Zelta Grauds, 2013), 19.

future generations.[10] The publications are provoking discussion in the national press. Furthermore, the painful and painstaking process of excavating these buried pasts is becoming a trope in the cultural arts of these countries, especially in novels, poems, theater, films, and photography.

Some of the circumstances conducive to this recovery work are subtler and more psychological in nature. The curious phenomenon whereby symptoms of a repressed experience manifest themselves long after the pathogenic event took place was first observed in wartime patients diagnosed with shell shock, war neurosis, and PTSD. Psychological latency and delay can also be seen in collectivities, such as families, towns, cities, regions, nations, and ethnic groups. Between the two wars, an understanding began to emerge of how the fragile human organism, after experiencing a sudden physical shock, attempts to recover and return to a stable, integrated equilibrium or "homeostatic state." In some regions of the West, this new line of bio-medical research eventually ushered in modern psychosomatic medicine and elucidated some of the mechanisms through which psyche and soma interact.[11] Analogously, following a trauma the psyche responds by seeking stability, sanity, and solace. A self-protective need to expel memories of the lived trauma from consciousness, and the numbing of recollections surrounding the experience, are common, modern psychology has found.

These psychodynamics may help explain why the work of psychological reconstruction in Central and Eastern Europe has of late become feasible. This initiative is being led by a generation of young researchers passionate to learn about their countries' suppressed pasts. The first fruits of the project are often authored by scholars early in their careers—individuals whose grandparents or other family members fought or died in the war. The young practitioners are a post-Soviet, post-Communist generation; they have a different relation to the past under study, including greater critical distance and their own set of memories and experiences. So far, older scholars—those who lived through the nightmares of Nazism and the Soviet occupation—are leading the way in locating autobiographical

---

[10] Hana Kubátová, "Guilt, Responsibility and Trauma: Restoring the Moral Self-Image in Postwar Slovakia," in this book. See also Myra Sklarew, *A Survivor Named Trauma: Holocaust Memory in Lithuania* (Albany: State University of New York, 2020).

[11] For an intriguing account of this development in broad cultural context, see Stefanos Geroulanos and Todd Meyers, *The Human Body in the Age of Catastrophe: Brittleness, Integration, Science, and the Great War* (Chicago: University of Chicago Press, 2018), esp. Chaps. 2 and 5.

primary source materials. Researchers born after 1990 appear likelier to perform the work of analyzing and synthesizing these materials.

At least one other development has encouraged this enterprise. In 2010, the Yale historian Timothy Snyder published *Bloodlands: Europe between Hitler and Stalin*.[12] Snyder's book became that rare academic phenomenon: a single-volume work of such scope and power that it altered the paradigm for an entire field of study. Snyder argued that between 1933 and 1945, the central "zone of death" in Europe was the area between Hitler's Germany and Stalin's Soviet Union. Conceptually, Snyder's book transcended a single-nation focus to develop an integrated regional, at times trans-continental, perspective. The killing fields of Central and Eastern Europe, between Berlin and Moscow and from Leningrad to Belgrade, encompassed Estonia, Latvia, Lithuania, western Russia, Belarus, Ukraine, Poland, Czechoslovakia, Hungary, and Yugoslavia. By emphasizing civilian mortality rather than battlefield combat deaths, Snyder in effect created a new unit of historical study, shifting the focus from better-known settings such as the skies over London, the deserts of North Africa, and the beaches of Normandy. Researched in recently opened archives in Russia, Poland, Ukraine, and East Germany, *Bloodlands* captivated scholarly and non-academic readers alike.[13]

Snyder's book has motivated scholars to explore other historical experiences in the Bloodland nations. At the same time, trauma was starting to emerge as a focus in historical scholarship of World War II. In 2013, for instance, Ville Kivimäki wrote a comprehensively researched doctoral dissertation on military psychiatry and wartime psychological injury in Finland, "Battled Nerves: Finnish Soldiers' War Experience, Trauma, and Military Psychiatry, 1941–44."[14] Two years later, Palgrave published *Traumatic Memories of the Second World War and After*, an essay collection edited by Peter Leese and Jason Crouthamel. That work is part of an ambitious multi-volume research project to study war and trauma

---

[12] Timothy Snyder, *Bloodlands: Europe between Hitler and Stalin* (New York: Basic Books, 2010).

[13] For a comparative global perspective on Snyder's material that appeared the same year as his book, see Christian Gerlach's *Extremely Violent Societies: Mass Violence in the Twentieth-Century World* (Cambridge: Cambridge University Press, 2010).

[14] Ville Kivimäki, "Battled Nerves: Finnish Soldiers' War Experience, Trauma, and Military Psychiatry, 1941–44" (PhD thesis: Åbo Akademi University, 2013).

transnationally in Europe across the twentieth century.[15] (The current volume, *Trauma, Experience and Narrative in Europe During and After World War II* is the fourth installment of this undertaking.) And in 2018, Oxford University Press published *Therapeutic Fascism: Experiencing the Violence of the Nazi New Order in Yugoslavia*, by Ana Antić, who did graduate work at Columbia University and now teaches at the University of Copenhagen. Antić's biographical profile is typical of the field's new generation of researchers. Her book uses "the history of psychiatry as an alternative history of the [Nazi] occupation," innovatively analyzing the newly available records of thousands of institutionalized patients to study the effects of wartime violence during the fascist and Communist periods of Balkan history.[16]

The Varieties of Trauma Experience

It is always exciting when a new field of research begins to take shape. Central and Eastern European trauma studies, however, should not simply apply ideas and insights from the scholarship on World War I shell shock to the later European conflict. Some features of psychic trauma may indeed remain consistent across both spatial and temporal fields, but in many other ways experiences of trauma differ greatly by time and place. Human responses to acute post-traumatic stress vary according to the nature of what Jeffrey Alexander has called "the original trauma-drama," that is, whether the precipitating event is a natural disaster, a car collision, a war, an act of domestic aggression, or some other phenomenon.[17] Whether the injury occurred suddenly and accidentally or over a longer time span and whether the victim was targeted intentionally can also influence how a person or group makes sense of the experience. As I have written elsewhere, the relation between the victim or sufferer and the agent or source inflicting the trauma can also shape the response.[18]

---

[15] Peter Leese and Jason Crouthamel, eds, *Traumatic Memories of the Second World War and After* (Cham: Palgrave Macmillan, 2016). See also Crouthamel and Leese, eds (2017); and Peter Leese, Julia B. Köhne and Jason Crouthamel, eds, *Languages of Trauma: History, Memory, and Media* (Toronto: University of Toronto Press, 2021).

[16] Ana Antić, *Therapeutic Fascism: Experiencing the Violence of the Nazi New Order in Yugoslavia* (Oxford: Oxford University Press, 2017).

[17] Jeffrey C. Alexander, *Trauma: A Social Theory* (Cambridge: Polity Press, 2012).

[18] Mark S. Micale, "Toward a Global History of Trauma," in Crouthamel and Leese, eds (2017), 304.

If, then, trauma is complexly and historically situated, how did the conditions of World War II in Central and Eastern Europe shape the experience of trauma? World War I last a little over four years, World War II five-and-a-half years. Both wars were fought on multiple fronts, and both centered on the western tip of the Eurasian land mass, with Germany as the key belligerent. For our purposes, that is about the extent of the similarities.

The Great War, with approximately 16 million fatalities, was the deadliest armed conflict in history—until World War II erupted, taking the lives of 70–85 million people. These figures include military personnel and civilians killed as well as deaths from war-related disease and famine. In contrast to the murderous stalemate in the maze-like trench system of France and Belgium from 1914 to 1918, World War II was a highly mobile conflict.[19] Especially in the early years of the war, overwhelming speed and force were key tactical features of the Nazi onslaught. Classic mass infantry armies were now accompanied by mobile artillery, reinforced with motorized tank divisions and air power. Although most associated in the public mind with the September 1939 invasion of Poland, the Nazi juggernaut tactic was also used to excellent effect in the 1940 Battle of France, in Rommel's panzer assaults in North Africa, and, beginning in 1941, in Operation Barbarossa, which drove 1000 miles to the outskirts of Moscow. The goal was to achieve quick territorial gains—and to inflict psychological terror. On the Western Front of World War I, the fighting and killing were terrifying but localized, whereas two decades later the impact was vastly wider. All nine countries "caught between Hitler and Stalin" suffered extreme and extensive violence.[20]

Another difference between the experience of the two world wars had to do with conflict in the air.[21] At the outset of World War I, aircraft was a new military technology and played limited, if colorful, roles. Balloons carried out reconnaissance, Zeppelin went on raids over London, Paris,

---

[19] Although, as Mark Edele rightly points out in the Coda to this book, the Eastern Front in World War I was also often a war of movement. See Norman Stone, *The Eastern Front, 1914–1917* (New York: Scribner, 1975). For this reason, a comparative historical and clinical study of the two fighting fronts, as well as the Middle Eastern theater, would be illuminating.

[20] Timothy Snyder, "Caught between History and Stalin," *New York Review of Books*, 30 April 2009.

[21] My emphasis throughout this chapter on the human experiencing of the war is indebted to Jay Winter's *The Experience of World War I* (London: Macmillan, 1988).

Antwerp, and Liege, and ace pilots engaged in one-on-one "dog fights." Two decades later, aerial warfare was a major component deployed by both Axis and Allied powers in all combat arenas. First directed against massed troops, military installations, and industrial sites, bombing in World War II soon targeted non-combatant populations, inflicting destruction deadlier and much more indiscriminate than anything witnessed a generation earlier. Americans tend to be most familiar with the London blitz and the bombing of certain other British and Dutch industrial cities but Hitler and Göring also targeted cities in the East and Southeast, including Moscow, Leningrad, Stalingrad, Lodz, Warsaw, and Belgrade. Later in the war, the Allies intensively bombed many German cities, including Berlin, Kassel, Cologne, Hamburg, Dresden, and Darmstadt.

The horrendous number of civilian deaths and casualties is arguably the single greatest difference between the two global confrontations. If World War I was characterized by the bloodbaths at well-known battle sites from Ypres to Gallipoli, World War II saw the invasion, occupation, and annexation of entire countries. The civilian death toll in the first war was eight million, roughly six million of them attributed to disease and famine. In the second war, 50–55 million civilians died—more than double the number of military deaths. By one estimate, in Poland alone three million Jews and between 1.8 and 1.9 million non-Jewish civilian Poles were fatalities of the Nazi occupation. According to a Soviet source, 21.2 percent of the Latvian population perished during the war.[22] Some of the worst wartime atrocities took place in villages, towns, and cities that were entirely civilian.[23]

Greater intermingling of soldiers and civilians brought opportunities for torture, murder, and rape. There were other kinds of victimization as well, including imposition of silence or neutrality, witnessing of violent acts, collaboration with the enemy, and consensual sex between men and women on opposite sides of the war. In the post-conflict period, these entanglements often played out in ways that were morally and psychologically damaging.

The role of women and children differed greatly from World War I to World War II. In the scholarship on shell shock, women and children figure as bereaved family members far removed from the site of the trauma.

---

[22] Zelče (2013), 18.
[23] For a listing of death tolls, see https://en.wikipedia.org/wiki/World_War_II_casualties (accessed 29 January 2021).

They are mothers, wives, offspring, and lovers of male soldiers who had been killed, maimed, or shell shocked.[24] More recently, in Hallett's and Moore's books, they are doctors and nurses. Pablo Picasso's epic painting *Guernica* of 1937 was as an early dramatization of the new war reality. During the Spanish Civil War of 1936–1939, which is often viewed as a kind of dress rehearsal for World War II, the Nationalists under Franco bombed civilian targets, including, on 26 April 1937, the inhabitants of the rural Basque village of Guernica. Picasso's iconic canvas depicts in an angular Cubist style the anguished, upturned faces of the victims—not male soldiers but women, children, horses, and cattle. Along with the elderly and disabled, women and children were much more deeply and complexly affected by violence in World War II. The concentration camp at Ravensbrück north of Berlin housed upwards of 132,000 women, mostly political prisoners, from Poland, the Soviet Union, Germany, Austria, and France. A huge number of civilians were transported westward to Germany and forced into slave labor, the majority of them young women. At Auschwitz, Treblinka, Sobibor, and other extermination facilities, huge numbers of Jewish women of all ages were murdered.

Recent scholarship has also documented that women were by no means just passive victims of fascist aggression. In every country involved in the war, women served in the auxiliary armed forces. In many places, they were active as spies, couriers, prison guards, and resistance fighters, in addition to playing other roles. Hundreds of thousands of women in Soviet Russia were military personnel, working as frontline soldiers, paratroopers, and even Nazi interrogators. Women in Russia and Romania served as combat pilots in the campaigns at Odessa and Stalingrad, and female Soviet snipers were celebrated. Over a hundred thousand women joined the anti-fascist forces in Yugoslavia.[25] Likewise, tens of thousands of German women in the East—guards, nurses, teachers, secretaries, wives,

---

[24] Suzanne Evans, *Mothers of Heroes, Mothers of Martyrs: World War I and the Politics of Grief* (Montreal: McGill-Queen's University Press, 2007).

[25] Sarah Helm, *If This Is a Woman: Inside Ravensbrück: Hitler's Concentration Camp for Women* (London: Little Brown, 2015); Dalia Ofer and Lenore J. Weitzman, eds, *Women in the Holocaust* (New Haven, CT: Yale University Press, 1998); Sophie Hodorowicz Knab, *Wearing the Letter P: Polish Women as Forced Laborers in Nazi Germany, 1939–1945* (New York: Hippocrene Books, 2016).

and mistresses—were accomplices in wartime atrocities.[26] Future psychological histories must integrate female choice and agency.

Another large and traumatized population was prisoners of war. Millions of soldiers on both sides were captured. The Geneva Convention restrained the Axis treatment of West European POWs considerably, but the Germans treated Soviet and Slavic prisoners with appalling neglect and brutality. Of an estimated 5.7 million Soviet prisoners seized by the Axis powers, 3.3 million died in captivity. During the winter of 1944–1945, thousands of Soviet prisoners, already weak, ill, and malnourished, were forced to undertake the infamous "Death Marches" during which many died of exhaustion or were shot.

Prisoners of the Soviet Union faced a heinous fate, too: following the September 1939 campaign, when the Nazis and Soviets briefly conspired to destroy and dismember Poland, the Soviet security officials, on Stalin's orders, arrested and then executed approximately 22,000 Polish officers, policemen, and intellectuals in the Katyn Forest and other killing sites.[27] Of the almost 100,000 Nazis captured after the pivotal Battle of Stalingrad, only 5000 survived the war. Many German captives were sent to Siberian labor camps where they died from cold, hunger, and exhaustion. Among both under-rationed troops and civilian populations, malnutrition and starvation played a far greater part in the suffering than during World War I. The 900-day Leningrad blockade, in which between 642,000 and one million civilians starved to death, is only the best known of such enforced famines.

Given these appalling facts, it should be clear why the term shell shock was never widely used to characterize psychological trauma in World War

---

[26] Anne Noogle, *A Dance with Death: Soviet Airwomen in World War II* (College Station: Texas A & M University Press, 1994); Jelena Batinić, *Women and Yugoslav Partisans: A History of World War II Resistance* (New York: Cambridge University Press, 2015); Wendy Lower, *Hitler's Furies: German Women in the Nazi Killing Fields* (New York: Houghton Mifflin Harcourt, 2013). A recent special themed issue establishes how myriad were the roles played by women in the war. See Sandra Trudgen Dawson, ed., "Women and the Second World War," *International Journal of Military History and Historiography* 39:2 (2019), 167–312.

[27] Anna M. Cienciala, Natalia S. Lebedeva and Wojciech Materski, eds, *Katyn: A Crime Without Punishment* (New Haven: Yale University Press, 2007), Part II, 121–205; Maria Kobielska, "Endless Aftershock: The Katyń Massacre in Contemporary Polish Culture," in Leese and Crouthamel, eds (2016), Chap. 9.

II.[28] Although decimating artillery barrages played a major role in the fighting—most famously in the Armageddon-like battles of Stalingrad and Berlin—exploding shells were no longer the signature battlefield experience. As a descriptor, shell shock was simply much too weak, semantically and symbolically, to account for the war experience.[29]

The phrase that Europeanists deploy most often to characterize the lethality of World War II is "the barbarization of warfare." The phrase was created by the Israeli-American historian Omer Bartov in the mid-1980s, specifically to describe warfare on the Eastern Front. It is sobering to reflect that up until trench warfare in World War I, European military conflicts typically involved disciplined professional soldiers marching in shoulder-to-shoulder formations, using bayonets, gun powder, and muskets in rural settings. What Bartov strove to capture was not just the mind-boggling numbers of war dead in the East, but a kind of total warfare that entailed several new practices undertaken simultaneously. These practices included the "blanket bombing" of civilian centers, mass execution of civilians by ground forces, inhumane treatment of POWs, large-scale labor enslavement, state-induced famines, and the racialization of mass violence.[30]

This brings us to yet another immense difference between the two wars, namely, the deadly role of ideology and race. World War I was the last Great Power conflict in European international relations in which Britain, France, Prussia/Germany, Russia, and Austria/the Austro-Hungarian Empire competed for continental dominance and overseas hegemony. By contrast, World War II featured titanic clashes between opposing political ideologies. In the Anglo-American view, the first phase of the war pitted the capitalist democracies of the Allies (Britain and its Commonwealth countries, France, Belgium, the Nordic nations, and

---

[28] In his chapter below, Robert Dale finds that the Russian term *kontuziia* comes close in meaning to the English "shell shock."

[29] Furthermore, in the 1920s, the term shell shock took on Futurist associations of speed, excitement, and modernity. See Tim Armstrong, "Two Types of Shock in Modernity," *Critical Quarterly* 42:1 (2000), 60–73.

[30] Omer Bartov, *The Eastern Front, 1941–1945: German Troops and the Barbarization of Warfare* (New York: St. Martin's Press, 1986). For reflections on Bartov's characterization, see George Kassimeris, ed., *The Barbarization of Warfare* (Washington Square, NY: New York University Press, 2006), especially Hew Strachan's "Time, Space and Barbarisation: The German Army and the Eastern Front in Two World Wars," 58–82 and Mary R. Habeck's "The Modern and the Primitive: Barbarity and Warfare on the Eastern Front," 83–100.

eventually the U.S.) against fascist Germany and Italy in Mediterranean North Africa and on the Western Front. In June 1941, with Hitler's turn eastward and his attack on the Soviet Union, a second epic collision broke out between fascist Germany and the Communist USSR as the totalitarian dictatorships of the political right and the political left fought to the death.

Unlike the Italian and Spanish versions of fascism, Hitler's worldview was highly racialized. The *Generalplan Ost*, or secret Nazi Master Plan for the East, called for the conquest, occupation, ethnic cleansing, and colonization of Central and Eastern Europe on a scale that beggars belief. Central and Eastern Europe has been historically multi-religious and multi-ethnic. Hitler regarded most of its inhabitants, including Jews, Slavic peoples, and Romani people, as inferior to the Anglo-Saxon races and especially to "Aryan Germans." Through war, Hitler aimed to obtain greater "living space" by conquering and colonizing areas east of Germany. Once subdued, these countries would be deprived of statehood, and multi-year plans of exploitation and cultural Germanization would commence.

Hitler's efforts at implementation created human suffering of a hitherto unseen and unimaginable scale: between 1939 and 1945, German soldiers abducted and forced into labor some 12 million men and women from the East European and Soviet territories. Rampaging through Wehrmacht-occupied territories of Central and Eastern Europe, Nazi *Einsatzgruppen* or other SS and police troops rounded up and shot over two million people. In the institutionalized and industrialized phase of the Holocaust, Nazi's corralled and killed around six million civilians in concentration camps, mostly located in Poland. These actions fairly meet the standard set in the 1980 edition of the *Diagnostic and Statistical Manual of Mental Disorders*: to qualify as psychologically traumatic, an event must be "generally outside the range of usual human experience."[31]

Then there was the postwar period. In much of the West, the years following the war brought recovering national economies, rising living standards, a new safeguarding of human rights, and the growing social benefits of the welfare state. Furthermore, after 1945 many Western Europeans and North Americans drew satisfaction from having won a quintessentially "good war." The human toll had been terrible, but, in a morally Manichean confrontation of absolute good and evil, they had prevailed.

---

[31] *Diagnostic and Statistical Manual of Mental Disorders*, Third Edition (Washington D.C.: American Psychiatric Association, 1980), 236.

For nations under the new Soviet sphere of influence, on the other hand, no return to prewar normalcy lay in store. Instead of liberation parades down Champs-Elysées or through Times Square, the cessation of the war in the East meant the replacement of one foreign dictatorship by another. Among the countries canvassed in this book, only Finland and Yugoslavia managed to escape a second captivity and obtain or regain political autonomy. As a consequence of the Molotov-Ribbentrop Pact of 1939, with its Secret Protocol setting out spheres of influence, the Soviet Union had occupied and annexed several countries, including Latvia, Estonia, and Lithuania as well as parts of Poland, Finland, and Romania. After Hitler broke the non-aggression pact, those countries became battlegrounds in the vast ideological war of extermination between Germany and the Soviet Union. After Hitler's defeat, the USSR occupied the Baltic countries and controlled East Germany, Poland, Romania, Bulgaria, Czechoslovakia, Hungary, Bulgaria, and Albania. Seeing those territories as a needed buffer zone of friendly Communist countries against the Soviet Union's historic enemies to the west, Stalin installed compliant authoritarian governments. By the mid-1950s, Soviet Russia consolidated these states into a collective ideological bloc, the Warsaw Pact, against Western nations, which had banded together to form the North Atlantic Treaty Organization. Although the new governments in Central and Eastern Europe were Communist rather than fascist, the totalitarianism of the right and of the left shared many operational features, including an extensive state police apparatus, the pervasive use of terror against their populations, national ideological indoctrination, the mass imprisonment of political opponents, and total control of public discourse, including the press.[32]

Carved out of the territorial remains of the German Kaisserreich, the Austro-Hungarian Empire, the Russian Empire, and the Ottoman Empire after World War I, Poland, Czechoslovakia, Hungary, and the Baltic Republics had enjoyed political independence for 20 years. After 1945, they were effectively re-subjugated. The governments and economies of Central and Eastern Europe's newly designated "Soviet republics" were controlled externally. Those professional elites and community leaders who had survived the war, and who might have served to revive the

[32] Carol Joachim Friedrich and Zbigniew Brzezinski, *Totalitarian Dictatorship and Autocracy*, second revised edition (Cambridge, MA: Harvard University Press, 1965 [1956]), Introduction: "The General Characteristics of Totalitarianism."

culture and history of their countries, were expelled. "Sovietization," especially during the 1950s, brought the confiscation of private properties, forced industrialization, and the collectivization of agriculture—resulting in the coercive resettlement and deportation of hundreds of thousands of inhabitants. People lived under the constant fear of surveillance by the state police forces and of arrest, interrogation, internment, or execution. If branded "an enemy of the people," a person could be arrested and imprisoned in the Soviet penal system. Many individuals simply disappeared and were never seen again.

The threat of military intervention in the face of resistance was constant. In Hungary in 1956 and Prague in 1968, the threat was carried out as Warsaw Pact forces harshly suppressed internal reform movements and reinstated neo-Stalinist policies. In short, decades after the extinction of the Nazi Empire, traumatizing conditions continued in the bloodlands. Omnipresent anxiety about a possible confrontation between NATO and the Warsaw Pact and about how that would play out in these regions of the continent added to the tension. After 1949, there was still another imponderable: fear of a nuclear exchange between the two "superpowers." Communist Central and Eastern Europe during the Cold War was no "safe space" for psychological healing.

TRAUMA IN THE AGE OF TOTALITARIANISM

Studying Central and Eastern Europe's psychiatric history should obviously be informed by our knowledge of shell shock, but it must also encompass much more. During and after World War II, widespread violence, including killing, permeated the lives of ordinary people across large swathes of Central and Eastern Europe. To be sure, the histories of the countries in these regions followed different courses and had varied outcomes, but the commonalities were great. The nations of the bloodlands were subjected to an interlinked process of invasion-conquest-deprivation-starvation-occupation-annexation-pacification-extermination-repression-indoctrination that extended over entire lifetimes and generations. All of these overlapping experiences were potential sources of trauma.

Today's clinical literature on PTSD may help us grasp the full range of these past situations. In the past decade, mental health professionals have formulated the sub-diagnosis of "Complex PTSD." Earlier theorists had viewed trauma as a single intensely adverse incident—a work accident, mugging, homicide, sexual assault, earthquake—that catches a person off guard. That experience might be devastatingly negative, but it was delimited in time and space. In Complex PTSD, sometimes called "chronic traumatic stress," a person is exposed repetitively to a traumatic or highly stressful situation from which there is no escape. In such cases, it is less one event than a chain of events or an entire environment that is pathogenic.

Harvard psychiatrist Judith Lewis Herman first brought to attention the phenomenon of cumulative emotional trauma in her classic book *Trauma and Recovery* (1992). Herman highlighted the physical and sexual abuse of women and children trapped in domestic relationships that were long-term and destructive.[33] More recent studies have investigated a Complex PTSD that is endemic in certain settings or institutions, such as prisons, war zones, or urban neighborhoods. Sociologists and social anthropologists apply the concept to ethnic and racial groups that historically have been traumatized, including Native American tribes, post-slavery African-Americans, Holocaust survivors, and people in apartheid and post-apartheid South Africa.[34]

Historians of Central and Eastern European will benefit from these new lines of clinical investigation. Current working notions of Complex PTSD, however, do not quite correspond with the past situations and circumstances that historians are studying. It is true that bloodlands violence was endemic, systemic, and long-term; indeed, it prevailed for over half a century and through multiple political regimes. The trauma arises not so much from witnessing or experiencing violence at every moment as from the ever-present fear that previously inflicted extreme violence will resume. PTSD research teaches that acute "anticipatory anxiety," especially when operating over a considerable time span, exerts a particularly corrosive effect. As historian of medicine Hans Pols has observed, "we must conceive of the subject somewhat differently when the trauma is continuing

---

[33] Judith Lewis Herman, *Trauma and Recovery* (New York: Basic Books, 1992).

[34] *Dodging Bullets: A Documentary Film on Historical Trauma*, Directed by Kathy Broere and Sarah Edstrom (2018); Lukoye Atwoli et al., "Trauma and Posttraumatic Stress Disorder in South Africa: Analysis from the South African Stress and Health Study," *BMC Psychiatry* 13:182 (2013), 1–12; Ron Eyerman, *Cultural Trauma: Slavery and the Formation of African American Identity* (Cambridge: Cambridge University Press, 2001); Joy De Gruy, *Post-Traumatic Slave Syndrome: America's Legacy of Enduring Injury and Healing* (Portland, OR: Uptone Press, 2005); Natan P. F. Kellermann, *Holocaust Trauma: Psychological Effects and Treatment* (Bloomington, IN: iUniverse Incorporated, 2009).

and on-going, and the real trauma is that there is no end in sight and no control over one's life and world."[35]

As an emerging project, the study of Central and Eastern European trauma is likely to depart from the study of shell shock in other ways, too. The intellectual history of trauma will probably figure less prominently as will the history of contrasting therapeutic practices (i.e., "disciplinary treatments" vs. verbal psychodynamic approaches).[36] The role played by social class in determining the symptom manifestations of war-related nervous disorders and in the institutionalization of patients, both well-explored topics in regard to shell shock in Britain, will be less relevant. Contrasting postwar government policies toward traumatized veterans, a topic rewardingly explored in regard to World War II, is also likely to attract less attention in the future.[37] Nor is there much danger of the 1939–1945 war on the Eastern Front being over-interpreted as, in Fussell's phrase, "a literary war."

Three groups that have been treated extensively in studies of shell shock will have to be presented differently in historical writing about the Eastern Front. I have in mind veterans, women, and children. The usual problems of returning war veterans, involving work, compensation, and stigmatization, are complicated when postwar Soviet occupation enters the picture. Issues of soldierly masculine identity will play out quite differently during and after World War II, most likely with less discussion of the "crisis of masculinity" theme.[38]

Similarly, in narratives of Central and Eastern European trauma, women will shift from being occasional, collateral victims of male combat to primary targets of structural civilian violence. They will appear in a greater range of roles, both passive and active, beyond traditional normative roles as nurturing caretakers and grief-stricken relatives.

---

[35] Email message from Hans Pols to Mark Micale, 5 March 2020.

[36] Antić (2017), which does devote a good deal of space to politics and psychiatric discourse, is an important exception.

[37] In Jolande Withuis and Annet Mooij's important edited volume *The Politics of War Trauma: The Aftermath of World War II in Eleven European Countries* (Amsterdam: Aksant, 2010), only one Central European country (Poland) receives coverage.

[38] See, however, Steven George Jug, "All Stalin's Men? Soldierly Masculinities in the Soviet War Effort, 1938–1945," Ph.D. thesis (University of Illinois at Urbana-Champaign, 2013); and Steven G. Jug, "Militarizing Masculinities in Red Army Discourse and Subjectivity, 1942–1943," *Masculinities: A Journal of Identity and Culture* 3 (February, 2015), 189–212.

The history of children must also receive more attention. In our own time, so-called "first responders" report time and again that the most personally devastating work they are called on to perform involves children, as at the Sandy Hook Elementary School shooting in Newtown, Connecticut in 2012. In the central and eastern regions of the European Continent, great numbers of children were orphaned in both world wars, but during the later war they were also victims (and sometimes survivors) of extreme violence, including in the Nazi extermination camps.[39] Children were also wartime offspring: Children Born of War (CHIBOW) is a fascinating international team project, funded by the European Union, that seeks to expand what we know about children born during World War II to women who became pregnant as the result of forced or consensual sex with enemy soldiers.[40] Building on the pioneering work of the American child psychiatrist Robert Coles, the field of childhood trauma has grown tremendously in the past generation; it offers another excellent opportunity for historians to engage medical psychology.

Other differences between historical writing about shell shock and future writing about trauma, I venture, will be less empirical than interpretative. Influenced by Eric Leed's work, shell shock studies have tended to attribute traumatic neurosis to the coming of modern industrialized warfare. In this interpretation, it was basically "the shock of the new" in military technology that assaulted the human nervous system.[41] This formulation works less well for World War II, which would seem to require a different hermeneutic. Hana Kubátová's essay below raises another challenge for the historian of bloodlands trauma. In light of the multi-ethnic and multi-religious character of these regions, and the much greater variety of victimized groups in World War II, first-hand accounts of events are likely to present contrasting or contradictory narratives, including significant differences between accounts by Jews and Gentiles. This situation differs from Western Europe, where autobiographical archives reflect

[39] Tuomas Laine-Frigren, "Traumatized Children in Hungary After World War II," in this book.

[40] See www.chibow.org (accessed 29 January 2021). I thank Oskars Gruzins of the University of Latvia for bringing this project to my attention. See also Sabine Lee, *Children Born of War in the Twentieth Century* (Manchester: University of Manchester Press, 2017), Chap. 3.

[41] Eric Leed, "Fateful Memories: Industrialized War and Traumatic Neurosis," *Journal of Contemporary History* 35:1 (2000), 85–100; Eric Leed, *No Man's Land: Combat & Identity in World War I* (Cambridge: Cambridge University Press, 1979), Chap. 5.

more homogenous national cultures.[42] There is also the question of how scholars themselves, who were born, raised, and trained on different sides of the Cold War divide, and in different countries, will approach and interpret psychological trauma. How do decades of state-mandated socialist/communist education (as opposed to Western capitalist-democratic schooling) influence the work of historians, both older and younger?

Somewhat more speculatively, I want to suggest that in "writing Central and Eastern European trauma," the actual affective content of the post-traumatic neuroses under investigation may differ from what was experienced in other times and places. Trauma is a singular noun but the psychological experience it designates is a shifting compound of many emotional ingredients, including stress, anxiety, fear, terror, dread, panic, helplessness, shock, sadness, and depression.[43]

The first of two emotions that I think may appear with special prominence in a psychiatric account of Central and Eastern Europe is guilt. Guilt over taking the life of another member of our species is universal. In an affecting episode in Remarque's *All Quiet on the Western Front* (1929), the young German soldier-protagonist Paul Bäumer, as he spends the night with an expiring young soldier, laments that he has bayoneted a Frenchman. Likewise, what today we refer to as "survivor's guilt" has been observed since ancient Greece and has been integrated into the symptom-synthesis that is PTSD.

In the bloodlands, there were other sources of acute remorse as well. Much soldier-on-civilian and civilian-on-civilian violence took place. Hand-to-hand aggression among combatants to secure a military goal or protect the homeland is one thing; but the killing of helpless or harmless non-combatants—"the slaughter of the innocents," to use the New Testament phrase—requires an altogether different mentality. *Einsatzgruppen* searched out and murdered Jews, Poles, Soviets, and Roma, including infants and the elderly, and then dumped the corpses in hastily dug mass graves. Even these presumably hardened executioners were said to report discomfort over their activities. As we know from Christopher Browning's acclaimed research, German police units composed of "ordinary" working-class, middle-aged German reservists worked

---

[42] See Kubátová, in this book.

[43] The ongoing work of Ruth Leys has shown a special awareness of trauma's affective variability. See Leys, *The Ascent of Affect: Genealogy and Critique* (Chicago: University of Chicago Press, 2017).

in Poland to round up Jews and other perceived enemies of the Third Reich for deportation to the death camps. Some people, according to Browning, were so troubled by what they were doing that they requested and received, transfers to other posts.[44]

"Perpetrator trauma" is a recent concept, formulated by legal scholars, to describe a severely bad conscience about committing or participating in an act of life-threatening violence.[45] Preferable to me is the notion of "moral injury." Conceptualized and coined by Jonathan Shay in the 1990s, moral injury is a haunting, profound shame about harming another human being that retrospectively violates the perpetrator's personal moral standards.[46] It is not a medical-pathological concept and is not part of the formal PTSD diagnosis, yet anyone familiar with the novels of Dostoevsky understands the destructive psychological effects that can arise, especially over a long time, from committing such acts.

The second affective phenomenon that is likely to figure more prominently is, I think, nostalgia. By nostalgia, I do not mean just a vague and wistful yearning for a bygone era or a sweet literary melancholy about "lost time." In his recent study *What Nostalgia Was: War, Empire, and the Time of a Deadly Emotion*, Thomas Dodman reminds us that in Europe nostalgia was once experienced as a more debilitating and even deadly disease.[47] The nostalgia of Central and Eastern European survivors of World War II is of this sort. It is a kind of pathological longing, lasting the remainder of one's lifetime, for an entire world that can never be revisited or reconjured because it was destroyed. From the Bolshevik Revolution of 1917 until the end of their lives, most Russian émigrés were never able to return to their homeland. Post-1945, the Jews of Berlin and Warsaw could not go back to their prewar neighborhoods and resume their prewar lives; the people and places constituting those worlds had been obliterated.

---

[44] Although, alas, this was only a small minority of people, as Browning makes clear. See Christopher R. Browning, *Ordinary Men: Reserve Police Battalion 101 and the Final Solution in Poland* (New York: Harper Collins, 1992).

[45] Saira Mohamed, "Of Monsters and Men: Perpetrator Trauma and Mass Atrocity," *Columbia Law Review* 115:5 (2015), 1157–216; Raya Morag, "On the Definition of the Perpetrator: From the Twentieth to the Twenty-First Century," *Journal of Perpetrator Research* 2:1 (2018), 13–9.

[46] Jonathan Shay, *Odysseus in America: Combat Trauma and the Undoing of Character* (New York: Simon & Schuster, 2010), Chap. 20. See also Susan Derwin, "Moral Injury: Two Perspectives," in Leese and Crouthamel, eds (2016), Chap. 3.

[47] Thomas Dodman, *What Nostalgia Was: War, Empire, and the Time of a Deadly Emotion* (Chicago: University of Chicago Press, 2018).

Death tolls tally the loss of individual lives; but beyond these "human losses" is the less quantifiable loss of entire towns, cities, and countries— the loss of landscapes, histories, and identities. On the Eastern Front, "total war" equaled total loss, to an exponentially greater degree than on the Western, or Middle Eastern, or Mediterranean fronts in either world war.[48] Because of the millions of displaced persons in these regions, any future historian of trauma will have to grapple with the psychological legacies of uprooting and the phenomena of exile memory and traumatic subjectivity.

Finally, writing Central and Eastern European trauma may well require a conceptual reorientation. If I read it correctly, the core subject being analyzed in the extant historiography of shell shock is the individual male combatant—the soldier in the trenches, or behind the lines, or writing home, or praying, or in a medical ward, or back home struggling with the war's emotional aftermath. As narrated by scholars thus far, the larger supra-individual contexts for the shell shocked soldier are families, veterans, and governments.

On this point, too, the nations of the former bloodlands present a fundamentally different historical picture. Study of psychological trauma in Central and Eastern Europe during the age of the dictators is preeminently the study of collectivities. Cataclysmic campaigns of mass violence were directed not just against the armed forces of foreign nations but against civilian groups and communities: Slavic peoples, Jews, communists, gypsies, gay people, black people, vagrants, Jehovah's Witnesses, the physically disabled, the mentally handicapped, the psychiatrically troubled—the whole gallery of collective Others demonized in fascist ideology.

Scholars will have to work out what the greater role of collective traumatization in Central and Eastern European history means. It seems clear that the overlapping concepts of "social trauma" and "cultural trauma"— especially as these categories have been formulated by the sociologist team of Jeffrey Alexander, Ron Eyerman, Neil Smelser, Bernhard Giesen, and Piotr Sztompka—will be pertinent.[49] In the process of this exploration,

---

[48] At the conference that preceded this book—"Aftershocks: War-Related Trauma in Northern, Eastern, and Central Europe," University of Tampere, Finland, 26 October 2018—loss was a theme of extensive group discussion.

[49] The best introduction to the concept remains Jeffrey C. Alexander, Ron Eyerman, Bernhard Giesen, Neil J. Smelser, and Piortr Sztompka, *Cultural Trauma and Collective Identity* (Berkeley: University of California Press, 2004), which includes an essay by Sztompka on trauma and post-Communism in Eastern Europe. See also Alexander (2012); Eyerman

historians may forge new interdisciplinary alignments with the social sciences. "The Second War and after" is also richer terrain for exploring the intergenerational transmission and transmutation of traumatic memory and identity than World War I and its aftermath. I hope the publication of *Trauma, Experience and Narrative in Europe During and After World War II* will encourage discussion of these and many other matters.

In this essay, I have mostly written about violence, death, and destruction. I want to end with an observation about opportunity, democracy, and the future. With the many contrasts I have tried to draw above between the psychological milieu of 1914–1918 and 1939–1945, the latter event has always appeared the darker and deadlier of the two conflicts. On one important point, though, this is not the case. The corpus of commentary on Western Front shell shock during the past 40 years has related a tragic and compelling story from a hundred years ago to an audience of scholars, novelists, and filmmakers as well as to general readers interested in military history. For all its quantity and quality, however, this scholarship has not really informed or altered the national self-identity of Britons, Belgians, the French, or Germans.

The nascent scholarly initiative to reconstruct the traumatic history of Central and Eastern Europe, however, is emerging under very different circumstances, and at a propitious time. It is a historiographical project that corresponds with a political transformation. Despite the recent setbacks in political freedom—and often after centuries of foreign rule and outright repression—most people in Central and Eastern Europe now enjoy more liberties than they have in historical memory. They have opportunities to discover, document, narrate, teach, and interpret "what really happened" during and after World War II, and they can conduct these vital cathartic activities in the public sphere. Instead of national identities based on silence and suppression, they can strive to forge a more open, honest, and non-pathological way of dealing with their past.

There is no way of knowing what the multifarious mental health impacts of the combined Nazi and Soviet traumas of 1939–1990 will be. This is a

(2001); Ron Eyerman, *Is This America?: Katrina as Cultural Trauma* (Austin: University of Texas Press, 2015); Ron Eyerman, *Memory, Trauma, and Identity* (Cham: Palgrave Macmillan, 2019); and Piotr Sztompka, "Cultural Trauma: The Other Face of Social Change," *European Journal of Social Theory* 3:4 (2000), 449–66. Historian Wulf Kansteiner provides a theoretical critique of the concept in "Genealogy of a Category Mistake: A Critical Intellectual History of the Cultural Trauma Metaphor," *Rethinking History: The Journal of Theory and Practice* 8:2 (2004), 193–221.

region of humanity's recent past about which our factual knowledge is now increasing rapidly but that we have mastered neither intellectually nor emotionally. If there were ever a place to recall William Faulkner's famous line—"The past is never dead. It's not even past"—it is here. Furthermore, the unprecedented opportunity for new democracies in this part of the world since the early 1990s has suffered major setbacks: there have been disturbing right-wing turns to nationalism in Poland, Hungary, and Turkey. As I write this essay, hundreds of thousands of pro-democracy protesters in the capital of Belarus are seeking to oust the dictator Alexander Lukashenko, who has been in power since the mid-1990s. Most tragic has been Russia's wholesale reversion to authoritarianism under Vladimir Putin. What is more, as Hans Pols and I have tried to demonstrate elsewhere in regard to another region of the world, the memorialization of historical traumas can itself be manipulated for malign political purposes.[50]

Notwithstanding these realities, this much seems apparent: in Central and Eastern Europe, more than any earlier time, the post-totalitarian present offers new opportunities for undertaking the requisite "trauma work." The process cannot be accomplished by academic historians alone, or by politicians and intellectuals without the involvement of many others. Nor will the task be completed in a single generation. The ten original studies in this volume are early admirable attempts at carrying out some of the important work required.

---

[50] Mark S. Micale and Hans Pols, eds, *Traumatic Pasts in Asia: History, Psychiatry, and Trauma from the 1930s to the Present* (New York: Berghahn, 2021), Introduction.

PART II

Case Studies

Testing the Silence: Trauma and Military Psychiatry in Soviet Russia and Ukraine During and After World War II

Robert Dale

INTRODUCTION

This chapter calls for a re-examination of how historians understand war-related trauma in the Red Army during World War II, and among Soviet veterans in the first postwar decade. Since the opening of the Soviet party-state's archives in the 1990s, many of the Stalinist regime's ideological claims have been thoroughly interrogated; many aspects of the Soviet experience once considered inaccessible or unknowable have begun to be reconstructed. What follows attempts to re-interpret the trauma of combatants in a similar spirit, offering a more nuanced interpretation of how mental trauma was understood by late Stalinist society. The official narrative, deeply embedded in Soviet military psychiatry, that Soviet soldiers

R. Dale (✉)
School of History, Classics, and Archaeology, Newcastle University, Newcastle-upon-Tyne, UK
e-mail: Robert.Dale@newcastle.ac.uk

© The Author(s), under exclusive license to Springer Nature Switzerland AG 2022
V. Kivimäki, P. Leese (eds.), *Trauma, Experience and Narrative in Europe after World War II*, Palgrave Studies in the History of Experience, https://doi.org/10.1007/978-3-030-84663-3_3

escaped the war on the Eastern Front without falling victim to the neuroses that affected the bourgeois West, and that the collectivist spirit and egalitarian class structure of the Red Army prevented traumatic reactions, is ripe for re-evaluation. The idea that "Russians possessed a superior cultural framework for coping with extreme circumstances"[1] can be hard to dispute given the hardships and horrors Soviet soldiers experienced on the frontlines, and veterans' relatively successful reintegration into civilian life.[2] Against the backdrop of the increasing politicization, even sacralization, of the Great Patriotic War's memory in post-Soviet Russia, advancing arguments about the extent of Soviet war trauma could be caricatured as disrespectful, intended to diminish veterans' heroism.[3] Similarly, the notion that the Soviet Union and its medical practitioners had little or no conception of psychological trauma, and only provided limited and frequently inadequate care, treatment, and assistance for psychiatric casualties, is firmly entrenched in western historiography. Nevertheless, the resilience of Soviet soldiers in the face of mass death and extreme violence needs revisiting. This chapter argues that Soviet war trauma was neither enveloped in a deafening silence, nor completely shrouded in social stigma. Building on earlier work on psychiatric research in postwar Leningrad,[4] I argue that the Soviet psychiatric profession and wider society had a much clearer conception of trauma than the scholarship has previously indicated. Closer examination of evidence of individual breakdown on the frontlines and in the wake of war reminds us that Soviet soldiers were anything but immune to the destructive, destabilizing and disquieting effects of war. Late Stalinist society managed the aftermath of wartime violence and

---

[1] Catherine Merridale, "The Collective Mind: Trauma and Shell shock in Twentieth-Century Russia," *Journal of Contemporary History* 35:1 (2000a), 39–55 (cit. 47).

[2] On the reintegration of demobilized veterans, see Mark Edele, *Soviet Veterans of the Second World War: A Popular Movement in an Authoritarian Society, 1941–1991* (Oxford: Oxford University Press, 2008), and Robert Dale, *Demobilized Veterans in Late Stalinist Leningrad: Soldiers to Civilians* (London: Bloomsbury, 2015).

[3] On the memory of the Great Patriotic War, see Nina Tumarkin, *The Living and the Dead: The Rise and Fall of the Cult of World War II in Russia* (New York: Basic Books, 1994); Roger Markwick, "The Great Patriotic War in Soviet and Post-Soviet Collective Memory," in *The Oxford Handbook of Postwar European History*, ed. by Dan Stone (Oxford: Oxford University Press, 2012), 692–712; Mark Edele, "Fighting Russia's History Wars: Vladimir Putin and the Codification of World War II," *History & Memory* 29:2 (2017), 90–124.

[4] Dale (2015), 120–29; idem, "'No Longer Normal': Traumatized Red Army Veterans in Postwar Leningrad," in *Traumatic Memories of the Second World War and After*, ed. by Peter Leese and Jason Crouthamel (Cham: Palgrave Macmillan, 2016), 119–41.

destruction remarkably successfully, but this should not blind us to the enormous material damage, emotional dislocation, and the psychological fallout of war.

This research tests the boundaries of the social, cultural and medical silences that supposedly surrounded Soviet war trauma. It explores neglected and underappreciated evidence about the extent of wartime and postwar psychological trauma among serving soldiers and demobilized veterans. Below the surface veneer of Stalinism's orderly transition from war to peace, war trauma was a significant medical, social and cultural problem. Grief, nightmares, fear, anxiety, emotional turmoil and an array of psychiatric conditions remained taboo, but they were nevertheless part of the postwar landscape. This is not to challenge the notion that war trauma was culturally constructed, or that Soviet society had its own extensive experience of dealing with the aftermath of violence, and its own vocabularies, diagnoses and treatment for trauma. Although Soviet war-related trauma was deeply conditioned by Russian culture and Stalinist politics, which provided coping mechanisms, there were still many people disturbed by their wartime experiences whose voices can be detected in the sources.

Given the intensity and murderousness of violence on the Eastern Front, one might anticipate that war's damaging psychological effects would be written large in Soviet archival records. As Ana Antić's chapter eloquently demonstrates, there was no direct correlation between exposure to extreme violence or the scale of wartime suffering and public articulation of psychological pain. Official sources often poorly articulate many Stalinist social and cultural practices, and the mentalities that underpinned them. Silences at the level of state policy or official public culture, as Catherine Merridale reminds us, often created "a barrier to the discussion of individual traumatic symptoms."[5] Although traumatic reactions to the Soviet wartime experience were abundant, they were frequently concealed. As Merridale writes, "Trauma, in the Red Army, was virtually invisible. [...] shock, and the distress of all that the men witnessed at the front was virtually taboo."[6] Trauma scholars, more generally, have considered trauma to be an "unclaimed experience," inaccessible to victims and researchers

---

[5] Merridale (2000a), 47.
[6] Catherine Merridale, *Ivan's War: The Red Army 1939–45* (London: Faber & Faber, 2005), 15.

alike, because traumatic experiences are unassimilated.[7] Cultural historians have long acknowledged the inadequacy of language to describe the horrors of modern warfare.[8] As the oral historian Anika Walke puts it, "The basic assumption here is that our cultural frameworks, and specifically our language, are inadequate to make sense of the experience."[9] Indeed, one of the central premises of the chapters gathered in this volume is that the available terms, diagnoses and vocabularies to articulate, as well as the social and cultural forums in which to share individual and collective trauma, were unequal to the task.

Trauma makes itself known precisely through silences. The relative silence around Soviet war trauma should not be confused with an indifference to war's psychological damage. Evidence of individual psychological breakdown on the frontlines or after demobilization is abundant. Numb personal silences, myths of stoic heroism and official silences, however, have frustrated a more sustained analysis of war trauma. These silences, and their social and cultural meaning, need careful interpretation. Silences, as Jay Winter observes, are better understood not as complete voids characterized by the absence of sound, but rather as "the absence of conventional verbal exchanges." Silences are a "socially constructed space in which and about which subjects and words normally used in everyday life are not spoken."[10] The boundaries of the spoken, the unspoken and the unsayable are maintained, observed and enforced in complicated ways. In the Soviet case, these silences might be consensual, contributing to the construction of accepted shared narratives that structured everyday life,[11] or strategic, communicating social values, enforcing conformity, or

---

[7] Cathy Caruth, *Unclaimed Experience: Trauma, Narrative and History* (Baltimore, MD: Johns Hopkins University Press, 1996), 4–7; Ruth Leys, *Trauma: A Genealogy* (Chicago: University of Chicago Press, 2000).

[8] For example, Paul Fussell, *The Great War and Modern Memory* (Oxford: Oxford University Press, 1975), 169–70.

[9] Anika Walke, *Pioneers and Partisans: An Oral History of Nazi Genocide in Belorussia* (Oxford: Oxford University Press, 2015), 33.

[10] Jay Winter, "Thinking about Silence," in *Shadows of War: A Social History of Silence in the Twentieth Century*, ed. by Efrat Ben Ze'ev, Ruth Ginio and Jay Winter (Cambridge: Cambridge University Press, 2010), 3–31 (cit. 4); idem, "Representations of War and the Social Construction of Silence," in *Fighting Words and Images: Representing War across the Disciplines*, ed. by Elena V. Baraban, Stephen Jaeger and Adam Muller (Toronto: University of Toronto Press, 2012), 27–45 (cit. 29).

[11] Winter (2010), 23.

providing political direction.[12] It was not that Red Army veterans avoided psychological pain and mental suffering, but that disquieting reminders of the horror of extreme violence and mass death could not be easily accommodated within public discourse. Silence represented the lack of an acceptable public discourse to frame trauma rather than the absence of war's psychological damage.

If we examine different social spaces, probe unexplored published and archival sources or even return to familiar sources with a critical awareness of the need to listen more carefully to subtle expressions of trauma, it is possible to test the limits of this supposed silence. In doing so, trauma emerges as more widely understood and discussed in Stalin's final years than is commonly appreciated. This chapter explores three main bodies of primary source material, examined in turn. Some of these sources are relatively well known—their general nature if not the specific examples familiar to subject specialists—while others are discussed for the first time. After an examination of the current state of the historiography dealing with Soviet war trauma, centered largely but not exclusively on Russia, the chapter begins by examining published medical and psychiatric research about Soviet soldiers' psychological trauma. These forms of evidence have been analysed by other scholars, but if read with sensitivity they reveal much about Soviet conceptions of trauma. The focus is on the leading publications *Voenno-meditsinskii zhurnal* (Military Medical Journal) and *Nevropatologiia i psikhitariia* (Neuropathology and Psychiatry). Far from ignoring war trauma, medical researchers studied traumatic reactions among soldiers and veterans in a sustained and nuanced manner. Psychiatrists, however, did not have a monopoly on how trauma was understood and constructed. In a second section, the chapter examines the vernacular languages of trauma expressed in combatants' letters, diaries and memoirs. Soldiers and veterans were prepared to employ the language of trauma in specific social circumstances. They listed instances of concussion (*kontuziia*), described psychological or emotional pain and identified themselves as traumatized more frequently than has been acknowledged. These were not transparent articulations of trauma, but representations of wartime damage enmeshed with assertions of privilege, martial masculinities and Stalinist identities. A third and final section

---

[12] Ketil Knutsen, "Strategic Silence: Political Persuasion between the Remembered and the Forgotten," in *Beyond Memory: Silence and the Aesthetics of Remembrance*, ed. by Alexandre Dessingué and Jay Winter (London: Routledge, 2016), 125–40.

examines how traumatized veterans were treated and cared for by local medical institutions, exploring medical treatment and care beyond research settings. Much of this material is drawn from the archival files of the Ukrainian Ministry of Health. It reveals much about how war trauma was experienced, shaped, represented and treated in different places, institutions and contexts within the Soviet Union. Together these sources reveal that the impact of war trauma was felt far beyond individual soldiers' private mental worlds.

HISTORIOGRAPHICAL CONTEXT

The traumatic reactions experienced by Soviet veterans of World War II do not have an extensive historiography. Many social histories of the Red Army and Soviet soldiers' frontline experiences make little or no reference to trauma or combat breakdown.[13] Historians of Soviet veterans of World War II have often acknowledged psychological trauma, but few, with the exception of Merridale, have systematically examined the impact of trauma on veterans' postwar lives. By contrast, in other national and historical contexts, particularly the trench warfare on the Western Front between 1914 and 1918, discussions of trauma, or, more specifically, shell shock have proliferated.[14] We know as much about the complexities and subtleties of late imperial Russian neuropsychiatry and the trauma of soldiers of the Russo-Japanese War and World War I as we do about the psychiatric casualties of the Great Patriotic War.[15] Several scholars have reconstructed

---

[13] Alexander Hill, *The Red Army and the Second World War* (Cambridge: Cambridge University Press, 2017); Roger R. Reese, *Why Stalin's Soldiers Fought: The Red Army's Military Effectiveness in World War II* (Lawrence: University Press of Kansas); Brandon M. Schechter, *The Stuff of Soldiers: A History of the Red Army in World War II Through Objects* (Ithaca, NY: Cornell University Press, 2019).

[14] For example Peter Leese, *Shell Shock: Traumatic Neurosis and the British Soldiers of the First World War* (London: Palgrave Macmillan, 2002); Fiona Reid, *Broken Men: Shell Shock, Treatment and Recovery in Britain, 1914–30* (London: Continuum, 2010); Jason Crouthamel and Peter Leese, eds, *Psychological Trauma and the Legacies of the First World War* (Cham: Palgrave Macmillan, 2016); Tracey Loughran, *Shell shock and Medical Culture in First World War Britain* (Cambridge: Cambridge University Press, 2017).

[15] A. B. Astashov, "Voina kak kul'turnyi shok: Analiz psikhopatologicheskogo sostoianiia Russkoi armii v pervuiu mirovuiu voiny," *Voenno-istoricheskaia antropologiia: Ezhegodnik 2002* (Moscow: ROSSPEN, 2002), 268–81; Paul Wanke, *Russian/Soviet Military Psychiatry, 1904–1945* (London: Routledge, 2005), 5–41; Laura L. Phillips, "Gendered Dis/ability: Perspectives from the Treatment of Psychiatric Casualties in Russia's Early Twentieth

the theoretical frameworks and administrative structures through which Soviet military psychiatry operated during the war, although these studies often reveal little about actual frontline practice.[16] The prevailing interpretation is that the Red Army and its medical services had little or no conception of trauma. To quote Merridale again, "Stress, let alone a complicated diagnosis like PTSD, post-traumatic stress disorder, was as foreign to the Red Army's medical orderlies as the hysterical indispositions of the bourgeoisie."[17] It was not that soldiers escaped mental damage, but that only the most extreme cases were likely to be recognized as such. Elena Seniavskaia, who has written extensively on the psychology of frontline soldiers, acknowledges the difficulties of soldiers' postwar adaptation and notes that after the Great Patriotic War "the unavoidable post-traumatic syndrome did not deepen into a crisis of spiritual values, as has often happened in history after unjust or senseless wars."[18] Scholarly interest in psychological trauma among combatants has been stronger in relation to veterans of more recent conflicts in Afghanistan and Chechnya. In the context of these unpopular military defeats, post-Soviet society has more willingly accepted that war exposed soldiers to horrific experiences, which proved deeply traumatic. Discussions of an Afghan or Chechen Syndrome have resonated beyond researchers and trauma scholars.[19]

Century Wars," *Social History of Medicine* 20:2 (2007), 333–50; Jan Plamper, "Fear: Soldiers and Emotion in Early Twentieth-Century Russian Military Psychology," *Slavic Review* 68:2 (2009), 259–83; Martin A. Miller, "Psychiatric Diagnosis as Political Critique: Russia in War and Revolution," in *Russian Culture in War and Revolution, 1914–22, Vol 2: Political Culture, Identities, Mentalities and Memory*, ed. by Murray Frame, Boris Kolonitskii, Steven G. Marks and Melissa K. Stockdale (Bloomington: Slavica, 2013), 245–56.

[16] Wanke (2005), 57–108; R. Gabriel, *Soviet Military Psychiatry: The Theory and Practice of Coping with Battle Stress* (Westport, CT: Greenwood Press, 1986); Albert R. Gilgen, *Soviet and American Psychology During World War II* (Westport, CT: Greenwood Press, 1997).

[17] Merridale (2005), 232.

[18] E.S. Seniavskaia, *Istoriia voin Rossii XX veka v chelovecheskom izmerenii: problemy voenno-istoricheskoi antropologii i psikhologii* (Moscow: Rossiiskii gosudarstvennyi gumanitarnyi universitet, 2012), 120.

[19] Karen Petrone, "Coming Home Soviet Style: The Reintegration of Afghan Veterans into Soviet Everyday Life," in *Everyday Life in Russia: Past and Present*, ed. by Choi Chatterjee, David L. Ransel, Mary Cavander and Karen Petrone (Bloomington: Indiana University Press, 2015), 350–67; Ben A. McVicker, "Afghantsy: The Social, Political, and Cultural Legacy of A Forgotten Generation," Ph.D. thesis (University of Toronto, 2018); Rodric Braithwaite, *Afgantsy: The Russians in Afghanistan, 1979–89* (London: Profile, 2012), 314, 321–2; Seniavskaia (2012), 120–9; Sergei Alex Oushakine, *The Patriotism of Despair: Nation, War and Loss in Russia* (Ithaca, NY: Cornell University Press, 2009); Maya Eichler,

"Instead of focusing on the limits and constraints that trauma imposes on one's symbolic capacity—instead of exploring the unclaimed, the unsaid, and the unrepresentable," Sergei Oushakine's work on Chechen war veterans in provincial Siberia has demonstrated how much can be learned by examining the "mechanisms and forms that capture the individual or collective experience of the traumatic."[20] Although the circumstances and historical context were different, the increased willingness for mental pain to be discussed within post-Soviet society, including among veterans themselves, may cross-fertilize research into the traumatic experiences and reactions of Soviet World War II veterans.

Western interpretations of Russian psychiatric practice, particularly those shaped by Cold War assumptions, frequently draw upon misplaced notions of the backwardness and/or brutality of Russian/Soviet science. New research, however, takes Soviet psychiatry seriously, examining and explaining the development of the psychiatric profession and mental health-care provision in the context of a revolutionary state and society.[21] How Soviet psychiatric practices, conditions and diagnoses developed over time, particularly under the pressures of Stalinism, have been reinterpreted.[22] Benjamin Zajicek, in particular, has reconstructed the theoretical underpinnings of Stalin-era psychiatry and demonstrated how Soviet

Militarizing Men: Gender, Conscription and War in Post-Soviet Russia (Stanford, CA: Stanford University Press, 2012), 121–6; Elisabeth Sieca-Kozlowski, "The Post-Soviet Russian State facing War Veterans' Psychological Suffering: Concept and Legacy," *The Journal of Power Institutions in Post-Soviet Societies* Issue 14/15 (2013), https://doi.org/10.4000/pipss.3995 (last accessed 13 January 2021); Fedor Nikolai and Igor' Kobylin, "'Sgushchenka kak lekarstvo ot stressa': voennaia psikhologiia i armeiskie praktiki preodoleniia strakha," *Novoe literaturnoe obozrenie* 162 (2020), 158–70, https://www.nlobooks.ru/magazines/novoe_literaturnoe_obozrenie/162_nlo_2_2020/article/22083/ (last accessed 13 January 2021).

[20] Oushakine (2009), 6.

[21] Irina Sirotkina, "Toward a Soviet Psychiatry: War and the Organization of Mental Health Care in Revolutionary Russia," in *Soviet Medicine: Culture, Practice and Science*, ed. by Frances L. Bernstein, Christopher Burton and Dan Healey (DeKalb: Northern Illinois University Press, 2010), 27–48; Maria Cristina Galmarini-Kabala, "Psychiatry, Violence, and the Soviet Project of Transformation: A Micro-History of the Perm´ Psycho-Neurological School-Sanatorium," *Slavic Review* 77:2 (2018), 307–32.

[22] Benjamin Zajicek, "Soviet Madness: Nervousness, Mild Schizophrenia, and the Professional Jurisdiction of Psychiatry in the USSR, 1918–1936," *Ab Imperio* 4 (2014), 167–94; idem, "Soviet Psychiatry and the Origins of the Sluggish Schizophrenia Concept, 1912–1936," *History of the Human Sciences* 31:2 (2018), 88–105; Gregory Dufaud, "Vyzov fiziologii: Sovetskaia psikhiatriia v 1930-e gody," *Ab Imperio* 4 (2014), 136–66.

society confronted the psychiatric and psychological consequences of World War II. Drawing on a wide range of sources, Zajicek offers a model of how to reread published and archival psychiatric texts.[23] Soviet psychiatry was anything but a paragon of therapeutic care; under-resourced institutions and over-worked staff were only able to provide basic treatment. Its impulses, however, were not exclusively totalitarian. The punitive use of psychiatry against dissidents, which was common from the 1960s onwards, did not characterize the entire Soviet period. Less invasive and more patient-centred approaches to mental disorders had their place in treating certain groups of patients at specific historical moments.[24] In light of this new scholarship, a re-examination of Soviet war trauma experienced during and after World War II now seems possible. We should not assume that serving soldiers and war veterans, among the most privileged groups in late Stalinist society, were subject to the same abuse of psychiatry as dissidents.

Studies of war-related trauma, as this volume testifies, are no longer restricted to the trauma experienced by combatants. The traumatic memories of civilians who experienced the horrors of the Siege of Leningrad or occupation regimes are now better understood.[25] Oral historians have observed that trauma had the capacity to generate group solidarity and grand narratives of heroic survival, but also that exposure to death and violence prompted difficult personal memories throughout survivors' lives, even when official narratives denied long-term psychological damage.[26] Several scholars have explored how children caught in the war zone,

---

[23] Benjamin Zajicek, "Scientific Psychiatry in Stalin's Soviet Union: The Politics of Modern Medicine and the Struggle to Define 'Pavlovian' Psychiatry, 1939–1953," Ph.D. thesis (University of Chicago, 2009), 168–227.

[24] Zhores A. Medvedev and Roy A. Medvedev, *A Question of Madness*, trans. Ellen de Kadt (London: Macmillan, 1971); Sidney Bloch and Peter Reddaway, *Russia's Political Hospitals: The Abuse of Psychiatry in the Soviet Union* (London: Gollancz, 1977); Alexander Podrabinek, *Punitive Medicine* (Ann Arbor, MI: Koroma Publishers, 1980); Robert van Voren, *On Dissidents and Madness: From the Soviet Union of Leonid Brezhnev to the "Soviet Union" of Vladimir Putin* (Amsterdam: Rodopi, 2009); Rebecca Reich, *State of Madness: Psychiatry, Literature, and Dissent after Stalin* (DeKalb: Northern Illinois University Press, 2018).

[25] Pavel Vasilyev, "Alimentary and Pellagra Psychoses in Besieged Leningrad," in *Food and War in Twentieth Century Europe*, ed. by Ina Zweiniger-Bargielowska, Rachel Duffett and Alain Drouard (Farnham: Ashgate, 2011), 111–21; Alexis Peri, *The War Within: Diaries From the Siege of Leningrad* (Cambridge, MA: Harvard University Press, 2017), 191–8.

[26] Alexandra Wacther, "'This Did Not Happen': Survivors of the Siege of Leningrad (1941–1944) and the 'Truth About the Blockade'," in *Civilians Under Siege from Sarajevo*

who lost family, were exposed to mass death, extreme violence and wholesale destruction, or experienced occupation, evacuation or concentration
camps, were traumatized.[27] As Maria Cristina Galmarini-Kabala writes,
"the concept of psychic trauma was frequently used by Soviet child psychiatrists in the years between 1945 and 1949 in order to find causal
explanations for children's deviant behaviors."[28] Children who had lived
in occupied territory for extended periods often exhibited traumatic symptoms, including depression, apathy, insomnia, obsessive compulsive behaviour, phobias, intense anxiety, speech disturbances and other symptoms,
which some specialists recognized as psychological problems prompted by
negative war experiences.[29] In practice, childhood psychological trauma
was frequently ignored or went untreated, discussed only in opaque for-
mulaic allusions. Nevertheless, as Anne Livschiz reminds us, the post-
Soviet memoirs of wartime children frequently contain "the admission
and descriptions of crippling and pervasive psychological trauma, something that survivors had to live with all their lives about which they could
neither talk about nor receive help for."[30] Research on the traumatic experiences, reactions and memories of Soviet civilians, particularly of women
and children, demonstrates that silences can be broken, and that a reas-
sessment of war trauma among soldiers is overdue.

SCIENTIFIC DISCOURSES ABOUT WAR TRAUMA

Confronted by the psychological and psychiatric damage wrought by a
brutal war of extermination, Soviet military psychiatry was not silent about
the capacity of extreme violence to incapacitate and disturb individual

to *Troy*, ed. by Alex Dowdall and John Horne (London: Palgrave Macmillan, 2018), 37–60;
Walke (2015), 207–16.

[27] Juliane Fürst, "Between Salvation and Liquidation: Homeless and Vagrant Children and
the Reconstruction of Soviet Society," *Slavonic and East European Review* 86:2 (2008),
232–58; Lisa A. Kirschenbaum, "The Meaning of Resilience: Soviet Children in World War
II," *Journal of Interdisciplinary History* 47:4 (2017), 521–35; Catriona Kelly, *Children's
World: Growing up in Russia 1890–1991* (New Haven, CT: Yale University Press, 2007),
245, 421–2.

[28] Maria Cristina Galmarini-Kabala, *The Right to be Helped: Deviance, Entitlement, and the
Soviet Moral Order* (DeKalb: Northern Illinois University Press, 2016), 188.

[29] Julie K. de Graffenried, *Sacrificing Childhood: Children and the Soviet State in the Great
Patriotic War* (Texas Station, TX: University Press of Kansas, 2014), 24–7.

[30] Ann Livschiz, "Growing up Soviet: Children in the Soviet Union, 1918–1958," Ph.D. thesis (Stanford University, 2007), 569–70.

soldiers. Although it has been suggested that psychiatric trauma was virtually invisible in the wartime Red Army, the military's medical and psychiatric services, as rudimentary and imperfect as they were, regularly
encountered and treated traumatized individuals. These experiences
informed a significant body of published scientific research examining the
etiology, treatment and prevalence of traumatic reactions to wartime experiences. Much about the scientific response to trauma was problematic.
Published medical research which addressed Soviet war trauma contained
much that could be challenged and criticized. The focus was often on
developing organizational structures capable of delivering psychiatric provision, plans that were at best difficult to implement, rather than analysis
of psychiatric treatment and care. Such exercises in central planning were
conducted in a parallel universe to, and in disregard of battlefield conditions.[31] Few recommendations filtered down to frontline medics, who
were over-burdened, under-resourced and lacked specialist training. Few
societies, including our own, have a distinguished record when it comes to
understanding, diagnosing and treating trauma. Soviet military medicine,
during and after the war, was not alone in falling short of its own standards. Nevertheless, a significant number of psychiatrists and medical
researchers took evidence of traumatic reactions to wartime experiences
seriously. Instead of silence and indifference, a close reading of published
medical research reveals sustained interest in war trauma, as well as a surprisingly open debate about its forms, causes and treatment.

There was, or course, an official line. This was Stalinism after all. Well
before the German invasion of the Soviet Union in June 1941, Viktor
Petrovich Osipov, director of the Leningrad Military Academy, had predicted that the Red Army would avoid a wave of future psychiatric casualties. Soldiers and armies with a higher political and class consciousness, he
argued, were better prepared to combat their natural biological, emotional
and nervous reactions to wartime experiences.[32] Other influential psychiatrists, such as V.A. Gorovoi-Shaltan, stressed the important role of class
unity and the political education provided by the party and Komsomol in

---

[31] D.N. Shogam, "O lechebno-evakuatsionnom obsluzhivanii kontuzhennykh v armeis-
kom raione," *Voenno-meditsinskii zhurnal,* no. 12 (December 1946), 8–15.

[32] V.P. Osipov, "Osnovy raspoznavaniia psikhozov i psikoticheskikh sostoianii v praktike
voennogo vracha," in *Voprosy psikhiatricheskoi praktiki voennogo vremeni,* ed. by V.P. Osipov
(Leningrad: Narkomzdrav SSSR, 1941), 11.

fostering resilience among soldiers.[33] Ideologized and politicized statements about the capacity of Soviet soldiers to endure physical and psychological hardships were expressed throughout the war and in its aftermath. In late 1947, for example, *Nevropatologiia i psikhiatriia* published an essay by G.G. Karanovich entitled "Thirty Years of Psychiatric Organization in the Soviet Union," which praised Soviet psychiatry's achievements since the October Revolution. He argued that psycho-neuroses were extremely rare among soldiers admitted to neuro-psychiatric institutions, and that wartime circumstances had not created special categories and forms of military psychoses. He maintained that "The high moral condition of the soldiers of the Soviet Army, their firm belief in the justness of the war, pursued in the name of freedom from the yoke of fascism, deep patriotism and unlimited love for their socialist motherland appeared to be the best prophylactic against neuro-psychiatric illnesses during the Great Patriotic War."[34] Soviet psychiatry's successes in managing trauma were, at least in the official analysis, attributed to the conditions created by Soviet socialism. These were contrasted with a higher prevalence of psychiatric disturbances among combatants from capitalist countries, who, unprotected by patriotism's prophylactic qualities, were reportedly experiencing higher levels of fear and psychiatric breakdown. A popular primer on modern forms of neurosis, written by V.N. Miasishchev and published in 1956, observed that during World War II, "according to statistical data, in the USA every fifth serviceman had visited a neuro-psychiatric institution."[35]

Statements about the comparatively low number of psychiatric casualties in the Red Army, and the role of Soviet social conditions in averting traumatic reactions, were commonplace in the specialist literature during and after the war. However, the psychiatric profession's response to war trauma was more complicated than these nods to official propaganda suggest. For something considered comparatively rare in the Red Army, trauma was nevertheless widely discussed in medical and psychiatric textbooks and journals. Much of this research, although by no means all, worked within official materialist and Pavlovian paradigms for mental illness which sought explanations for traumatic reactions in physiological

---

[33] V.A. Gorovoi-Shaltan, "Psikhonevrozy voiny: Postonovka voprosa i osnovnye istochniki," in Osipov, ed. (1941), 120.

[34] G.G. Karanovich, "Tridtsatiletie psikhiatricheskoi organizatsii v Sovetskom Soiuze," *Nevropatologiia i psikhiatriia* 16:6 (November–December 1947), 15–25 (cit. 22).

[35] V.N. Miasishchev, *Sovremennye predstavleniia o nevrozakh* (Moskva: Izdatel'stvo Znanie, 1956), 15.

changes to the brain, nervous or immune systems. Some researchers questioned the seriousness of the problem, citing evidence of simulation, while others documented successful treatments and positive stories of swift recovery, claims which require further interrogation. Nevertheless, traumatic reactions to wartime service and exposure to mass violence were on the scientific agenda. Volume 26 of the official medical history of the Great Patriotic War, published in 1949, devoted over 300 pages of research to wartime nervous disorders.[36] This was no accident. On 26 March 1946, the USSR Council of Ministers passed legislation which commissioned a generously funded and ambitious multi-volume history of wartime medicine intended to collate the lessons of Soviet military medicine.[37] *Voenno-meditsinskii zhurnal* subsequently published a scientific plan for the project, developed by its editorial college, which invited submissions on hundreds of topics. Although primarily concerned with physical injuries and focused on the wartime research and practice of doctors, surgeons, nurses, epidemiologists and therapists, the plan also sought to highlight the efforts of psychiatrists to return soldiers to action.[38] Contributions were solicited on the treatment of *kontuziia* of the brain, literally a concussion or contusion, the treatment of "post-traumatic disorders of hearing and speech" and aspects of the treatment and physiology of traumatic shock.[39] *Kontuziia* was the favoured term for frontline psychiatric injuries, but the term implied physical damage to the brain caused by the concussive force of exploding shells or rapid changes in air pressure. Shells or exploding bombs were understood to cause material changes to the brain and nervous system which manifested themselves in disturbed psychiatric states. In practice, the diagnosis was applied to soldiers caught in shellfire or who broke down under battlefield conditions, irrespective of whether their symptoms could be attributed to physical brain injury. The term

[36] S.N. Davidenkov and V.A. Gorovoi-Shaltan, eds, *Nervnye bolezni: Osobennosti ikh vozniknoveniia, techeniia, preduprezhdeniia i lecheniia vo vremia voiny*, in *Opyt sovetskoi meditsiny v velikoi otechestvennoi voine, 1941–1945 gg.*, ed. by E.I. Smirnov, Vol. 26 (Moscow: Medgiz, 1949).

[37] "O nauchnoi razrabotke i obobshchenii opyta sovetskoi meditsiny za vremia Velikoi Otechestvennoi voiny 1941–45 g.g." *Pravda*, March 27, 1945, 1; State Archive of the Russian Federation (hereafter GARF) f. R-4446, op. 51, d. 3528, ll. 12–10.

[38] "Ot redaktsionnoi kollegii truda 'Opyt sovetskoi meditsiny v Velikoi Otechestvennoi voine, 1941–1945 gg.'," *Voenno-meditsinskii zhurnal*, no. 3 (March 1946), 4–5.

[39] "Plan izdaniia truda 'Opyt Sovetskoi meditsiny v Velikoi Otechestvennoi voine 1941–1945 gg.'," *Voenno-meditsinskii zhurnal*, no. 3 (March 1946), 5–12.

might be loosely translated as shell shock, but without the specific associations of British World War I military psychiatry. Far from avoiding discussion of war-related trauma, Soviet psychiatric research maintained an interest in wartime psychiatric disorders and approached these conditions with relatively little overt ideological interference. Reshaped by the demands of war, the higher status and growing strategic importance of science, Soviet researchers enjoyed much greater intellectual autonomy during and immediately after the war.[40] Relative freedom from Stalinist bureaucratic control, combined with better access to international scholarship, contributed to the range of responses to trauma published in scientific journals.

Far from denying war's traumatizing effects, a number of articles surveying the state of postwar Soviet psychiatry or evaluating psychiatry's wartime contribution acknowledged that psychiatric and psychologic damage was a "medical-sanitary consequence of war." A lengthy editorial in *Nevropatologiia i psikhiatriia*, for example, noted that as soon as the war began the problem posed by "closed injuries to the brain" had been recognized, prompting the creation of specialized hospitals for neuropsychiatric, neurosurgical and complex-concussion cases. The term "closed injuries" referred to internal brain damage, as opposed to open wounds where the brain or skull had been penetrated by bullets or shrapnel.

The editors celebrated the remarkable statistic that between 50 and 60 percent of injured soldiers with neuro-psychiatric diagnoses were returned to military service. This was a credit to the practical efforts of psychiatrists, but also to the "huge quantity of work related to psychiatric disorders of closed trauma to the brain." Many of the leading Soviet psychiatrists were listed as studying psychiatric problems connected with wartime injuries, including dealing with "the problem of reactive conditions" and liquidating "the medical-sanitary consequences of the war."[41] In February 1947, *Voenno-meditsinskii zhurnal* published a detailed examination by A.V. Snezhnevskii of the wartime experience of frontline psychiatric hospitals. Snezhnevskii would go on to enjoy notoriety as the director of the USSR Academy of Medical Sciences' Institute of Psychiatry throughout the heyday of punitive psychiatry under Brezhnev, and the key progenitor

---

[40] On the changing status of science during and after the war, see Nikolai Krementsov, *Stalinist Science* (Princeton, NJ: Princeton University Press, 1997), 95–128.

[41] "'Tridtsat' let sovetskoi nevrologii i psikhiatrii," *Nevropatologiia i psikhiatriia* 16:5 (September–October 1947), 3–18 (cit. 16–7).

of the diagnosis of "sluggish schizophrenia," which was used to justify the punitive use of psychiatry against dissidents.[42] In contrast, this article was remarkable for taking war-related trauma seriously, recognizing that the hospitalization of traumatized combatants was a major problem. During periods of active operations, especially of offensive actions, *kontuziia* cases quadrupled. At such moments, all wards of the hospital were pressed into service and approximately 80 percent of patients admitted were considered psychiatric casualties of some form. Even in quieter periods, psychiatric hospitals continued to treat soldiers suffering from the delayed effects of *kontuziia*, or who were being readmitted for further examination, often after fits, stammering or bouts of disordered consciousness. These unfortunates were estimated to be a fifth of all concussion cases. Such cases were not always well understood. As Snezhnevskii observed, "Shortcomings in our clinical knowledge of air concussion [*vozdushnoi kontuzii*] and the imperfection of our diagnostics of functional adaptability usually appear as the reason for mistakenly sending these patients [back] to [their] military units." Approximately 60 percent of new cases returned to their units, although about a quarter of patients required evacuation to hospitals behind the lines. Most patients recovered within six months, but around 8 percent were discharged from the military. However, the number of soldiers with reactive conditions, or forms of neurosis as a result of *kontuziia*, was considered to be only 2 percent. This was contrasted with the findings of Henderson and Moore whose research was reported to reveal that reactive neuroses were 35 times higher in English military hospitals.[43]

Another article evaluating the state of postwar psychiatry noted that a wartime increase in psychiatric illness had been avoided, but the distribution of illnesses had changed. More specifically, the quantity of injuries to the central nervous system, as well as the number of reactive conditions (including both those with psychogenic and somatic causes) had increased. It identified the psychological health of disability (*psychogigiena invalidnosti*) as the most pressing task facing the discipline. It stressed that "There is a large number [of people] in a post-traumatic condition [*postkontuzionnykh sostoianii*], due to the huge scale of the past war, who demand from

---

[42] Reich (2018), 23–59.

[43] A.V. Snezhnevskii, "Opyt raboty frontovogo nevropsikhiatricheskogo gospitalia v velikuiu otechestvennuiu voiny," *Voenno-meditsinskii zhurnal*, no. 2 (February 1947), 23–31 (cit. 23–7). This was presumably a reference to J.L. Henderson and Merrill Moore, "The Psychoneuroses of War," *New England Journal of Medicine* 230:10 (March 1944), 273–7.

us a developed program of special measures. An accurate record of the disabled [*invalidov*], medical-prophylactic measures, social events, work placements, and so on, will undoubtedly significantly reduce the severity of the problem in the coming years."[44] Look below the surface and it can be seen that parts of the psychiatric profession acknowledged that wartime experiences, in certain circumstances, prompted ongoing psychiatric trauma, the causes of which could be physical damage to the nervous system or psychogenic factors.

The scientific literature offered a remarkably varied series of explanations for war-related psychiatric conditions, anything but a general Stalinist line. In early 1946, for example, L.M. Ratgauz and B. Bamdas published a remarkable article in *Voenno-meditsinskii zhurnal* which investigated, and sought to explain, unusual instances of extreme fatigue among military pilots after sorties. They described how pilots became exhausted, increasingly withdrawn and depressed. Some reported poor sleep, headaches, irritability, instability, anxiety, and tension during flight, a declining desire to fly, conflict in their everyday life and a range of biological changes. The article acknowledged that shortages of oxygen at altitude, as well as the consumption of alcohol while off duty, might have weakened nervous systems.[45] The well-informed reader might have discerned a dialogue and disagreement with an article published in the same journal in the summer of 1945 which explained instances of neurosis among pilots as the physical effects of repeated exposure to prolonged periods of reduced oxygen at altitude. It argued that "there is not any kind of basis to consider this a professional pathology connected with the danger of flying during wartime."[46] Ratgauz and Bamdas disagreed, arguing that pilots' fatigue and depression could be attributed to the traumatic effects of excessive emotional strain. They noted that fear was an integral part of pilots' combat experiences. Flying was a risky endeavour, undertaken alone, which created sustained emotional stress and, from a biological perspective, a variety of new psychological reactions. They noted the views of an anonymous Hero of the Soviet Union who considered that "a pilot not capable of repressing the feeling of fear in their first combat flight could not

[44] A.O. Edel'shtein, "Sovetskaia psikhogigena na sovremennom etape," *Nevropatologiia i psikhiatriia* 16:2 (March–April 1947), 9–13 (cit. 11–12).

[45] L.M. Ratgauz and B. Bamdas, "O reaktsiiakh letchika na boevoi polet," *Voenno-meditsinskii zhurnal*, no. 1–2 (January–February 1946), 27–34.

[46] O.S. Marshalkin, "Profilatika astenii vegetativnykh nevrozov u letchikov-vysotnikov," *Voenno-meditsinskii zhurnal*, no. 7–9 (July–August 1945), 34–8 (cit. 37).

become a good combat pilot." Individuals varied in their levels of resilience and nervous constitutions. Some soldiers might fly a hundred sorties without experiencing a reaction, others might fly seven or eight before encountering problems. Some soldiers might identify these individuals as cowards and malingerers, but the article was in no doubt that the emotional pressures on pilots were extreme and potentially damaging. The solution was to prompt an emotional shift, through rest, sport and physical culture, and an emphasis on adequate sleep. As the authors noted, "It is very important to give the pilot after a sortie time to respond, to react to emotional stress."[47] Pilots were, of course, anything but representative; they enjoyed better access to medicine than common infantrymen. Acknowledging that "Stalin's falcons," a group celebrated as exemplars of Stalinist masculine heroism,[48] could be broken down by repeated exposure to extreme fear, suggests that silence did not envelop war trauma.

The published psychiatric research discussed traumatic reactions to wartime experiences more openly and in more varied and interesting ways than has been understood. Although the official scientific position was that psychiatric disturbances were the product of physical damage or changes to the brain and nervous system caused by explosions, many researchers painted a more complicated picture of the manifestations of trauma and their causes. A close reading of the learned journals indicates a remarkable diversity, and a very fragile consensus, around war trauma. There was, for example, a strand in the scholarship which accepted that wartime psychiatric disorders had an emotional or psychological dimension. An article by A.N. Mindadze, published under the title "About emotional reactions in the conditions of military operations," stated that "war is a grandiose psychological experiment" that had complicated and diverse effects. The article was based on the author's observations of the conditions created by frontline aerial bombardment. He noted that concussion (*kontuziia*) and emotional commotion were frequently conflated. According to his research, *kontuziia* was the term systematically applied, but often mistakenly. The article offered several detailed patient histories of soldiers caught in aerial bombardments whose conditions were considered emotional rather than physiological. Mindadze related the case of a patient he treated at a medical evacuation point in the direct aftermath of

[47] Ratgauz and Bamdas (1946), 27–34.
[48] On the special status of pilots, see K. E. Bailes, "Technology and Legitimacy: Soviet Aviation and Stalinism in the 1930s," *Technology and Culture* 17:1 (1976), 55–81.

an attack. The soldier was in a state of complete detachment, standing against a wall looking at a fixed point. He returned to his self after about six hours but continued to exhibit traumatic symptoms. Further aerial raids caused extreme fear; the patient became pale and his whole body shook. He suffered from insomnia and nightmares.[49] Exposure to fear, Minadadze argued, manifested itself in many different ways, including pallor, cold sweats, a widening of pupils, tremors, a quickening or slowing of the pulse. Although those individuals with the most resilient nervous systems might be able to "localize their emotional suffering," even completely healthy people might suffer emotional reactions to military service.[50] Another paper published in the same issue of *Nevropatologiia i psikhiatriia* explored instances of visual hallucinations which developed as a form of delirium after *kontuziia*. One soldier, concussed in the autumn of 1942 and again in February 1943, lost the power of speech, the ability to hear and periodically his consciousness. He subsequently felt weak, experienced headaches and dizziness and was discharged from the army in June 1943, after which he began to experience visions. These consisted of seeing manifestations of horses, goats, dogs and various people. At night he often experienced scenes from the frontlines, including a recurring vision of explaining how to handle grenades to soldiers.[51]

Acceptance that frontline experiences could be traumatic and that psychiatric illnesses might have psychological or emotional aetiologies was not universal. Much of the scientific discussion about trauma linked disturbed psychiatric states to physical illnesses and injuries or explored the connection between trauma and other psychiatric conditions. Psychiatrists, as other historians have noted, were keen to connect unexplained psychological or psychiatric reactions with physical conditions such as hypertension.[52] In a detailed patient history published in 1947, V.L. Zvereva described a soldier who had been lightly shell shock (*kontuzhenyi*) in 1941. Although he had not lost consciousness, he had temporarily lost his hearing, and for two weeks he suffered from a tremor and stutter. He fully recovered but suffered a relapse in June 1945 after "suffering a serious

[49] A.A. Mindadze, "Ob emotsional'nykh reaktsiakh v usloviiakh boevoi obstanovki," *Nevropatologiia i psikhiatriia* 16:2 (March–April 1947), 37–41 (cit. 39).

[50] Ibid., 41.

[51] A.N. Molokhov, "O zritel'nykh galliutsinatsiiakh u rezidual'nykh travmatikov," *Nevropatologiia i psikhiatriia* 16:2 (March–April 1947), 26–30 (cit. 28).

[52] Merridale (2000a), 47; idem, *Night of Stone: Death and Memory in Russia* (London: Granta, 2000b), 304.

psychogenic trauma." After this, he would suddenly awake during the night feeling worried or frightened. His heart beat more quickly, "like a hammer in his chest," and his arms and legs shook. Although the author noted that the soldier was experiencing anxiety and depression, and that psychological factors were contributing factors, their ultimate explanations were sought in raised blood pressure.[53] Instances of war trauma were also conflated with, and treated as, schizophrenia.[54] One article, for example, explored the connection between schizophrenic disorders and wartime traumas. However, it noted that less than 7 percent of cases (20 out of the 300 studied) developed after *kontuziia* or head injuries. It concluded that these instances were the product of a weakening of organic systems. Yet, it should also be noted that the research was unclear as to precisely how and why cases of schizophrenia occurred on the battlefield, and it called for more detailed and specialized investigations.[55] This and other articles provide a reminder that many psychiatric processes remained very poorly understood, and that many psychiatrists were at a loss to explain the conditions presenting before them.

Discussions of war trauma also centred upon instances of what was termed "deaf mutism," which in either partial or total form was connected to *kontuziia*. The conventional wisdom held that disturbances to hearing and speech were the result of physical changes to the brain and nervous system. Nevertheless, in December 1945, *Voenno-meditsinskii zhurnal* published a remarkable article by Ia. M. Sviadoshch, a junior researcher, which challenged the materialist interpretations of leading authorities. He argued that "all cases of functional deaf-mutism among the concussed relate to psychogenic (hysterical) reactions." The differing distributions of hysterical fits and deaf mutism across different armies suggested that a physical commotion of the brain and nervous system was not the root cause. Psychological factors provided a better explanation. As he explained, "Concussion from the explosion of an artillery shell or aerial bomb appears to be a factor more favorable for [explaining] the development of psychogenic reactions on the battlefield because they give material for hysterical fixations in view of somatic disturbances conditional on physical trauma

[53] V. L. Zvereva, "K klinike psikhicheskikh narushenii pri gipertonnicheskoi bolezni," *Voenno-meditsinskii zhurnal*, no. 6 (November—December 1947), 48–54 (cit. 49).

[54] Merridale (2005), 232.

[55] B.G. Gurvich, "Osobennosti klinicheskoi kartiny i techaniia shizofrenii, vyiavlennoi travmami voennogo vremeni," *Nevropatologiia i psikhiatriia* 16:2 (March–April 1947), 62–5.

and emotional reactions which cause a fit of fear," revealed through the loss of speech and hearing.[56] Although expressed in a convoluted form, perhaps for protection, this was a radical idea. One of the recommended solutions for treating speech disturbances for psychiatric casualties was through a detailed program of physiotherapy and exercises, leading to the pronunciation of key words and sentences. The vocabulary chosen for this crude form of speech therapy, which included phrases such as, "the task of the Red Army is to attack," "it is necessary to destroy the enemy" and "the Soviet people are gladdened by the Red Army's victory," is nevertheless a reminder that discussions about trauma were wrapped up with ideology and wider ideas about martial masculinities.

In the immediate aftermath of World War II, Soviet psychiatry pursued a more open discussion of the causes, prevalence and treatment of war-related trauma than might have been anticipated. For a few years, before Stalinist control of science was reasserted, a wider range of ideas about trauma circulated, as a scientific consensus emerged.

Soldiers' Own Expressions of Trauma

The language of psychological pain and suffering, however, circulated far beyond the rarefied theoretical discussions of a relatively small community of professional psychiatrists discussing trauma in seminars, the clinics of research institutions or the pages of learned journals. The medical profession did not have a monopoly on making sense of traumatic war experiences or explaining the ways in which these manifested themselves in psychiatric conditions. Finding acceptable vocabularies to describe mental breakdown proved difficult for psychiatrists and wider society; nevertheless, expressions of trauma can be discerned beyond the boundaries of professional scientific discourses. Far from experiencing wholesale repression of information about psychiatric or psychological damage, in certain social situations, and in the documents these generated, veterans showed themselves freely prepared to describe mental injuries and psychological problems, often in language echoing that of medics.

The memoirs of veterans written during the Soviet period make little or no reference to difficult or disquieting experiences, let alone lasting traumatic damage. Under Khrushchev, the restrictions on what could be

---

[56] Ia.M. Sviadoshch, "O partsial'noi i total'noi forme istericheskoi glukhoty i glukhonemoty," *Voenno-meditsinskii zhurnal*, no. 12 (December 1945), 23–5 (cit. 25).

written were briefly relaxed, but discussions of trauma within memoirs sat uncomfortably alongside official patriotic narratives. As Roger Markwick explains, "The state-sanctified depiction of the war, embodied in massive historical works and numerous, even more massive memorials, prohibited any challenge to the hegemonic, heroic-patriotic narrative of the war."[57] Prevented from publishing honest memoirs in the immediate aftermath of the war, most veterans waited decades for the opportunity to document traumatic experiences. Shaped by the political atmosphere and public culture in which they were writing, many veterans internalized comforting official myths, echoing them in their own life writing.[58] The collapse of the Soviet Union, however, created a space for more realistic accounts of war to emerge. The sterile official formulas of late socialist memoirs, and the politicization of war memories, have not disappeared, but memoirs published after 1991 have been more willing to confront the fear, confusion and trauma of frontline life. As Markwick writes, "Blood, filth, fear, ineptitude, revenge, cruelty, and sexual harassment are often depicted [...] to a degree that was near impossible in the largely sanitized Soviet memoirs."[59] Against a cultural backdrop where the damaged veterans of Afghanistan and Chechnya were familiar characters on the big and small screens, Soviet veterans of World War II perhaps found it easier to acknowledge, in fiction and in memoirs, traumatic aspects of their own experience.[60] Postwar cultural products, as Ville Kivimäki observes in his contribution to this volume, could be triggers for posttraumatic memory, but they could also facilitate discussion of psychological pain.

Post-Soviet memoirs readily discussed feelings of fear and the emotional sensations of battle and combat.[61] Frontline action, as the artillery officer Isaak Kobylyanskiy described, could induce intense "bodily" fear: "It appeared instantly when you heard the ever increasing hissing of

[57] Roger D. Markwick, "Post-Soviet Russia Memoirs of the Second World War," in *War Stories: The War Memoir in History and Literature*, ed. by Philip Dwyer (New York: Berghahn, 2016), 143–67 (cit. 144).

[58] Catherine Merridale, "Culture, Ideology and Combat in the Red Army, 1939–45," *Journal of Contemporary History* 41:2 (2006), 305–24 (cit. 308); idem (2005), 322–3.

[59] Markwick (2016), 146.

[60] Andrei Gelasimov, *Thirst*, trans. Marian Schwartz (Las Vegas, NV: Amazon Crossing, 2011); *Zhazhda* [Thirst] (dir. Dmitrii Tyuruin, 2013); *Moi svodnyi brat Frankenstein* [My Step-Brother Frankenstein] (dir. Valerii Todorvskii, 2004).

[61] Gabriel Temkin, *My Just War: The Memoir of a Jewish Red Army Soldier in World War II* (Novata, CA: Presidio Press, 1998), 176.

murderous metal, and when shells or bombs exploded close at hand. The explosions deafened you and cast you about like a piece of grain. This kind of fear deprives you of your will."[62] Boris Bogachev's revealing memoir also acknowledges this paralysing fear in the face of artillery fire, "I felt alone and helpless on that stormy field of fire. My heart was thumping. My nerves were taut. I expected death at any minute. [...] Could that shell be the one that would end your fragile existence? This anticipation was horrible."[63] Bogachev and his comrades turned to alcohol to deal with nervous tension, fatigue and "to distract [them] from negative thoughts."[64] Even for healthy young men the strain told: "I was only nineteen and I found it very difficult to bear the huge physical and psychological tension of battle." Things must have been harder still for "middle-aged soldiers of nearly fifty with three or four small children at home."[65] In the words of the artillery officer Petr Mikhin, "as time passed and thousands of deaths and horrible wounds happened to those around you, the grief and emotional toll eventually exhausted a man psychologically." Men serving on the frontlines for months, even years, without leave eventually reached a point of complete nervous and physical collapse, verging on insanity. Mikhin described how exhaustion and the stress of knowing "a bullet or a piece of shrapnel always found a man sooner or later" pushed him and a comrade towards a breakdown.[66] Surviving a closely fought action, his fellow officer Morozov "covered his face with his large hands, burst into sobs and broke out in a loud desperate wail: 'I can't take this anymore! I can't! I caaaaan't!"[67] Both were given ten day's leave at a sanatorium in Odessa to restore their health.

Bogachev openly described the recurring nightmares about combat and traumatic experiences that were seared on his consciousness. For a long time after the war, he dreamt about "a tank attack with assault troops on the tank armour; the enemies moving toward me, and my automatic

---

[62] Isaak Kobylyanskiy, "Memories of War: Part 2: On the railroads, the battle on the outskirts of Vishnyovy hamlet, 'mysterious are the ways of the Lord,' fear, and about blocking detachments," *The Journal of Slavic Military Studies* 16:4 (2003), 147–56 (cit. 152).

[63] Boris Bogachev, *For the Motherland! For Stalin! A Red Army Officer's Memoir of the Eastern Front* (London: Hurst & Company, 2017), 188.

[64] Ibid., 263.

[65] Ibid., 197.

[66] Petr Mikhin, *Guns Against the Reich: Memoirs of an Artillery Officer on the Eastern Front* (Barnsley: Pen and Sword, 2010), 127.

[67] Ibid., 132.

gun won't fire; enemy aircraft bombs are being dropped on me… I used to wake up in a cold sweat."[68] In another parallel with the experiences of Finnish veterans explored in Kivimäki's chapter, traumatic memories intruded on dreams.

The image of the remains of one dead comrade, "his bright red naked body torn in two halves and his protruding white ribs," remained with him for the rest of his life. Over half a century later, he still avoided "looking at bloodied animal carcasses with protruding white ribs" at the butchers.[69] In his memoirs, Nikolai Nikulin recalled how in the spring of 1942 he encountered a heap of corpses, abandoned after the previous autumn's battles, revealed by the thawing snow. "After all the passing years, this frightening picture is imprinted on my consciousness forever, and on my subconscious still more firmly: I acquired here a constantly recurring dream—piles of corpses alongside railway embankments."[70] Nikulin was never invalided out as a psychiatric casualty, but fighting between December 1941 and May 1942, around the village of Pogost'e in the Leningrad region, had a profound impact on his future psychological health: "For me Pogost'e was the turning point [in my] life. I was killed and broken down."[71] After this point Nikulin was never the same again. "Exactly after Pogost'e an unhealthy compulsion to wash my hands ten times a day, and frequently wash my underwear manifested itself."[72]

Boris Bogachev's, Petr Mikhin's and Nikolai Nikulin's eloquent memoirs are not typical, but they are not alone in offering a more psychologically complicated picture of frontline service and the damaging effects of war. For these men, and others, it was suffering and witnessing extreme violence that proved traumatic. Discussions of the traumatizing effects of enacting violence on others remain deeply taboo. Compilations of veterans' biographies or service careers, pieced together by relatives or institutions with links to veterans, increasingly note whether an individual experienced *kontuziia*, whether the individual returned to active service or was discharged.[73] A major multi-volume collection of veterans' reminiscences published between 2003 and 2011, the first 14 volumes of which

---

[68] Bogachev (2017), 269.

[69] Ibid., 79.

[70] Nikolai Nikulin, *Vospominaniia o voine* (Moscow: ACT, 2014), 62–63.

[71] Ibid., 57.

[72] Idid., 58.

[73] Zakhar Prilepin, Marina Stepnova, Leonid Iuzeforivh et al., *Kak my perezhili voiny: Narodnye istorii* (Moscow: Izdatel'stvo AST, 2016), 501, 505, 523, 582.

contained the accounts of nearly 700 veterans of World War II, paid close attention to instances of *kontuziia*.[74] Respondents appear to have been encouraged to comment on their injuries, including instances of *kontuziia*, both in the sense of being concussed or knocked unconscious by shellfire as well as through experiencing wider damage to sensory apparatus and nervous systems. These veterans understood *kontuziia* to be a largely physical injury, caused by the explosive force of mines, shells and bombs exploding near soldiers or their vehicles. Some individuals described the impact of concussion as minimal, stressing how they continued to fight without serious consequences.[75] Zoia Dobrovol'skaia, a rare female infantry soldier, described her experience of "shell shock" in particularly masculine terms. "I bore my concussion on my feet; after three days my sight and hearing were restored and lying in hospital might not have been in vain, but I thought it would pass. I was under bombardment hundreds of times over four years, mercifully, everything passed, only the noise in my head didn't pass."[76] For many veterans, mental breakdown remained something to be understood in physical terms, a product of psychiatric theory and medical practice that stressed the material basis of trauma, as well as a postwar culture which stressed the resilience and heroism of Soviet soldiers.

Others, however, described more serious damage to their nerves that required medical treatment, even hospitalization. The experience of physical injury, particularly that of being caught in a major explosion, could have traumatizing effects. In the spring of 1945, Sergei Vladimirskii was knocked unconscious by the force of an anti-tank weapon. He spent 12 days in a medical unit while he regained the power of speech.[77] On 5 December 1941, Anatolii Svolokov's tank was hit. When he regained his consciousness, he was confronted with a traumatic spectacle and his senses remained disturbed. "Surrounding me was a horrifying picture: the radio operator was dead with shrapnel in his head, the tank didn't have a tower,

[74] *Ot soldata do generala: Vospominaniia o voine*, Vol. 1–16 (Moscow: Izdatel'stvo MAI, 2003–15).

[75] Nikolai Fedorovich Levchenko, "Unichtozhenie brodskoi gruppirovki," *Ot soldata do generala: Vospominaniia o voine*, Vol. 4 (Moscow: Izdatel'stvo MAI, 2004), 161–3.

[76] Zoia Ivanovna Dobrovol'skaia, "Kak ia na kone vyekhala na peredovuiu," *Ot soldata do generala: Vospominaniia o voine*, Vol. 5 (Moscow: Izdatel'stvo MAI, 2005), 155–93 (cit. 188).

[77] Sergei Aleksandrovich Vladimirskii, "V moei polevoi sumke—krasnoe znamia," *Ot soldata do generala*, Vol. 4 (2004), 119–29 (cit. 128).

blown up bodies lay around the tank, it was frighteningly cold. It's a miracle I came around, I spent three months shell shock, hearing nothing and not speaking."[78] After a period of medical treatment, just behind the frontline or in evacuation hospitals, many soldiers recovered from temporary losses of hearing, speech and memory, and were able to return to active service. In the worst cases, however, severe *kontuziia* resulted in the medical discharge and demobilization of soldiers.[79] Fedor Kamenev, for example, initially spent 14 days recovering from his trauma in a hospital located in a railway wagon. Upon returning to civilian life, he was diagnosed with *kontuziia* by a Medical Labor Expert Commission and classified as a Group II war invalid.[80]

As the final generation of combatants reach the end of their lives, the barriers to voicing trauma have faded as veterans and their families seek to bear witness to wartime heroism. Although we should guard against anachronistically reading back widespread trauma during and after the war based on these sources, this last generation of Soviet veterans would not be the first cohort of veterans of modern industrialized warfare to discover that disquieting and disturbing memories resurfaced late in life.

Discussions of war's damaging psychological effects, however, were not just the product of hindsight or personal reflection. Although I've previously argued that veterans refused to identify themselves as victims and acknowledge war's psychological damage,[81] there is increasing evidence that some veterans in specific circumstances were prepared to employ the language of victim trauma. On 1 June 1945, Major I.S. Pavlov wrote a letter of complaint to Stalin, which began by explaining the hardships of four years of frontline sacrifice: "Many people lost their minds in this struggle and didn't endure until the joyous victory. But those who survived are exiting from this war pretty tattered, with a shattered organism, with a disordered nervous system, with many material and moral hardships and with serious mental traumas [*s tiazhel'ymi dushevnymi travami*], with

[78] Anatolii Ivanovich Svolokov, "Byli trizhdy v okruzhenii," *Ot soldata do generala*, Vol. 5 (2005), 520–23 (cit. 522).
[79] Ivan Nikolaevich Mironovich, "Ia byl prostym soldatom," *Ot soldata do generala: Vospominaniia o voine*, Vol. 12 (Moscow: Izdatel'stvo MAI, 2008), 292–6 (cit. 293).
[80] Fedor Alekseevich Kamenev, "Ia sluzhil razvedchikom otriada," *Ot soldata do generala*, Vol. 5 (2005), 322–6 (cit. 324).
[81] Dale (2015), 122.

the hope of healing them in the motherland."[82] This was an unusual letter, not least because it was addressed to Stalin. Pavlov was not relating a personal traumatic experience, but over its five pages was expressing frustration that, after four years of service, returning soldiers, especially officers, were not automatically awarded medals.[83] This emotive language about wartime psychological damage was deployed in the hope that it would resonate with the reader, strengthening the claim for recognition. More commonly, veterans listed instances of contusion (*kontuziia*) alongside physical injuries, to bolster letters of appeal for privilege, material assistance or medical treatment. Physical and mental injuries were not hidden but were listed, in order to demonstrate entitlement to housing, better employment, welfare payments or prosthetics.[84] Far from evidence of a fragile wounded masculinity, physical and psychological injury was highlighted as evidence of heroic manly suffering. These were not transparent articulations of trauma, but self-interested representations intended to elicit a response from the authorities. To be effective, however, references to *kontuziia* relied upon an assumed understanding of what it was, and its potential impact upon the individual.

Sometimes veterans cited *kontuziia* as an explanation, or perhaps even as an excuse, for rule-breaking or their wider predicaments. In 1951, Kovalchuk, a mechanical engineer in Kyiv's Ukrkabel factory, offered a number of defences for his failure to participate in political education classes, including the fact that he had been "concussed twice and it is difficult to make my brain work."[85] In April 1953, M.N. Berezniak, a veteran from Orel, wrote to the reception room of the USSR Supreme Soviet appealing against being sacked for workplace drunkenness. Although he admitted to drinking 150 ml of vodka the previous day, he claimed that his boss had mistaken a fit for drunkenness. In 1943, he was conscripted into the Red Army, "participated in battles, was concussed [*kontuzhen*], and started to suffer fits."[86] He was not alone in drawing a link between wartime frontline concussion and postwar psychiatric illness. In April 1949, the Supreme Soviet's Reception Room investigated the case of I.P. Pervago,

[82] Russian State Archive of Socio-Political History (hereafter RGASPI), f. 558, op. 11, d. 891, l. 29.

[83] RGASPI, f. 558, op. 11, d. 891, l. 30–3.

[84] GARF, f. R–7523, op. 55, d. 23, l. 60.

[85] Serhy Yekelchyk, *Stalin's Citizens: Everyday Politics in the Wake of Total War* (Oxford: Oxford University Press, 2014), 94.

[86] GARF, f. R–7523, op. 55, d. 55, ll. 4–5.

a disabled veteran from Moscow, who had appealed in person for material aid. He cited psychiatric illnesses and regular admission to the Kashchenko psychiatric clinic as an explanation for why he was unable to hold down regular employment. The ensuing investigation confirmed that his psychiatric problems appeared after concussion at the front, after which he was unable to find stable work, something that pushed him and his family towards poverty.[87] The connection between disturbing wartime experiences and postwar mental illness were, however, not always upheld. A.V. Zakharov, a Group I war-invalid who had written to the Supreme Soviet to complain about being refused psychiatric care, was, after an examination of his case, accused of simulating his condition. According to the examining doctors, Zakharov's schizophrenia was "not connected with his time at the front." The doctors suspected that he had been in German captivity and therefore could not be considered a legitimate war invalid.[88] Veterans' recourse to the language of psychological damage did not guarantee a positive response, let alone sympathy.

When veterans employed the word *kontuziia* in their letters, appeals and petitions, they assumed that the authorities knew and understood the term, at least in a general sense. The references to trauma were often opaque and fleeting, little more than a sentence, a passing phrase, even a solitary word, but these were not silences. The language of trauma not only circulated within the psychiatric profession and among groups of frontline veterans but much more widely within society. Vernacular languages of trauma, however, are no easier to decipher than professional discourses. When veterans used the term *kontuziia,* their precise meaning, and the exact nature of their traumatic injury, were not always clear. They used the word in different ways to those of medical professionals, with different purposes, intentions and meanings. *Kontuziia* was often used as shorthand for a wider range of traumatic experiences and symptoms, all implied by a single word. It prospered as a term precisely because of this malleability and capacity to accommodate a range of meanings. Jay Winter's observation that "'Shell shock' was a term of mediation, but one with a quicksilver and shifting character," could equally apply to *kontuziia.*[89]

---

[87] GARF, f. R-7523, op. 55, d. 30, ll. 66–71.
[88] GARF, f. R-7523, op. 55, d. 41, ll. 12–13.
[89] Jay Winter, "Shell shock and the Cultural History of the Great War," *Journal of Contemporary History* 35:1 (2000), 7–11 (cit. 7).

TREATING TRAUMA AFTER DEMOBILIZATION

How veterans' war-related trauma manifested itself once they had been demobilized is difficult to discern from either published psychiatric texts, which were frequently based on wartime research, or ex-servicemen's memoirs. The long-term impact of traumatic experiences and wartime injuries needs to be sought in other sources. How the war's psychiatric casualties were treated within the community, and what happened to soldiers who experienced delayed traumatic reactions after demobilization, require further investigation. As Benjamin Zajicek reminds us, the overwhelming majority of Soviet psychiatric patients were treated as regular outpatients at psychiatric dispensaries.[90] As I have previously argued on the basis of Leningrad, traumatized veterans can be discerned in many parts of the archives. Veterans with psychiatric disorders, and the social problems they created, frequently left traces in the files of the various institutions with whom they interacted. Nevertheless, how the war's traumatic aftermath was handled within civilian medical institutions is unclear. On the basis of the archival materials examined below, many for the first time, caring for veterans with war-related trauma represented a serious and ongoing challenge for the Ukrainian Ministry of Health and its hospitals. Although, the official line remained that the Soviet Union escaped widespread trauma, on the evidence of Soviet Ukraine war-related trauma was a visible and intractable problem. Amidst the "bloodlands" of World War II, where the nature of war was qualitatively different, and removed from the political centres of Moscow and Leningrad, the problems of war trauma appear to have been discussed more openly.[91]

Between 23 and 26 January 1946, the Ukrainian Ministry of Health's administration for hospitals for invalids of the Great Patriotic War held a conference in Kyiv which addressed how medical care, prosthetics, skills training and employment could be organized for the war disabled. The proceedings' focus, in line with Soviet policy towards disabled soldiers, was directed towards treating physical injuries and labor arrangement (*trudoustroistvo*).[92] However, V.P. Protopopov, a member of the Ukrainian Academy of Sciences, presented a paper entitled "The organization of

---

[90] Zajicek (2009), 168–86.

[91] Here I borrow the term bloodlands from Timothy Snyder, *Bloodlands: Europe between Hitler and Stalin* (New York: Basic Books, 2010).

[92] Tsentral'nyii derzhavnii arkhiv vishchikh organiv vladi ta upravlinnia Ukraini (hereafter TsDAVO), f. 342, op. 14, d. 2335, ll. 1–185.

psychiatric assistance for invalids of the Patriotic war." It stressed that psychiatric dispensaries should be the starting point for treatment, but patients with more serious psychoses were to be sent to psychiatric hospitals or colonies, depending on the nature of their condition. Crucially, this document recognized that these patients included veterans suffering from traumatic psychoses, forms of epilepsy, as well as "traumatic neuroses" of organic, reactive and psychogenic forms.[93] The next paper, which also examined postwar neurology, neurosurgery and psychiatry, commented on the challenges presented by disturbances to speech caused by contusion (*kontuzionnye rasstroistva rechi*), noting their extreme complexity and the large number of "ingredients" that went into their development.[94] Treating veterans with traumatic reactions to wartime experiences remained a noticeable part of the work on the Ukrainian Ministry of Health's hospitals for war invalids. According to a report detailing the medical treatment of war invalids in 1946, altogether 3557 individuals, 6.2 percent of hospital admissions, were treated for psycho-neurological illness, which rose to 4712 (or 7.2 percent) in 1947.[95] Although the absolute numbers of traumatized soldiers represented only a small fraction of total cases, the wider psychological damage wrought on combatants, their families and communities was much greater. These hospitals, however, were neither silent about trauma nor entirely constrained by official materialist explanations.

As the annual medical report for the Ukrainian Republican Neuro-Psychiatric Hospital for Invalids of the Great Patriotic War for 1946 revealed, treating traumatized soldiers was a significant part of its work. This institution was based upon the structures of a hospital which had been evacuated to Tambov during the war and which, in July 1944, returned to Kyiv. From 1 January 1946, it was reorganized as a special facility for war invalids with neuro-psychiatric diagnoses.[96] Over the course of 1946, the hospital treated 937 patients admitted from across the Ukrainian republic, 77.2 percent of whom with the most severe (Group I and II) disability classifications. Disentangling what patients were being treated for is difficult, since those with various conditions were grouped together, but 372 patients (39.6 percent) were treated for "closed wounds

[93] TsDAVO, f. 342, op. 14, d. 2335, ll. 76–8.
[94] TsDAVO, f. 342, op. 14, d. 2335, ll. 79–87 (cit. 86).
[95] TsDAVO, f. 342, op. 14, d. 2428, l. 9.
[96] TsDAVO, f. 342, op. 14, d.2368, l. 1.

of the skull," internal damage rather than open fractures or penetrative wounds, the category which included the traumatic after-effects of concussions.[97] For the years 1944 and 1945, approximately 59 percent of patients were admitted with *kontuziia* or forms of neurosis.[98] The average length of treatment for patients with post-traumatic conditions, such as hysterical reactions, was calculated as 28 days.[99] This case load was not, however, predicted to fall; *kontuziia*-related disorders, it was feared, would increase in 1947, even if other psychiatric complaints might decrease. As the report noted, "It is necessary to consider that part of these patients have been demobilized, and not considering the capabilities and 'resilience' [*ustoichivosti*] of their nervous system, did not finish their treatment, occupying themselves [rather] with arranging their affairs." Hasty discharge, it was feared, would result in a significant increase in the number of readmissions and recurring cases.[100]

The same institution's annual report for 1947 confirmed these fears. It drew attention to the ideas of Academician Giliarovskii, an expert on the nervous system, who had observed a phenomenon which he called, "nervous demobilization of the personality." During times of intense pressure, individuals proved capable of holding themselves together; only when the situation relaxed did their psychological problems resurface. The hospital noted that many patients' problems began with demobilization and hospital admittance. These patients found it hard to adjust to the different tempo of life on a ward.[101] This was a tacit acknowledgement that the transition from war to peace would result in an increase in psychiatric cases as the immediate stress of wartime service dissipated. As it entered its third postwar year, the hospital anticipated being full. The psycho-neurological department, for example, was experiencing "a significant increase in the weight [of its patient load], on account of an increase in the registration of patients with fixed post-traumatic changes in personality, patients with psychopathologic behavior and those with alcoholic dependence [...]"[102] Although psychiatric casualties were supposed to be treated in dispensaries in the community, the report noted that "The hospital, as before,

[97] TsDAVO, f. 342, op. 14, d.2368, l. 10.
[98] TsDAVO, f. 342, op. 14, d.2368, l. 23.
[99] TsDAVO, f. 342, op. 14, d. 2368, l. 11.
[100] TsDAVO, f. 342, op. 14, d. 2368, l. 24.
[101] TsDAVO, f. 342, op.14, d. 2461, l. 8. On Giliarovskii's theory of "Nervous demobilization" more generally see Zajicek (2009), 197–211.
[102] TsDAVO, f. 342, op. 14, d. 2461, l. 30.

continues to remain the only form and aspect of treatment for invalids of this profile on the right bank [of Ukraine]."[103] In 1947, Kyiv's psycho-neurological research institute continued to treat war invalids with psychiatric problems, 6.9 percent of whom were admitted for "phenomena" that appeared after concussion. Although the number of war invalids was beginning to fall, its report stressed the pressures on psychiatric services for the war disabled. It noted that "in the city of Kyiv alone there are around 3,000 invalids of the patriotic war of a psycho-neurological profile who need periodic treatment and a whole range of measures to raise their employability."[104] In-patient services would also be required. In 1947, according to a Ukrainian Ministry of Health report, 37.5 percent of all hospital admissions for psycho-neurological illnesses were repeat admissions, a significant increase on the 11.6 percent in 1946.[105] As time passed, the mental aftermath of war did not appear to be healing.

It was not only specialist psychiatric institutions caring for war invalids that dealt with the traumatic effects of wartime experience and injury. Although disabled veterans were supposed to be treated in a dedicated unit, a lack of facilities meant that the war-disabled were often cared for alongside other patients.[106] The report of a hospital for war invalids in the city of Lubny in the Poltova oblast for 1950 noted that it treated 212 patients with neurological conditions, including five cases of "post-concussion syndromes."[107] The case of one patient described in this report illustrates the challenges of treating manifestations of war trauma in less specialized facilities. Kharchenko had been ill since 1945 because of *kontuziia*. He was treated in 1949 but discharged once his condition improved. He was readmitted in March 1950, but was shortly discharged, "due to family circumstances," before he could complete his treatment and without his condition improving.[108] In many cases trauma was not easily resolved. Far from disappearing, war trauma left subtle traces which, with careful research, it is possible to begin to uncover. The records of medical institutions dealing with the physical injuries also noted damaging psychological effects. The boundaries between physical injury and psychological trauma were often blurred. The 1947 annual report of the

---

[103] TsDAVO, f. 342, op. 14, d. 2461, l. 31.
[104] TsDAVO, f. 342, op. 14, d. 3143, ll. 91–2.
[105] TsDAVO, f. 342, op. 14, d. 2428, l. 10.
[106] TsDAVO, f. 342, op. 14, d. 1940, l. 26.
[107] TsDAVO, f. 342, op. 14, d. 2607, l. 46.
[108] TsDAVO, f. 342, op. 14, d. 2607, l. 50.

Ukrainian maxillo-facial hospital for war invalids noted the complexities of treating soldiers with serious wounds who had already undergone repeated operations. These individuals needed special attention, including neuro-psychiatric support. Veterans who had completely lost their sight were often depressed and required "systematic discussions about the possibilities for study and employment" before depression would lift.[109] As a report from Kyiv's city hospital for disabled veterans observed, patients who had undergone long periods of hospitalization became detached from society. Where individuals felt themselves to be actively engaged, rather than discarded on the margins, their treatment and reintegration was more effective.[110] The files of the Ukrainian Ministry of Health demonstrate that the traumatic impact of war left tangible traces, which continued to resonate in the immediate wake of war. Medical institutions and their staff encountered and discussed the war's psychiatric casualties and were concerned that trauma was becoming more apparent, rather than less so.

CONCLUSION

Soviet society, then, neither denied the possibility that the war could have damaging psychological and psychiatric effects, nor ignored its traumatic effects. Far from having no conception of war-related trauma, Soviet society possessed varied understandings of how wartime service could be traumatic. Psychological trauma was not surrounded by silence, it was just understood differently and discussed in different ways dependent on social and cultural context. Throughout the war and its immediate aftermath, Soviet psychiatry studied post-traumatic reactions to wartime injury in surprising depth and from a variety of different perspectives. There was significant interest in the reactive conditions that developed after *kontu-ziia*, and a variety of explanations and treatments for these disorders circulated. What the published psychiatric literature indicates is not a lack of interest in trauma but, rather, a very fragile scientific consensus. The language of trauma, however, circulated far beyond the professionalized discourses of medical researchers. Soldiers, and the wider communities to which they returned, had their own vernaculars for trauma and psychological suffering that co-opted professional psychiatric terms to describe their own experiences. Discussions of trauma were not the preserve of the

[109] TsDAVO, f. 342, op. 14, d. 2459, ll. 13–14.
[110] TsDAVO, f. 342, op. 14, d. 2445, l. 30.

seminar room or a research institute's clinic. Hospitals continued to treat veterans mentally damaged by their experiences in the years and decades that followed, although war's psychological aftermath was anything but contained within medical institutions.

The traces left by war-related trauma, then, can be found in different spaces, where they were expressed in different languages. This is not to argue that Soviet society treated traumatized soldiers well, or that trauma was universally recognized as a problem. While Stalinist society wrestled with the challenges of postwar reconstruction, there was little opportunity to dwell on war's psychological damage. This was a society that faced enormous immediate problems and discouraged introspection whenever possible. Individual psychiatric trauma, however, was not completely off limits. If we look beyond the official propaganda, war trauma found regular and repeated expression during and after the war, in ways which penetrated the silence supposedly woven around it. These instances of trauma were almost certainly only part of a wider and deeper set of traumatic experiences which often went unspoken. The sources analyzed in this chapter allow us to begin to listen more precisely for expression of trauma. Nevertheless, much work remains in order to reveal other social and cultural spaces in which multiple forms of war-related trauma left their traces.

CHAPTER 4

Experiencing Trauma Before Trauma: Posttraumatic Memories, Nightmares and Flashbacks Among Finnish Soldiers

Ville Kivimäki

INTRODUCTION

The psychiatric diagnosis of posttraumatic stress disorder (PTSD) entered the standard American *Diagnostic and Statistical Manual of Mental Disorders* in 1980 and the World Health Organization's *International Classification of Diseases* in 1992.[1] The diagnosis has been an attempt to create a universal, objective psychiatric description of the psychological consequences of traumatic stress, and to thus medically standardize the observation and treatment of traumatized patients. The key premises

---

[1] *Diagnostic and Statistical Manual of Mental Disorders*, 3rd ed. (Washington, DC: APA, 1980), 236–8; *The ICD-10 Classification of Mental and Behavioral Disorders: Clinical Descriptions and Diagnostic Guidelines* (Geneva: WHO, 1992), 148–9.

V. Kivimäki (✉)
Faculty of Social Sciences, Tampere University, Tampere, Finland
e-mail: ville.kivimaki@tuni.fi

© The Author(s) 2022
V. Kivimäki, P. Leese (eds.), *Trauma, Experience and Narrative in Europe after World War II*, Palgrave Studies in the History of Experience, https://doi.org/10.1007/978-3-030-84663-3_4

behind PTSD are, first, that there exist traumatic events that cannot be processed within the normal spectrum of human experiencing; second, that those events as such can cause long-term psychological consequences for the victim; third, that these consequences take the form of "traumatic memory;" and fourth, that its symptoms form a distinctive disorder separate from other mental disorders.[2]

As Peter Leese points out in his introduction to this volume, PTSD as a combination of psychiatric knowledge is a historically constructed concept. As several studies on the genealogy of PTSD have demonstrated, its birth in the United States was bound to the politicized atmosphere surrounding the Vietnam War in the 1960s and 1970s. A new generation of psychiatrists started to advocate a concept of war trauma which would be medically valid but also socially just and morally acceptable. Finally, and after heated debates, this advocacy gave birth to the diagnosis of PTSD.[3] It has also been pointed out how PTSD's "objective" scientific premises are embedded in a particular Western culture of mental illness and individual subjectivity, whereas human responses to potentially traumatizing events are diverse, historically and culturally conditioned, and often do not correlate with the diagnostic criteria of PTSD.[4] Historians have joined in

[2] For the "inner logic" of PTSD, see Richard McNally, "Conceptual Problems with the DSM-IV Criteria for Posttraumatic Stress Disorder," as well as Allan Young, "When Traumatic Memory Was a Problem: On the Historical Antecedents of PTSD," both in *Posttraumatic Stress Disorder: Issues and Controversies*, ed. by Gerald M. Rosen (Chichester: Wiley, 2004).

[3] Most importantly, see Allan Young, *The Harmony of Illusions: Inventing Post-Traumatic Stress Disorder* (Princeton, NJ: Princeton University Press, 1995); and further Wilbur J. Scott, "PTSD in DSM-III: A Case in the Politics of Diagnosis and Disease," *Social Problems* 37:3 (1990), 294–310; Michael G. Kenny, "Trauma, Time, Illness, and Culture: An Anthropological Approach to Traumatic Memory," in *Tense Past: Cultural Essays in Trauma and Memory*, ed. by Paul Antze and Michael Lambek (New York: Routledge, 1996), 151–71; Patrick J. Bracken, "Hidden Agendas: Deconstructing Post Traumatic Stress Disorder," in *Rethinking the Trauma of War*, ed. by Patrick J. Bracken and Celia Petty (London: Free Association, 1998), 38–59; Derek Summerfield, "The Invention of Post-traumatic Stress Disorder and the Social Usefulness of a Psychiatric Category," *British Medical Journal* 322 (2001), 95–8; Simon Wessely, "Twentieth-century Theories on Combat Motivation and Breakdown," *Journal of Contemporary History* 41:2 (2006), 269–86.

[4] Derek Summerfield, "Cross-cultural Perspectives on the Medicalization of Human Suffering," in Rosen, ed. (2004), 233–45; Peter D. Yeomans and Evan M. Forman, "Cultural Factors in Traumatic Stress," in *Culture and Mental Health: Sociocultural Influences, Theory, and Practice*, ed. by Sussie Eshun and Regan A. R. Gurung (Chichester: Wiley-Blackwell, 2009), 221–44.

the critique of PTSD's timeless validity: it is not possible to take the current psychiatric paradigm as universal knowledge that can be applied as such to past experiences.[5]

In the humanities, in cultural studies, and in social sciences concerned with the concept of trauma, there is thus a strong constructivist focus on the idea of posttraumatic memory and its changing manifestations. From this perspective, trauma and PTSD are seen as discursively produced conglomerations of psychiatric knowledge. Yet my concern in this chapter is not to underline the historical and cultural sensitivity of trauma's conceptualizations, although I have done so elsewhere.[6] In the critique of the universality of the PTSD paradigm, it has been natural to emphasize temporal changes and cultural variations in human reactions to violence. As an example, one of the most thorough and historically informed works in the field has been *Shell Shock to PTSD: Military Psychiatry from 1900 to the Gulf War* (2005) by psychiatrists Edgar Jones and Simon Wessely, in which they concluded: "Our findings imply that the pathology of war syndromes is not static. Culture, along with advances in treatments, the discovery of new diseases, new diagnostic tools and the changing nature of warfare, plays a significant role in shaping patterns of symptoms." Interestingly, though, Jones and Wessely also observed a considerable overlap in the recorded symptoms from different wars, stretching from the 1850s to the 1990s. There was no clear-cut PTSD to be found in the past sources; yet there was also remarkable coherence in symptoms that kept

[5] Jay Winter and Emmanuel Sivan, "Setting the Framework," in *War and Remembrance in the Twentieth Century*, ed. by Jay Winter and Emmanuel Sivan (Cambridge: Cambridge University Press, 2000), 15–6; Paul Lerner and Mark S. Micale, "Trauma, Psychiatry, and History: A Conceptual and Historiographical Introduction," in *Traumatic Pasts: History, Psychiatry, and Trauma in the Modern Age, 1870–1930*, ed. by Mark S. Micale and Paul Lerner (Cambridge: Cambridge University Press, 2001), 6–9, 20–7; Wulf Kansteiner, "Genealogy of a Category Mistake: A Critical Intellectual History of the Cultural Trauma Metaphor," *Rethinking History* 8:2 (2004), 193–221; Frank Biess, *Homecomings: Returning POWs and the Legacies of Defeat in Postwar Germany* (Princeton, NJ: Princeton University Press, 2006), 73–4; Svenja Goltermann, *Die Gesellschaft der Überlebenden: Deutsche Kriegsheimkehrer und ihre Gewalterfahrungen im Zweiten Weltkrieg* (München: DVA, 2009), 18–22.

[6] Ville Kivimäki, "Languages of the Wound: Finnish Soldiers' Bodies as Sites of Shock during World War II," in *Languages of Trauma: History, Memory, and Media*, ed. by Peter Leese, Julia B. Köhne and Jason Crouthamel (Toronto: University of Toronto Press, 2021a), 70–96.

appearing in all the studied conflicts over the timespan of 140 years.[7] Similarly, historian Eric T. Dean has shown how the soldiers of the American Civil War in 1861–65 suffered from traumatic and posttraumatic symptoms long before the invention of these concepts in psychiatry.[8] In accordance with Dean, I will claim that by an adjustment of perspective it is possible to see continuity and constancy in the very same source materials that reveal change and variety in human reactions to extreme stress and violence.

In short, my criticism of the critique of PTSD is that it tends to reduce the question of posttraumatic memory to an analysis of medico-political construction of a *psychiatric* concept. This is useful and important in its own right, but it directs attention away from the *experiences* of trauma. I agree that the diagnostic principles and medical treatments available at a given time do influence the experience of a mental disorder. But in contrast to studies that emphasize the role of psychiatric knowledge in the genesis of trauma,[9] I consider this a secondary influence when compared to the experiences of violence (which are a culturally and socially conditioned phenomena, as well). Consequently, in this chapter I will study the manifestations of traumatic memory among the Finnish soldiers of World War II in the 1940s and 1950s, at a time when traumatic memory (and even less PTSD) was not recognized in Finnish psychiatry or in the culture at large. I will demonstrate that the following central tenets of traumatic memory can be found in wartime and postwar sources: these recurrent memories are outside the person's control; they intrude into the mind in vivid flashbacks, dreams, or re-experiencing; and they can (re)appear even years after the traumatic event.[10] It is important to note that I am not

---

[7] Edgar Jones and Simon Wessely, *Shell Shock to PTSD: Military Psychiatry from 1900 to the Gulf War* (Hove: Psychology Press, 2005), 199–208, cit. 208.

[8] Eric T. Dean, Jr., *Shook over Hell: Post-traumatic Stress, Vietnam, and the Civil War* (Cambridge, MA: Harvard University Press, 1999).

[9] For fine examples in this vein of research, see Young (1995); Ruth Leys, *Trauma: A Genealogy* (Chicago: University of Chicago Press, 2000); Didier Fassin and Richard Rechtman, *The Empire of Trauma: An Inquiry into the Condition of Victimhood* (Princeton, NJ: Princeton University Press, 2009); Ulrich Koch, *Schockeffekte: Eine historische Epistemologie des Traumas* (Zürich: Diaphanes, 2014); Anne Freese, *Gewalt – Deutung – Selbstoptimierung: Eine Geschichte der posttraumatischen Belastungsstörung seit dem Vietnam-Syndrom* (Stuttgart: Franz Steiner, 2018).

[10] Cf. *DSM-5: Diagnostic and Statistical Manual of Mental Disorders*, 5th ed. (Washington, DC: APA, 2013), 271, 275. For an introduction to the problem of traumatic memory, see Richard J. McNally, *Remembering Trauma* (Cambridge, MA: Belknap Press, 2003).

claiming any universal diagnostic validity for PTSD that could allow it to be applied as such in historical studies. What I want to show, nevertheless, is that the phenomenon of posttraumatic memory can be empirically found and studied in sources from earlier times, too. By so doing, I will argue that traumatic symptoms are not simply born out of changing psychiatric paradigms and conceptualizations, but that the "culture" that shapes and produces the symptoms must be understood much more broadly. In the end, I am proposing the concept of experience as a move forward in the historical analysis of human reactions to trauma.

I consider this a relevant approach to a wider understanding of human reactions to the mass-scale violence of World War II. There have been some preliminary attempts to apply PTSD in analyzing post-1945 histories[11]—and the concept of trauma is, of course, an often-used metaphor for the devastating memory of the war and the Holocaust. But the study of experiencing the violence of 1939–45 and the possible role of posttraumatic memory in this respect—as it manifested in the specific historical conditions of the time—necessitate much closer scrutiny, as Mark Micale underlines in his chapter. This is especially true for Eastern and Central Europe, where most of the violence in Europe took place and where societies and individual lives alike were most profoundly affected by war. Finland was not among these "Bloodlands" as famously phrased by Timothy Snyder.[12] In fact, Finland remained an exceptional country in war-waging Europe with regard to the distribution of war-related fatalities since nearly all of the Finns who died in the war were military personnel.[13] Nevertheless, the relevance of the Finnish case in studying posttraumatic experiences of violence lies in showing how these experiences could have a long-lasting effect on people's lives, although there was no psychiatric or public discourse that recognized them. In Finland, trauma existed even

---

[11] Alice Förster and Birgit Beck, "Post-Traumatic Stress Disorder and World War II: Can a Psychiatric Concept Help Us Understand Postwar Society?" in *Life after Death: Approaches to a Cultural and Social History of Europe During the 1940s and 1950s*, ed. by Richard Bessel and Dirk Schumann, (Cambridge: Cambridge University Press, 2003); Niels Birbaumer and Dieter Langewiesche, "Neuropsychologie und Historie – Versuch einer empirischen Annäherung: Posttraumatische Belastungsstörung (PTSD) und Soziopathie in Österreich nach 1945," *Geschichte & Gesellschaft* 32:2 (2006), 153–75.

[12] Timothy Snyder, *Bloodlands: Europe Between Hitler and Stalin* (London: Bodley Head, 2010).

[13] Ville Kivimäki, "Sankariuhri ja kansakunta – Suomalaiset sotakuolemat 1939–1945," in *Suomalaisen kuoleman historia*, ed. by Ilona Pajari et al. (Helsinki: Gaudeamus, 2019), 280–3.

before its medical invention, and this was also arguably the case elsewhere in war-torn countries and regions. My chapter thus mirrors the very similar findings made by Robert Dale in his previous chapter on psychological injuries in the Red Army during World War II.

CONTEXT, QUESTIONS, AND SOURCES FOR TRAUMATIC MEMORY

Finland became independent of the Russian Empire on 6 December 1917. Only a small number of Finnish volunteers had participated in the battles of World War I, practically all of them on the Eastern Front. In January–May 1918, a short but bloody civil war raged in Finland, fought mostly between two amateur militias: the Red Guards and the "White" Civil Guards. Most of the fighting consisted of short skirmishes between light infantry, and there were no artillery barrages or prolonged trench battles akin to what was experienced on the Western Front. It is safe to say that most of the horrors of modern warfare in 1914–18, including the outbreak of war-related mental breakdowns, remained unfamiliar to a majority of the Finnish population. The most traumatic experiences of the Civil War were the summary executions perpetrated by both sides of the conflict and the terribly high prison-camp fatality rate of the defeated Reds following the end of the war.[14]

Finnish psychiatry of the 1920s and 1930s had close ties to German psychiatry. The interwar period saw the establishment of large asylums for the treatment of mental illnesses, which were seen as hereditary and constitutional psychopathologies. Actually, the role of psychological (or "environmental") explanations for mental diseases *diminished* considerably from the turn of the century up to the interwar era.[15] It is noteworthy that both psychoanalysis and clinical psychology were still in their infancy in Finland: the former made its breakthrough only in the 1950s and the first professor of psychology at the University of Helsinki was appointed as late as 1951—up until then psychology had been taught under the

---

[14] For a concise history of the conflict in English, see *The Finnish Civil War 1918: History, Memory, Legacy*, ed. by Tuomas Tepora and Aapo Roselius (Leiden: Brill, 2014).

[15] Helena Hirvonen, *Suomalaisen psykiatriatieteen juuria etsimässä: Psykiatria tieteenä ja käytäntönä 1800-luvulta vuoteen 1930* (Joensuu: University of Eastern Finland, 2014), 206–10.

discipline of philosophy.[16] Some German post-1918 discussions on the nature and proper handling of "war neurosis" were noted in passing in Finnish psychiatric discussions of the 1930s, but this did not amount to a wider recognition of traumatic memory. The generation of Finnish psychiatrists who would come to have the responsibility of treating the military psychiatric patients in 1939–45 had adopted a German doctrine which rejected the idea of traumatic neurosis; the reasons for soldiers' mental breakdowns were to be looked for elsewhere. During World War II, altogether about 18,000 Finnish soldiers ended up in military psychiatric care. Yet their conditions were not perceived as symptomatic of mental trauma, but were treated as signs of psychopathology, nervous weakness, deficient intelligence, or earlier mental illness.[17]

This short overview is designed to underline the fact that the occurrence of traumatic memory among the Finnish soldiers and war veterans could not be derived from a medical culture that might have produced or fostered posttraumatic symptoms. A popularization of psychiatric concepts was not uncommon in Finland: at the turn of the twentieth century, "neuroses" and "neurasthenia" escaped from the professional medical vocabulary into lay language and encouraged ordinary people to examine their own nerves for signs of fragility and exhaustion.[18] But for trauma, this was not the case in the 1940s and 1950s, so the soldiers or war veterans would not have been encouraged to express their mental agony in terms of traumatic memory.

[16] Juhani Ihanus, "Psykologia," in *Suomen tieteen historia 2: Humanistiset ja yhteiskunta-tieteet*, ed. by Päiviö Tommila (Porvoo: WSOY, 2000), 451–5.

[17] Ville Kivimäki, *Battled Nerves: Finnish Soldiers' War Experience, Trauma, and Military Psychiatry, 1941–44* (PhD thesis in Nordic history: Åbo Akademi University, 2013). Virva Liski's study on war invalids on the "White" side of the Civil War is about to bring some new light to this issue. It appears that there was some recognition of war-related mental disorders among the *older* generation of Finnish psychiatrists, as long as the invalids had served in the victorious White troops, which had a glorified position in the post-1918 Finnish society. Yet the phenomenon remained quite marginal and confined to the professional discipline of psychiatry. Furthermore, mirroring a similar development in Germany, the attitudes grew less tolerant during the 1930s and the younger generation of Finnish psychiatrists rejected the idea of traumatic neurosis altogether; see Virva Liski, "'Vain veri yksin ei ole invaliditeetin merkki': Henkiset invalidit ja psyykkisesti sotavammaiset valkoisessa Suomessa 1918–1939," *Historiallinen Aikakauskirja* 119:2 (2021), 195–207.

[18] Minna Uimonen, *Hermostumisen aikakausi: Neuroosit 1800- ja 1900-lukujen vaihteen suomalaisessa lääketieteessä* (SHS: Helsinki, 1999); Anssi Halmesvirta, *Vaivojensa vangit: Kansa kysyi, lääkärit vastasivat – historiallinen vuoropuhelu 1889–1916* (Jyväskylä: Atena, 1998), 247–78.

I will study Finnish soldiers' traumatic memories as seen in three different instances. In the first part of the analysis, I will focus on posttraumatic memory in military hospital care during the war. My aim here is to acquire an overview of the prevalence and nature of these symptoms among the psychiatric soldier-patients. To this end, I am using a cluster sample of 315 military psychiatric patient files from the years 1941 and 1944. In addition to the statistical sample, I have also studied a large number of unsystematically chosen patient files: all in all, the work here is based upon the reading of over 550 military psychiatric patient files from 1939 to 1945.[19] For my doctoral dissertation in 2013, I conducted both a statistical analysis of the symptoms recorded in the patient files as well as a close reading of individual files in order to understand details and contexts for each case.[20] Individual patient files are usually terse when it comes to patients' subjective experiences but reading through several hundred files can compensate for this by offering a polyphonic archive of short but intense expressions of trauma.

In the second part, I will examine Finnish soldiers' dreams in the immediate postwar era, with the aim of analyzing the intrusive re-experiencing of violent memories in war-related nightmares. My source here is the survey "From War to Peace" ("Sodasta rauhaan"), which was collected from war veterans in Northern Finland in 1999–2000. One of the questions on the survey form focused on dreams: "Did the war follow you into your dreams? What kind of war dreams did you have and for how long?" As with the patient files, although the answers to the question were typically brief, this was balanced by the size and coverage of the data: the survey collected 1058 responses in total.[21] Many respondents simply stated whether they had had war-related dreams or not—but many also described their most memorable nightmares and offered an estimate as to how long they had had war dreams or if they were still having them. It must be noted that these are dreams recorded in writing more than 50 years after the end of World War II. Thus, they are not "authentic," immediate dream descriptions, if there is such a thing. But even though we cannot trust the details and precision of each individual dream reminiscence, the overall

[19] The patient files are stored at the National Archives of Finland (NAF), at the patient archive of each respective military hospital. The patients' names have been changed.
[20] Further details of the sample are described in Kivimäki (2013), 84–5, 479–85.
[21] National Archives of Finland in Oulu (NAF Oulu), "From War to Peace" Survey 1999–2000. I am grateful to Soja Ukkola for first pointing out this material to me more than ten years ago.

picture of the postwar "nightmare years," mediated through several hundred survey replies, is coherent and reliable.[22]

Third and last, I will use the same dream reminiscences as above to discuss the posttraumatic nature of the postwar culture at large. This is of course a vast field for research, and I will limit myself to only one question: How did the dream narrators relate their nightmares to war novels and war movies in the 1940s and 1950s? It has been hypothesized that the introduction of television sets, video recorders, and certain cinematic techniques in Vietnam-war movies "popularized" flashback memories as a symptom of trauma in the final decades of the twentieth century, whereas they would have been rare in earlier times.[23] Several dream reminiscences in the "From War to Peace" survey actually do find a connection between war-related nightmares vis-à-vis war movies and novels as early as in the 1940s and 1950s, but, as I will argue, this relation is not at all straightforward to the point where the movies and novels could be said to have "produced" the flashback-like symptoms. In addition to the above-mentioned survey, I have also used here one particular war-dream reminiscence from the collections of the Finnish Literature Society Archives (FLSA), which underlines the multilayered intertwinement of traumatic experiences, cultural products, and posttraumatic symptoms.[24]

TRAUMATIC MEMORY IN MILITARY PSYCHIATRY

In December 1943, Private Peter Ö., an unmarried fisherman born in 1921, was hospitalized at the 1st Military Hospital in Helsinki for jaundice. He had been conscripted in the autumn of 1941 and was sent to the front in January 1942. The following April, an artillery shell exploded close to him, killing his good friend in a direct hit. After this shocking experience, Peter Ö. started to have uncontrollable fear and tremor fits.

---

[22] For a more thorough discussion of war-related dreams and their sources, see Ville Kivimäki, "Nocturnal Nation: Violence and the Nation in Dreams during and after World War II," in *Lived Nation as the History of Experiences and Emotions in Finland, 1800–2000*, ed. by Ville Kivimäki, Sami Suodenjoki and Tanja Vahtikari (Cham: Palgrave, 2021b), 297–318.

[23] Edgar Jones et al., "Flashbacks and post-traumatic stress disorder: the genesis of a 20th-century diagnosis," *British Journal of Psychiatry* 182 (2003), 158–63.

[24] Originally, FLSA started as a folklore archive, collecting and preserving the national heritage of Finnish folk poetry, but it has since grown into a unique memory organization collecting and studying all kinds of oral history materials.

His sleep turned miserable, and he often had a nightmare where a gun was pointed at him. Now, at the military hospital, Peter Ö. had a mental breakdown: first he ran away, ripping off his clothes, and later lay on his bed immobile and unresponsive. Transferred to the psychiatric unit of the 10th Military Hospital in the Pitkäniemi mental asylum, Peter Ö. appeared mentally exhausted and depressed. Interviewed about what had happened to him in the earlier hospital, he said that the sound of an air-raid alarm during the heavy Soviet bombing raids against Helsinki in February 1944 had triggered horrible nightmares for him, in which he re-lived his past war experiences: the very real sound of artillery shells, air bombardments, and his fellow soldiers mutilated by bayonets. The nightmares were accompanied by a bad headache, and any loud noise in the hospital made him nervous and caused him to tremble. Peter Ö.'s roommates said that he regularly talked about rifles and shells while asleep. He was dismissed from the hospital in April 1944 with a diagnosis of neurasthenia, *reactiones psychogeneae*, and was deployed to auxiliary service at the home front.[25]

Peter Ö.'s case is close to being a textbook example of a contemporary diagnosis of chronic PTSD as represented in the latest version of the *Diagnostic and Statistical Manual of Mental Disorders*. He had clearly been exposed to a traumatic event involving actual or threatened death or serious injury; he suffered from a number of intrusion symptoms as if the traumatic event was recurring; there was persistent avoidance of stimuli associated with the trauma; there were negative alterations in cognition, mood, arousal, and reactivity associated with the traumatic event; the duration of the disturbance was more than one month; and all this caused clinically significant distress or impairment in social, occupational, or other important areas of functioning.[26]

The remarkable thing here is, of course, that the PTSD entered official psychiatric diagnostics only after the Vietnam War in 1980. Although the concepts of traumatic memory and delayed psychological symptom presentation, central to the present PTSD paradigm, had their early origins in the classic writings of Sigmund Freud, Pierre Janet, Jean-Martin Charcot, and others,[27] these ideas were neglected by the Finnish psychiatry of the time, as described above. Consequently, Finnish military psychiatrists were

[25] NAF, 10th Military Hospital Patient File Archive, date of arrival 1 March 1944, folder 68, patient file 3043 (3254).

[26] *DSM-5* (2013), 271–2.

[27] See Leys (2000), passim; Young (1995), 13 ff.

not at all inclined to observe and record their patients' "posttraumatic" symptoms; they were sharply focused on quite different factors such as heredity, intelligence, psychopathology, and nerves.[28] Thus, Peter Ö.'s final diagnosis was based on neurasthenia and *reactio psychogenea*, already recognized as quite ambiguous medical terms at the time, and both of which referred to his constitutional weaknesses.

Yet it is obvious that Peter Ö.'s was not a singular case. Undefined and unrecognized in the 1940s, the posttraumatic symptoms associated with traumatic violence—nightmares, general nervousness and irritation, memory problems, depression, tearfulness, delusions—nevertheless surfaced frequently among Finnish soldiers. In Table 4.1, I have collected the ten most frequently recorded symptoms in the cluster sample of 315 military psychiatric patient files during June–December 1941 and January–September 1944.

It is important to note the shortcomings of such a categorization. First of all, there were differences in military hospitals' accuracy and scrupulousness in writing down their patients' symptoms. Furthermore, categories such as "tremor," "general nervousness," or "disorientation"

Table 4.1 Symptoms recorded in the military psychiatric patient files: combined samples of 1941 and 1944 (n = 315, frequencies in percentages)

	Percent among all patients
1. Sleeplessness, tiredness, restless sleep	60.7
2. General nervousness and/or irritation	53.8
3. Tremor	45.3
4. Depression, depressive reticence	35.8
5. Headache	35.5
6. Memory loss	31.1
7. Dizziness, nausea	28.0
8. Disorientation, general confusion	25.8
9. Uncontrollable fear or terror	25.2
10. Tearfulness	24.8

Source: National Archives of Finland (NAF), the sample of patient files from the Finnish military hospitals' psychiatric units in 1941 and 1944

[28] On the slow entry of the traumatic memory paradigm to military psychiatry, see Young (2004), 130–2; also, Wessely (2006).

include symptoms with very different gravities. Some of the symptom categories, such as "sleeplessness, tiredness, restless sleep," are quite elastic: although most records note a difference between, for instance, exhaustion and nightmares, not a few use such ambiguous terms as "lack of sleep" without further specification, thus hindering a more nuanced differentiation between the symptoms. The recording of symptoms at the hospitals was not "objective," so that all the symptoms might be noticed equally readily. Instead, the psychiatrists, following their training and tenets, paid more attention to things they considered medically relevant for the patient's condition—and ignored other signs of disorder. Consequently, "posttraumatic" symptoms may have been considered irrelevant or might not have been noticed at all, although it is also possible that some doctors would have found them curious and thus worth noting.[29]

Notwithstanding these shortcomings, the table provides a sufficiently precise general overview of the frequency of the patients' most common symptoms. While it is not a list of diagnostic criteria in any medical sense, we can see many features of posttraumatic memory embedded in and between the symptoms. The most frequent group of symptoms—sleeplessness, tiredness, restless sleep—was very common indeed, visible in over 60 percent of the patients. Based on the reading of individual patient files, that usually translates to nightmares or the inability to fall or stay asleep because of some troubling war-related memories. The broad categories of "general nervousness and/or irritation" and "uncontrollable fear or terror" often talk about the same phenomenon of being disturbed by one's earlier war experiences. Similar to "depression and depressive reticence" and "tearfulness," they may also connotate a temporary or lasting change of behavior or character following the traumatic experience. The category of "memory loss," and partly also "disorientation and general confusion," can be seen as related to problems of dissociation. Witnessing severe and continuous violence could lead to a fracture in relating to the surrounding reality: the experienced world turned unreal or was completely wiped from memory.[30]

The figures above provide a quantitative outline of the prevalence of posttraumatic symptoms in the totality of the military psychiatric patient files. Yet each and every case was different, and the soldiers' traumatic experiences and their symptoms combined in various ways. It will therefore prove useful to examine another example of how "trauma before trauma" could appear in wartime medical records:

Lance Corporal Veikko M., an unmarried worker born in 1918, spent three weeks at the front in the Winter War without any mental problems. When Finland joined Operation Barbarossa in June 1941, he served as a tank driver. During the Finnish offensive in the summer of 1941, two of his fellow crewmen were badly wounded by a direct hit, and their blood covered the interior of the tank. Even though Veikko M. survived and continued to carry out his assignment, he began to feel nervous and claustrophobic and could drive the tank only with its hatches open. Later, in December 1941, he was wounded in the arm by a rifle shot. The wound did not heal properly, and Veikko M. spent long periods in military hospitals. Taken into custody for drunk and disorderly conduct in February 1944, he became psychotic and experienced the police cell as a tank, the walls of which were about to crush him. When released, he was in a state of shock, was experiencing tremors and was sent to the psychiatric unit of the 10th Military Hospital in Pitkäniemi. Depressed and apathetic, Veikko M. explained that his "nerves" had been in bad shape ever since his tank was hit in 1941; he was sleepless, his hands shook, and everything frightened him. He was also using quite a lot of alcohol and had problems adapting to military discipline. Given seven electroshock treatments over a two-week period in April 1944 and with his condition somewhat "improved," Veikko M. was diagnosed with *constitutio et reactio psychopathica* and sent to serve in the special fortification detachments for "nervous convalescents."[31]

It is neither necessary nor possible to medically diagnose Veikko M. in retrospect. For the purpose of this chapter, it is enough to note the posttraumatic qualities of his case. He was clearly haunted by the experiences of surviving a direct hit and witnessing the severe wounding of his comrades. Consequently, he suffered from various psychological, psychosomatic, and social symptoms, which had not eased over the two and a half years subsequent to the traumatic experiences. The use of alcohol as an attempt to alleviate the situation—and its negative impact—also fits the picture of coping with trauma. The incident at the police cell can be seen as a recurrence of the original traumatic event in the tank. Yet, as Veikko M.'s patient file demonstrates, those posttraumatic elements of his

---

[31] NAF, 10th Military Hospital Patient File Archive, date of arrival 17 March 1944, folder 357, patient file 3131.

experience and his symptoms, which now seem so obvious, were not recognized as etiological causes of his condition—the diagnosis pointed
instead to his personal psychopathology.

The wartime psychiatric patient files reveal the acute immediacy of violent experiences, similar in their symptoms to those Soviet cases documented by Robert Dale in his chapter. In addition to war-related
nightmares and sleep disturbances, the soldiers were sometimes thrown
back onto their traumatic memories in a wide-awake state and with such
overwhelming force that it resembled re-living the experience as if it were
happening again. For the limitations described earlier, the statistical analysis of psychiatric patient files does not allow for pinpointing the exact prevalence of posttraumatic symptoms among the soldier-patients. Yet the
frequency shown in several symptom categories in Table 4.1 is evident.
Furthermore, it is worth stressing that posttraumatic symptoms were by
no means limited to military psychiatric patients. In order to be sent to a
military hospital, a soldier had to be in such bad condition that he was
clearly useless for military service—and the official policies in this respect
were also notoriously random. Different war-related psychological (and
psychosomatic) troubles were widespread among ordinary soldiers who
never visited a medical officer; these troubles also included various post-
traumatic symptoms.[32]

Haunted Dreams

Of the diagnostic criteria for PTSD, one of the most typical symptoms for
persistent re-experiencing of the traumatic event is the nightmare: "recurrent distressing dreams in which the content and/or effect of the dream is
related to traumatic event(s)."[33] As an example of this important manifestation of posttraumatic memory, I will now look at Finnish ex-soldiers'
dreams in the postwar era. Just as with the appearance of posttraumatic
symptoms within the wartime patient files, I want to emphasize here that
the prevalence of war-related nightmares in the 1940s and 1950s cannot
be attributed to any "therapy culture"[34] that could have encouraged the
expression of violent memories in dreams. As was noted earlier, there was

[32] Kivimäki (2013), 170–7.
[33] DSM-5 (2013), 271.
[34] Frank Furedi, *Therapy Culture: Cultivating Vulnerability in an Uncertain Age* (London:
Routledge, 2004).

no support for the idea of traumatic memory among Finnish psychiatrists at the time. Freudian psychoanalysis, which could have fostered an interest in dreams, was a real latecomer to Finnish psychiatry, making its breakthrough only in the 1950s and 1960s.[35]

At the end of the 1990s, over 50 years after the end of World War II, the advisory committee on war-veteran matters in Northern Finland decided to collect information and reminiscences from surviving war veterans in the Oulu and Lapland Provinces. At this time, the Finnish "memory boom" with regard to World War II had lasted for over a decade, and the war stories of 1939–45 had been eagerly consumed in both public and private spheres of life.[36] The committee decided that it would also be useful to gather information on the transition from war to peace immediately after the war had ended. The mid-1990s had finally seen some public discussion of the war veterans' mental health issues, their problems in returning to civilian life, and some of these themes were now included in the survey "From War to Peace," which was taken in 1999–2000.[37] I am focusing here only on one question in the long, 17-page survey form: "Did the war follow you into your dreams? What kind of war dreams did you have and for how long?"

At the turn of the millennium, the great majority of the survey's respondents belonged to the youngest Finnish age cohorts that had been conscripted into military service during World War II: only 297 respondents of the total of 1058 had been born before 1920. It was thus natural that the chain of events, which had most strongly influenced the informants' dreams after the war, centered on the experience of the Finnish retreat and desperate defensive battles carried out against the Red Army in June–July 1944. The opening phase of these battles was especially characterized by an overwhelming Soviet superiority in terms of artillery, tanks, infantry, and air power. The Finnish Army was forced to conduct a hasty and partly

---

[35] Yrjö O. Alanen, Johannes Lehtonen and Pekka Tienari, "Psykiatrinen tutkimus," in *Seitsemän vuosikymmentä suomalaista psykiatriaa*, ed. by Kalle Achté, Jaakko Suominen and Tapani Tamminen (Helsinki: Suomen psykiatriyhdistys, 1983), 49–55.

[36] See, for example, Tiina Kinnunen and Markku Jokispilä, "Shifting Images of 'Our Wars': Finnish Memory Culture of World War II," in *Finland in World War II: History, Memory, Interpretations*, ed. by Tiina Kinnunen and Ville Kivimäki (Leiden: Brill, 2012), 436–82; Ville Kivimäki, "Between Defeat and Victory: Finnish Memory Culture of the Second World War," *Scandinavian Journal of History* 37:4 (2012), 482–504.

[37] NAF Oulu, From War to Peace, E:2–3 includes preparatory materials, instructions, and statistical summaries of the survey.

chaotic retreat, although in the end the Red Army was not able to break through the last lines of defense. This was a bitter and violent struggle that included many traumatic experiences: immense concentrations of Soviet firepower against thinly manned Finnish lines; heavy tank assaults; constant threats of airstrikes; panicky withdrawals and a fear of being taken captive by the Soviets. Of all the phases of World War II in Finland, the summer of 1944 left the strongest and most traumatic imprint on the immediate postwar years.[38]

"Very often, at first," was the answer a man born in 1922 gave to the survey question of whether he had had war-related dreams after the war: "I was often woken up by a 'Uraah'-cry, which made me search for a machine pistol. [The battle of] Ihantala [in 1944] still sometimes returns to my dreams."[39] In a similar tone, another veteran born in 1915 reminisced: "At the beginning I often had a dream of a site where I was the only survivor of our machinegun crew. Being afraid of getting wounded or taken captive, I continued the fight alone, but now I haven't had those dreams anymore."[40] A man born in 1926 belonged to the youngest age cohort that was conscripted into military service during the war and as an 18-year-old recruit he had been wounded in July 1944: "Yes, especially my fear of airplanes follows me in my dreams very frequently. I often have a dream where there are thousands of planes in the sky, especially at night. This might be because of the low-flying Russian ground-attack aircraft, which buzzed above us."[41] "Yes, the war did affect my nerves, I had nightmares. For example, I would be in a difficult situation and want to get away, but I could never escape as fast as I needed to," a fourth man, born in 1923, responded to the same question: "I always woke up before they caught me. Often my weapon didn't work, so flight was the only option. This went on for about a year almost every night. Then the nightmares became less frequent before they finally stopped."[42]

These examples are representative of the laconic style and content of the responses. The survey form which held a total of 123 different questions, but only limited space for each answer, did not invite the respondents to write down long and detailed dream accounts. Many chose to

---

[38] For an overview of these events in English, see Pasi Tuunainen, "The Finnish Army at War: Operations and Soldiers, 1939–45," in Kinnunen and Kivimäki, eds (2012), 159–68.

[39] NAF Oulu, From War to Peace, B:8 N:o 02733.

[40] NAF Oulu, From War to Peace, B:2 N:o 02014.

[41] NAF Oulu, From War to Peace, A:11 N:o 03168.

[42] NAF Oulu, From War to Peace, B:41, unnumbered survey form.

answer with a simple yes or no. Because most respondents were already very old and frail, they often chose to answer only part of the question litany. This makes it difficult to provide any exact statistical summary regarding the prevalence of war-related dreams. Yet the survey makes clear that war nightmares were a widespread phenomenon, easily recognized and experienced by a great number, if not the majority, of the survey's respondents. Many relate their nightmares to the immediate postwar years. Then the grip of nightly terrors started to ease around ten years after the war. For some, nevertheless, the nightmares were still a frequent disturbance over 50 years after the war—and for some of the respondents the nightmares had started again in old age or were triggered by an incident that somehow resembled the original traumatic event.[43]

The Finnish war generation was also a nightmare generation. Psychologist Nils Sandman et al. have studied the prevalence of nightmares among the Finnish population between 1972 and 2007, pointing out that frequent nightmares were clearly more common among the men and women who had experienced the war, than for members of the younger generations.[44] It is safe to say that the recurrence of violent wartime experiences in dreams was a prevalent phenomenon among Finnish ex-servicemen after the war. Based on the "From War to Peace" survey, these dreams were typically very straightforward. Instead of containing symbolically rich content or fantastic plots, war-related nightmares were brutal repetitions of the traumatic event: of being assaulted and wounded, losing one's comrade, fearing for one's life. This matches the findings of psychiatrist Bas Schreuder et al. regarding Dutch combat veterans' traumatic dreams, which were so realistic and "replicative" of the soldiers' original experiences that they could be considered posttraumatic re-enactments.[45]

---

[43] Kivimäki (2021b).

[44] Nils Sandman et al., "Nightmares: Prevalence Among the Finnish General Adult Population and War Veterans During 1972–2007," *SLEEP* 36:7 (2013), 1041–50. For similar findings in Germany, see Michael Schredl and Edgar Piel, "War-Related Dream Themes in Germany from 1956 to 2000," *Political Psychology* 27:2 (2006), 299–307.

[45] Bas J. N. Schreuder, Wim C. Kleijn and Harry G. M. Rooijmans, "Nocturnal Re-Experiencing More Than Forty Years After War Trauma," *Journal of Traumatic Stress* 13:3 (2000), 453–63; Bas J. N. Schreuder, Marjan van Egmond, Wim C. Kleijn and Anouschka T. Visser, "Daily Reports of Posttraumatic Nightmares and Anxiety Dreams in Dutch War Victims," *Journal of Anxiety Disorders* 12:6 (1998), 511–24.

Realistic, re-enactive nightmares thus come close to paralleling the so-called flashback memories, although they take place while asleep. Unlike "normal" memories of past events, flashbacks include strong, involuntary, and visual "revival" of the traumatic experience that keep recurring over and over.[46] In the diagnostic criteria for PTSD, flashbacks are mentioned as an example of "dissociative reactions" among the so-called intrusion symptoms, which include unwanted, upsetting memories, nightmares, flashbacks, and emotional distress or physical reactivity after exposure to traumatic reminders.[47]

Regarding flashbacks that appear in a wide-awake state, the theory considering them to be photographic, "iconic" memories of the original incident has been disproved.[48] But even if flashbacks do not represent traumatic experiences with objective accuracy, and contain distortions of what happened, they can still be seen as pointing to the subjective experience of trauma. Similarly, while we cannot really know whether the nightmares recollected in the "From War to Peace" survey are accurate replications of what the dreamer had witnessed when at war, they are clearly referential in this respect and point to actual experiences at the front, whether distorted or not. Besides the continuous repetitions of the same traumatic event, they also refer to a deep experience of vulnerability, impotence, and an inability to act upon the deadly threat. Under assault, a soldier is caught unguarded, he does not find his weapon, or the gun does not function properly: "Two dreams have followed me to this day: 1) The enemy is attacking, and I cannot make my weapon work; 2) I'm skiing downhill in a beautiful pine forest right into the middle of a swarm of enemies."[49] Such repetitive visions caused strong emotional arousal and a feeling of being thrown back into the war, night after night.

This type of traumatic memory focuses on dreamers' feeling of helplessness and being at the mercy of violent powers outside of their control. In nightmares, both the body and the mind are under constant assault. There is also a different kind of traumatic memory that represents a disturbing moral injury: the dreams that bring to mind acts of violence

[46] Michael Linden, "Spectrum of Persisting Memories and Pseudomemories, Distortions, and Psychopathology," in *Hurting Memories and Beneficial Forgetting: Posttraumatic Stress Disorders, Biographical Developments, and Social Conflicts*, ed. by Michael Linden and Krzysztof Rutkowski (London: Elsevier, 2013), 5–6.

[47] *DSM-5* (2013), 271.

[48] McNally (2003), 113–7.

[49] NAF Oulu, From War to Peace, B:8 N:o 01833.

committed by the dreamers themselves. The "From War to Peace" survey includes a handful of such reminiscences;[50] yet they represent only a tiny minority. Instead, the intrusive, posttraumatic element of the vast majority of war-related nightmares expressed itself in forcing the person to be a passive object of violence. To a great extent, this had to do with the circumstances of modern warfare. The soldiers in their trenches were targets of a multitude of invisible threats, from which they could not readily protect themselves: indirect shelling, sniper shots, machine-gun bursts, and air bombardments. These experiences resulted in victimhood dreams rather than in morally traumatic contemplations concerning a person's own wartime deeds.

Posttraumatic Flashbacks and Cultural Products

One particular question regarding posttraumatic flashbacks concerns their relation to cultural products. Originally, the term "flashback" was borrowed from the literature and film industry to studies on hallucinogenic drugs carried out at the end of the 1960s. Consequently, the term was used to describe the traumatic experiences of Vietnam veterans in the 1970s.[51] The historically conditioned nature of flashbacks has been studied in an article by Edgar Jones et al., where the authors compared the British Army war invalid records from six different conflicts, ranging from the Victorian Campaigns to the first Gulf War (1856–1991), in order to understand the historical epidemiology of flashback symptoms. In these sources, flashbacks were almost non-recorded up until the 1990s: in the Gulf War sample (n=400), 9.0 percent of the studied cases recorded flashback symptoms, whereas the second highest rate was recorded in the World War II sample (n=367) with 1.4 percent of the cases. The study underlined flashbacks as a historically and culturally sensitive phenomenon. In explaining the appearance of flashbacks in the 1990s, Jones et al. went on to contemplate the role played by "affordable television sets" and the subsequent introduction of video recorders, color motion pictures,

---

[50] One respondent had had to kill Soviet soldiers at close range and recalled their anguished faces, while another respondent had had to participate in a firing squad; see NAF Oulu, From War to Peace, B:49 N:o 00896 and B:64 N:o 00825, respectively.

[51] Fred H. Frankel, "The Concept of Flashbacks in Historical Perspective," *International Journal of Clinical and Experimental Hypnosis* 42:4 (1994), 321–36.

and flashbacks as a "frequent cinematic device" in Vietnam-war movies serving to popularize the symptom.[52]

Much in this debate depends on the definition of flashbacks. If we adopt a narrow concept of flashbacks as overwhelming visual experiences of being thrown back into the exact moment of trauma in an awake state, then it may indeed be rare to find them in historical archives. This does not necessarily mean that they did not exist; and as the examples of Peter Ö. and Veikko M. in this chapter have shown, at least something closely resembling wide-awake flashbacks can be found in Finnish sources from the 1940s as well. The rarity of flashbacks could also be explained by the scarcity of historical documents that might have recorded such subjectively experienced trauma symptoms in sufficient detail.[53] But it is also possible that a posttraumatic "re-run" or "replay" of the original incident[54] as a "correct" symptom of mental agony could indeed have become more common through popular cinematic culture, although I think this hypothesis would require much more evidence than has surfaced so far. Yet if we take a wider definition of flashbacks as visual, emotional intrusions of the violent past, when either asleep or awake—and notwithstanding the question of whether these images are photographic "copies" of the original incident—then this chapter has shown that flashbacks are not simply a post-Vietnam-War novelty employed in expressing traumatic memories, but that they were also a real phenomenon in the Finland of the 1940s and 1950s.

The question of posttraumatic memory vis-à-vis cultural products is an interesting one and the dream reminiscences in the "From War to Peace" survey offer some answers to it. I have tracked altogether ten respondents who make some reference to movies, television, or war novels when they write about their dreams.[55] All these answers share the same story: reading

[52] Jones et al. (2003), cit. 162; see also Jones and Wessely (2005), 174. As the British Army did not participate in the Vietnam War, the study displays a long gap between the first Gulf War and the previous conflicts, Malay (1948–60) and Korea (1951–53). Furthermore, even as Malay and Korea are treated as single conflicts in the study, they produced an insignificant number of cases (n=21), so we cannot really recognize a possible gradual change between World War II and the Gulf War in the occurrence of flashbacks. In the Victorian Campaigns (n=28) and the Boer War (n=400), no flashbacks were recorded at all; in World War I (n=640), only three cases of flashbacks were recognized.

[53] McNally (2004), 7–8.

[54] Leys (2000), 241.

[55] In addition to these ten respondents, one war veteran in the survey specifically mentions *not* being disturbed by war novels or watching television; and one comments on how he

a book or watching a movie might have reinvigorated war-related night-mares, but did not cause them in the first place. "Yes, there were night-mares too, but they were soon over. Only when *The Unknown Soldier* movie appeared did it cause battle dreams and nightmares the following night," a veteran reminisced.[56] Väinö Linna's *The Unknown Soldier* was an immensely popular war novel, dealing with frontline experiences in 1941–44, that was published in 1954 and filmed the following year. Five of the respondents in the "From War to Peace" survey mention war novels as a nightmare trigger, four mention war movies or watching television, and one mentions both books and television. It is worth noting that nov-els were just as common as visual materials in triggering war-related dreams: "[The war] followed [in my dreams] and still does, especially when I've read, or am reading, a war book. Always nightmares, there's a dangerous situation and one cannot escape. One has to yell, to warn others."[57] Books, movies, or TV-programs could re-launch nightmares even over 55 years after the war had ended.

Based on these ten responses, postwar cultural products could indeed be triggers for posttraumatic memory. But in contrast to the idea that the traumatized persons may have "borrowed" their symptoms from cultural representations, the direction of causality is rather the reverse. As I have shown earlier, posttraumatic nightmares and even flashback-like symp-toms are already to be found in the wartime materials—and the reminis-cences in the "From War to Peace" survey also point out that the war-related dreams were most disturbing immediately after the war. The postwar Finnish novels and movies can be seen as a delayed response to these traumatic experiences, not vice versa.

In the first instance, the troubled war experiences can be recognized in Finnish literature. As soon as the war in Finland ended in 1944–45, the men and women of the war generation started to publish their debut nov-els, where they discussed the challenges faced by young people in the midst of war and its aftermath: personal losses, moral decay, experiences of violence, rootlessness, and relationship problems. This genre consists of around a dozen novels published in 1944–50 and came to be known as

himself had edited a war-related book, something that had brought the nightmares back in the 1990s; see NAF Oulu, From War to Peace, B:46 N:o 01816 and B:9 N:o 02177, respectively.

[56] NAF Oulu, From War to Peace, B:35 N:o 00822.

[57] NAF Oulu, From War to Peace, B:27 N:o 00617 (original underlining).

"homecoming literature."[58] But while the genre includes specifically war-related stories and some flashback-like narrations, it is not really "trauma fiction" in the contemporary sense of the term. The war generation's troubled memory is a sub-theme, but the authors' main concern is rather to depict personal, social, and societal tensions in young people's readjustment to civilian life.[59]

Similar themes were important in Finnish postwar movies. In the 1940s, the films focused on moral decadence, alcoholism, juvenile delinquency, and other social problems within the postwar society. With respect to ex-soldiers' posttraumatic memories, things turn more interesting only in the 1950s when a handful of movies thematize in various degrees the disturbing memory of wartime violence.[60] As Ana Antić, Hana Kubátová, and Marta Kurkowska-Budzan show in their respective chapters for this volume, postwar fiction films have been a major cultural arena for depicting and processing troublesome wartime experiences—this was also the case in Finland.

In "Eyes in the Dark" (*Silmät hämärässä*, directed by Veikko Itkonen in 1952), a previously shell shocked sergeant suffers from the invisible shame of his experience and commits a crime after the war. The sergeant is haunted by a cry for help from his wounded officer, whom he had abandoned in the battle. In "The Days of Decision" (*Ratkaisun päivät*, directed by Hannu Leminen in 1956), a major has had to shoot one of his men for mutinous behavior. Wounded soon afterwards, the major also undergoes a "mental shock" which makes him mourn and ramble on about the incident while unconscious in the hospital. In "Little Ilona and Her Lambkin" (*Pikku Ilona ja hänen karitsansa*, directed by Jorma Nortimo in 1957)—a peculiar children's movie with rather dreadful depictions of war-related loss and maltreatment—one of the characters is a "shaken-up" and nervous ex-soldier, whose life the war has derailed. And in "Blood on Our Hands" (*Verta käsissämme*, directed by William Markus in 1958), a Finnish officer has to witness a chaotic retreat, the suicide of a wounded soldier, and being taken prisoner in the summer of 1944. Returning from Soviet captivity in the 1950s, the ex-officer ends up

[58] Risto Turunen, *Uhon ja armon aika: Suomalainen kirjallisuusjärjestelmä, sen yhteiskuntasuhteet ja rakenteistuminen 1944–1952* (Joensuu: University of Joensuu Press, 2003), 228–30.

[59] Pertti Lassila, "Min täällä teen, se kaikki kieroon vie," in *Ja kuitenkin me voitimme: Sodan muisto ja perintö*, ed. by Lauri Haataja (Helsinki: Kirjayhtymä, 1994), 141–57.

[60] Pekka Kaarninen, *Kotimaisen elokuvan maammekirja* (Vantaa: Avain, 2018), 188–202.

betraying his friend and killing a young boy in a car accident, an act he tries to conceal. In the final scene, the troubled man is walking to the police department to turn himself in. This image overlaps with a full-blown flashback to the last desperate battles at the front, as if the man is simultaneously being haunted by these sights and is about to be redeemed from them.[61]

What all four movies have in common is that past war experiences cast a shadow over the postwar life and behavior of either the film's protagonist or some other main character. In all four movies the violent events of 1944 cause troubled memories—and, actually, all of the films, except for "Eyes in the Dark," open with a dramatic scene that takes place at the front. The later battle scene in "Eyes in the Dark" is similar to those in the other three: a powerful enemy is attacking, there is heavy artillery fire and the Finns are forced to retreat. The films also make surprisingly strong reference to other traumatic experiences that were characteristic of the summer of 1944: the executions, air bombardments, tank assaults, shell shocks, being caught by the enemy, and having to leave behind one's wounded comrades. This was the same exact subject matter that terrorized war veterans' dreams as we have seen earlier. The nightmares were there first; and the novels and movies took them as their raw material, or mental canvas, in order to connect with the feelings and experiences of their audience.[62] This happened at roughly the same time in the 1950s, when a major portion of the dream reminiscences tell us that the nightmares began to be less frequent than immediately after the war.[63]

I think the best way to understand the link between the ex-soldiers' posttraumatic memories and the postwar cultural products is to see them in a dynamic relation. The tersely worded replies in the "From War to Peace" survey do not allow for a much closer scrutiny of this issue, but it

---

[61] As was noted earlier, Väinö Linna's novel *The Unknown Soldier* was filmed in 1955. Yet as the novel and the film take place entirely in wartime, they lack the same flashback-like quality as the four films discussed here, which are all situated in the postwar context. On the other hand, Linna's work definitely had the capacity to take its readers or viewers back to the war years, so it can perhaps be seen as a one long flashback for audiences in the 1950s.

[62] For a similar observation on Väinö Linna's work, see Ville Kivimäki, "Väkivallan kantajat: Tuntemattoman sotilaan posttraumaattisuudesta," in *Väinö Linna – tunnettu ja tuntematon*, ed. by Jyrki Nummi, Maria Laakso, Toni Lahtinen, and Pertti Haapala (Helsinki: WSOY, 2020), 195–211.

[63] Kivimäki (2021b).

is particularly visible in a singular dream reminiscence recorded in the collections of the FLSA:

At the end of June 1944, a 23-year-old Finnish officer, Kalervo A., was at rest behind the frontline when he was suddenly awoken by an approaching Soviet patrol. Kalervo A. and his fellows managed to fire first and killed the three Soviet soldiers. Following a common habit, Kalervo A. went to check the pockets of his fallen adversaries. One of the dead soldiers was also an officer, who had a picture of his wife in his pocket. As the fighting went on, Kalervo A. ignored the incident. Only after he was demobilized in November 1944, did he start to have recurrent nightmares, in which the encounter was vividly repeated. In addition, the woman in the photograph started to haunt Kalervo A.'s dreams, accusing him of murdering her husband. In the spring of 1945, Kalervo A. went to see a movie which depicted a boat that was carrying deceased persons to heaven. The boat's staff consisted of people who had committed suicide and who were thus not allowed to enter the kingdom of heaven. After the film, Kalervo A.'s nightmare grew to new dimensions: he saw himself in the boat and the wife of the dead Soviet soldier had to serve there as a kind of waitress, since she had committed suicide after hearing the news of her husband's death. Kalervo A. started to be afraid of falling asleep and, as the dream usually occurred around three o'clock in the morning, he could no longer get proper rest. As time passed, however, the nightmare became less frequent. Telling his story in 1994, Kalervo A. reported that he had had the dream for the last time in February 1983, following surgery. With regard to this final instance, he remembered telling his pursuer that since the killed officer had had a pistol in his hand, he had been forced to do what he did.[64]

Here, too, war dreams preceded the movie, but the film acted as a trigger that intensified the nightmare and gave it new content. I think that this kind of a reciprocal relation, where war-related traumatic experiences (or rather some fragments of them) influence cultural products in the postwar period, which then retroactively act upon the memories of those experiences, presents a dynamic way of studying trauma, emotions, and memory in the postwar culture.[65] This is not, of course, an automatic or

---

[64] FLSA, "Minuun sattui"—Mikkeli area war invalids' reminiscence collection 1994, Kalervo A., 7–10.

[65] Frank Biess, "Feelings in the Aftermath: Toward a History of Postwar Emotions," in *Histories of the Aftermath: The Legacies of the Second World War in Europe*, ed. by Frank Biess

mechanical process, whereby traumatic experiences get transferred to films and novels swiftly and in their entirety. What is transferrable (i.e., culturally expressible) depends upon a multitude of factors—and there are essential gaps, fractures, and silences in this process.[66] In every case, this is a more complicated, and thus more intriguing, setting than the idea that the "culture" simply produces (or not) flashbacks and other posttraumatic symptoms—the direction of influence is also the opposite.[67]

Finally, Kalervo A.'s story suggests one more observation to be made in relation to posttraumatic memory. Kalervo's dream was different from the vast majority of other dream reminiscences in that it dealt with the moral injury incurred in having killed an enemy soldier; as discussed earlier, the postwar nightmares in "From War to Peace" survey were, with few exceptions, victimhood dreams. Interestingly, in this respect Kalervo A.'s dream comes close to paralleling the acts portrayed in the films introduced above, three of which dealt with troubles occasioned by the act of killing.[68] It seems to me that the narratively rich character of both Kalervo A.'s dream and the fiction movies is well suited to contemplating the moral problem produced by committing violent acts, and the experiences of guilt and shame that that can cause. These are also recurrent themes in modern war movies and their depictions of "perpetrator trauma."[69] The blunt, repetitive dreams of being an object of violence did not have this same narrative capability of creating a plot or agency. At least in this respect they were less relatable, less story-like. There are neither sufficient sources nor enough space to take this question further here, but it may nevertheless be one

---

and Robert G. Moeller (New York: Berghahn, 2010), 30–48.

[66] Jay Winter, "Thinking about silence," in *Shadows of War: A Social History of Silence in the Twentieth Century*, ed. by Efrat Ben-Ze'ev, Ruth Ginio, and Jay Winter (Cambridge: Cambridge University Press, 2010), 3–31.

[67] Cf. Anton Kaes, *Shell Shock Cinema: Weimar Culture and the Wounds of War* (Princeton, NJ: Princeton University Press, 2009).

[68] "How does it actually feel to kill a human being," as the female protagonist asks of the ex-officer in "Blood on Our Hands," after they have run over the young boy. In "Eyes in the Dark," the sergeant is ashamed of not having saved his comrade—and then commits a murder after the war. In "The Days of Decision," the major sees nightmares of having shot his subordinate.

[69] On perpetrator trauma and films, see Julia B. Köhne, "Aesthetic Displays of Perpetrators in Joshua Oppenheimer's *The Act of Killing*: Post-Atrocity Perpetrator Symptoms, Re-enactments of Violence, and Perpetrator-Victim-Inversions," and Raya Morag, "Perpetrator Trauma and Current American War Cinema," both in Leese, Köhne and Crouthamel, eds (2021).

worthwhile considering at a later date: different cultural medias may underline and reinforce certain types of posttraumatic memory while neglecting others.

CONCLUDING REMARKS: CULTURE IN TRAUMATIC EXPERIENCE

In this chapter I have ended up balancing between two paradigms of understanding trauma, the constructivist one and the diagnostic one, without being satisfied with either of them. First of all, I started the chapter by criticizing the critique of the "objective" medical PTSD paradigm, as this constructivist standpoint focuses so strongly on the politico-medical "invention" of trauma and lacks interest in the traumatic dimension of the experiences of violence. Therefore, I have shown that posttraumatic memories and their intrusive symptoms can also be found and studied before the genesis of the medical concept of trauma—or in a culture that did not recognize trauma as a psychiatric disorder. On the other hand, it should be clear that I am not advocating any culture-free concept of trauma either. Historically changing cultural meanings, social realities, and medical knowledge matter in defining the space for the experience of trauma, even if this experience cannot be reduced to the sum total of these preconditions.[70]

In order to reconcile the unsatisfactory situation between the two paradigms, I would like to conclude with the following suggestion: the analysis of cultural factors could be brought closer to the primary experience. Instead of searching for trauma in diagnostic manuals (as important as this remains in its own right), there is a plenitude of culture at play in the immediate vicinity of traumatic experience. As bodily, sensory, and mental experiences, such practices of violence as drumfire, death squads, carpet bombing, bayonet assaults, or guerrilla warfare are also cultural phenomena, which produce distinctive experiences both for the victims and the perpetrators. Consequently, they also produce distinctive experiences of trauma, which are then further framed by varying medical paradigms in order to treat and conceptualize these experiences within different societal contexts.[71] There is, for instance, a transnational culture of having

---

[70] On films and perpetration, see also Ana Antić's chapter in this book.

[71] For a pathbreaking study on the interplay between the violent experiences of guerrilla warfare and the consequent idea of "Partisan hysteria" in Yugoslav psychiatry of the 1940s,

experienced indirect artillery fire that has been undergone by millions of men and women in the twentieth century. This experience has given birth to a multitude of novels, films, and art works, but it has also created a wilder and less articulated culture of mental shocks, bodily sensations, and posttraumatic nightmares.[72]

By situating the social and cultural study of trauma within experiences and in their direct circumstances, I think we can better understand the consequences of violence and possibly circumvent too weighty an emphasis on texts and discourses when defining traumatic experiences. It is possible that on this visceral level there is less cultural and historical variation in trauma responses than is the case in cultural representations and medical cultures of trauma.[73] Discussing emotions as embodied practices, Monique Scheer has propounded the following notion concerning the limits the body sets on cultural variation:

> *The body also provides the habitus with something to shape; it is not radically or arbitrarily modifiable, and it dictates the range of practices available. Clearly, no human society will develop a dance step that requires five feet or a musical instrument made for a hand with eight digits. [...] Yet, a bright line between nature and culture cannot be drawn on or in the body because human beings hardly leave anything about themselves or their environment untouched.*[74]

Something similar may apply to the case for traumatic experiences and posttraumatic memories. The processes of the human brain give structure to the ways in which potentially traumatic experiences take shape and the

---

see Ana Antić, *Therapeutic Fascism. Experiencing the Violence of the Nazi New Order* (Oxford: Oxford University Press, 2017), esp. Chap. 5.

[72] We have a rich research tradition concerning the cultural history and memory of World War I, where shell shock and other frontline experiences occupy a prominent place; see for example, Jay Winter, *Remembering War: The Great War Between Memory and History in the Twentieth Century* (New Haven, CT: Yale University Press, 2006). Yet a transnational history of experiencing artillery fire and other traumatic aspects of modern warfare in the twentieth century are, to my knowledge, missing; Ville Kivimäki, "Violence and Trauma: Experiencing the Two World Wars," in *Routledge Companion to Cultural History in the Western World*, ed. by Alessandro Arcangeli, Jörg Rogge, and Hannu Salmi (London: Routledge, 2020), 533.

[73] William M. Reddy, "The Unavoidable Intentionality of Affect: The History of Emotions and the Neurosciences of the Present Day," *Emotion Review* 12:3 (2020), 171–2.

[74] Monique Scheer, "Are Emotions a Kind of Practice (and Is That What Makes Them Have a History?): A Bourdieuian Approach to Understanding Emotion," *History and Theory* 51:2 (2012), 201.

manner in which the haunting cognition of them may avoid integration into normal biographic memory and contextual knowledge, thus leading to dissociation and intrusive memories of the event.[75] This would explain the appearance of posttraumatic symptoms and their relative coherence in a variety of historical and cultural settings—although I recognize that a truly comparative, transnational, and transcultural study of trauma responses is still a work in progress.[76] Yet there would still be considerable room for the socio-cultural analysis and explanation of trauma, too; just as Scheer points out, this would be a matter of an encounter between biology and culture, where both are inseparably intertwined. The brain and its processes are culturally preconditioned before the experience of trauma, and the brain also continues to experience and memorize along culturally conditioned paths after a traumatic incident. All this takes place in a historically specific context of social relations and societal circumstances.[77]

In returning now to the Finnish soldiers and war veterans in the 1940s and 1950s, the posttraumatic nature of their experiences seems clear to me. They were unwilling participants in the culture of modern warfare, which in the Finnish case materialized most concretely in the experience of artillery fire and trench combat. This was a different experience from fighting in far-away Vietnamese villages and rainforests in the 1960s and 1970s, the American experience of which was then seminal for the shaping of the PTSD paradigm.[78] But it was also a distinctively limited experience when compared to what occurred throughout most of Europe in 1939–45, where genocidal warfare, foreign occupations, forced resettlements and massive air operations against civilian targets introduced a variety of limitless violence and devastation. All of these different experiences of violence share things in common, hence we may speak of a culture of twentieth-century war trauma. The traces of this culture can be recognized across

---

[75] Cf. Chris R. Brewin, *Posttraumatic Stress Disorder: Malady or Myth?* (New Haven, CT: Yale University Press, 2003), Ch. 6 and 209–14.

[76] Laurence J. Kirmayer, Robert Lemelson, and Mark Barad, "Introduction: Inscribing Trauma in Culture, Brain, and Body," in *Understanding Trauma: Integrating Biological, Clinical, and Cultural Perspectives*, ed. by Laurence J. Kirmayer, Robert Lemelson, and Mark Barad (Cambridge: Cambridge University Press, 2007), 1–20.

[77] Rob Boddice, "The Cultural Brain as Historical Artifact," in *Culture, Mind and Brain: Emerging Concepts, Models, Applications*, ed. by Laurence J. Kirmayer et al. (Cambridge: Cambridge University Press, 2020), 369–76.

[78] For the perception of this experience by one of the leading protagonists of the PTSD paradigm, see Robert Jay Lifton, *Home from the War: Learning from Vietnam Veterans* (New York: Simon & Schuster, 1973).

national borders—and if it would be possible to conduct a comparative study of European dreams after World War II, I would expect to find a transnational culture of posttraumatic nightmares as well.[79] But it is just as important to pay attention to variations in traumatic experiences and their societal contexts during and after the war, which will partly explain the diverse national politics of memory and trauma within contemporary Europe.

[79] Cf. Peter Burke, "The Cultural History of Dreams," in idem, *Varieties of Cultural History* (Cambridge: Polity Press, 1997), 25–7; Kivimäki (2021b).

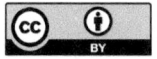

CHAPTER 5

Entangled Bystanders: Multidimensional Trauma of Ethnic Cleansing and Mass Violence in Eastern Galicia

Anna Wylegała

Introduction

The objective of the present chapter is to contribute to the discussion on individual and collective trauma by conceptualizing the multi-level trauma suffered by civilians during ethnic cleansing. Using the example of Eastern Galicia—a region that experienced ethnic cleansing on a massive scale during World War II, I will attempt to answer the following questions: what traumatizes those who witness mass and long-term ethnic violence (bystanders), what type of trauma it is, and what its long-term consequences are for the communities under study.

The level of ethnic violence in Eastern Galicia during World War II was unmatched. On the eve of World War II, Eastern Galicia was a multi-ethnic region that was part of the Second Polish Republic. It was primarily

A. Wylegała (✉)
Institute of Philosophy and Sociology, Polish Academy of Sciences,
Warszawa, Poland

© The Author(s) 2022
V. Kivimäki, P. Leese (eds.), *Trauma, Experience and Narrative in Europe after World War II*, Palgrave Studies in the History of Experience, https://doi.org/10.1007/978-3-030-84663-3_5

inhabited by Ukrainians, had a Jewish minority of approximately ten percent of the population, mainly in cities, and a strong Polish (politically privileged) minority, which, depending on the area, constituted about 25 percent of the population. In September 1939, Galicia was annexed by the Soviet Union (USSR). The almost two-year-long occupation was initiated with murders of Polish landowners and arrests of the members of Polish elites, but repression soon touched other population groups as well. It is estimated that Soviet authorities deported at least 350,000 Polish citizens (the highest estimates point to a million) to the Soviet interior and arrested at least 100,000 in the period 1939–1941.[1] Over 21,000 were killed in the so-called Katyń massacre, and at least 10,000 during the so-called prison massacres—the mass executions of political prisoners during the evacuation of Soviet prisoners at the beginning of the German-Soviet war in June 1941.[2]

During the German occupation, the Nazis killed at least 550,000 Jews, or 95 percent of the pre-war Jewish community, in Galicia and thus effectively committed a genocide of the Jewish population.[3] Galician Jews were murdered in extermination camps located in present-day Poland (mainly in Bełżec), but more than half of them were killed on the spot, in front of their neighbors.[4] The Holocaust in Galicia began immediately with the arrival of the Wehrmacht when a wave of pogroms swept through these lands, carried out by locals with the consent of German authorities.[5] During Operation Reinhardt—the major killing operation of the Holocaust in the General Government implemented in 1942–1943—Germans had the support of the Ukrainian auxiliary police, but they also employed ordinary civilians, Poles and Ukrainians, for a number of additional tasks.

Ethnic cleansing of the Polish population took place in Galicia almost concurrently with the Holocaust. It was carried out by Ukrainian

---

[1] Stanisław Ciesielski, Wojciech Materski and Andrzej Paczkowski, *Represje sowieckie wobec Polaków i obywateli polskich* (Warszawa: Ośrodek Karta, 2002); Keith Sword, *Deportation and Exile: Poles in the Soviet Union, 1939–48* (London: St. Martin's Press, 1994).

[2] Ksenya Kiebuzinski and Alexander Motyl, *The Great West Ukrainian Prison Massacre of 1941: A Sourcebook* (Amsterdam: Amsterdam University Press, 2017).

[3] Alexander Kruglov, "Jewish Losses in Ukraine, 1941–1944," in *The Shoah in Ukraine: History, Testimony, Memorialization*, ed. by Ray Brandon and Wendy Lower (Bloomington: Indiana University Press, 2008), 272–90.

[4] Patrick Desbois, *The Holocaust by Bullets: A Priest's Journey to Uncover the Truth behind the Murder of 1.5 Million Jews* (New York: Palgrave Macmillian, 2008).

[5] Kai Struve, *Deutsche Herrschaft, ukrainischer Nationalismus, antijüdische Gewalt: Der Sommer 1941 in der Westukraine* (Oldenbourg: De Gruyter, 2015).

nationalists, with the participation of Ukrainian locals: between 60,000 and 100,000 Poles died in Volhynia and Eastern Galicia in the period 1943–1946. Thousands of Ukrainian civilians were killed by Poles in acts of retaliation.[6] The majority of the remaining Polish population was resettled in Poland when the border between Poland and the USSR was redrawn at the end of World War II. However, the end of the war did not end the violence—the return of the Red Army to Galicia in the summer of 1944 set in motion the conflict between the Soviet authorities and the Ukrains'ka Povstans'ka Armiia (UPA) that would last for many years. This conflict resulted in the deportation of over 150,000 Ukrainians to the USSR and the death of thousands of Ukrainians accused of supporting partisans.[7]

The above brief summary of Galician history during World War II and its immediate aftermath shows that, over the course of the war, all major ethnic groups residing in the area were subjected to mass violence: both by the occupier and by their own neighbors. Moreover, they all witnessed violence inflicted on their neighbors—in some cases by the occupier, in others, by other neighbors. With the exception of Jews, members of all ethnic groups were also perpetrators of violence. People's positions in the social hierarchy of individual groups changed over time, but the violence continued. The present chapter focuses on the war experiences of civilian Poles and Ukrainians but excludes the Jewish experience for several reasons. First of all, Jews were subjects of a total annihilation that cannot be compared with even the most brutal mass violence committed towards their Polish and Ukrainian neighbors. Second, violence towards other ethnic groups appears in Jewish testimonies only occasionally. Most of the Jews who survived the Holocaust spent the crucial war years in hiding and thus were not direct witnesses to what was happening to the Poles and Ukrainians. After the war, in turn, they focused on the suffering of their own ethnic group, and not on the suffering of the others.

For methodological reasons, I would now like to make two essential statements of a methodological as well as an ontological nature. First,

---

[6] Grzegorz Motyka, *Od rzezi wołyńskiej do "Akcji Wisła": Konflikt polsko-ukraiński 1943–47* (Kraków: Wydawnictwo Literackie, 2011).

[7] For an overview of the underground activity, see Grzegorz Motyka, *Ukraińska partyzantka 1942–1960: działalność Organizacji Ukraińskich Nacjonalistów i Ukraińskiej Powstańczej Armii* (Warszawa: ISP PAN, Oficyna Wydawnicza Rytm, 2006); on the postwar deportations from Western Ukraine, see Tamara Vrons'ka, *Upokorennia strakhom: simeine zaruchnytstvo u karalnii praktytsi radianskoi vlady (1917–1953)* (Kyiv: Tempora, 2013).

despite focusing on the perspective of the witness, this chapter does not deny the fact that some Poles and Ukrainians also assumed the role of perpetrators—both during the Holocaust and during the Polish-Ukrainian conflict. Second, a bystander of the type of ethnic violence that took place in Eastern Galicia is not a person standing on the side-lines and uninvolved. Such a possibility is precluded by the very nature of this violence—happening so close to and frequently in front of local communities, often drawing them into a spiral of addictive violence. Michael Meng argued that in Central Europe it was impossible to remain outside of the Holocaust; not only Jews, but also their neighbors were constantly in the middle of the events—due to complicity, but also by means of the physical proximity of death.[8]

Polish researchers introduce special theoretical categories that allow for taking a new look at the bystander category—Elżbieta Janicka writes about participative witnesses (pl. *świadek uczestniczący*), Roma Sendyka about outsiders (pl. *postronny*).[9] Also Michael Rothberg's category of the implicated subject is very inspiring, defining some groups of bystanders as "implicated subjects [who] occupy positions aligned with power and privilege without being themselves direct agents of harm."[10] However, in this chapter I will claim that most of the regular bystanders to the Holocaust and other mass violence did not occupy positions of power. They were, rather, entangled witnesses, who might have benefited from the reality of the ethnic cleansing or not, but in fact were not given the choice of standing aside: they were thrown inside by the very fact of being born where they were. The notion of the "entangled bystander" describes the reality not only of the Holocaust, but also of other ethnic cleansings and outbreaks of mass violence against civilians by showing the fluidity of assigned

[8] Michael Meng, *Shattered Spaces: Encountering Jewish Ruins in Postwar Germany and Poland* (Cambridge, MA: Harvard University Press, 2011).

[9] Elżbieta Janicka, "Pamięć przyswojona: Koncepcja polskiego doświadczenia zagłady Żydów jako traumy zbiorowej w świetle rewizji kategorii świadka," *Studia Litteraria Historica* 3/4 (2014–2015), 148–224; Roma Sendyka, "Od świadków do postronnych: Kategoria bystanders i analiza 'podmiotów uwikłanych,'" in *Świadek: jak się staje, czym jest?*, ed. by Agnieszka Dauksza and Karolina Koprowska (Warszawa: Instytut Badań Literackich PAN, 2019), 61–82.

[10] Michael Rothberg, *Implicated Subject: Beyond Victims and Perpetrators* (Stanford, CA: Stanford University Press, 2019); see also Mary Fulbrook, "Bystanders: Catchall concept, alluring alibi or crucial clue," in *Probing the Limits of Categorization: The Bystander in Holocaust History*, ed. by Christin Morina and Krijn Thijs (New York: Berghahn Books, 2018), 15–35.

roles—from onlooker to perpetrator, from perpetrator to starer, from bystander to supporter, from supporter to victim. This chapter tells the story of people involved in shifting roles of mass violence and of how this violence traumatized them—from both the individual and the collective perspective.

I use three main groups of sources. The first group consists of memories and diaries created during and after the war, both published and archival materials, authored by Poles and Ukrainians. The second group includes oral history interviews from the Yahad-In Unum collection created by a French project documenting places of mass executions during the Holocaust in Central and Eastern Europe.[11] The third group of my sources contains over 150 interviews conducted within the project implemented in the Institute of Philosophy and Sociology of the Polish Academy of Sciences by my team and me during field studies in Eastern Galicia in 2017–2019 with people born in 1921–1939.

CIRCLES OF HELL: PROXIMITY OF VIOLENCE

To be a civilian in Eastern Galicia during World War II meant, above all, to be in constant proximity to death. It is an experience comparable to going increasingly deeper into a spiral of violence. Depending on the situation, the residents of Galicia watched various victims transported to death camps, beaten, humiliated, murdered in a number of ways, buried in mass graves; they smelled the stink of decaying bodies, they saw piles of corpses, they were forced to bury them, they looted in the ruins. Those who stood on the edge of the first circle only watched victims taken away or hurried into the unknown. In some cases, they knew that their neighbors were going to die, in others they only watched them disappear and learned about their fate much later.

At the beginning of 1940, during the first of the three deportations of Polish citizens to the USSR, entire village populations disappeared from Galicia. Dmytro Kup'iak, from the village of Jabłonówka (Yablunivka),[12] saw carriages riding towards the Polish colony at night and went with

---

[11] Website https://www.yahadinunum.org/, last accessed 6 June 2020.
[12] Throughout the text, I use pre-war Polish names in reference to the period 1939–1945, and Ukrainian names in reference to the postwar period. When a name is given for the first time, I provide the second name in brackets.

other villagers to take a look at empty Polish houses in the morning.[13] In Bóbrka (Bibrka), Yosif Patetskyi witnessed his neighbors being thrown out of their homes and loaded onto carts with their entire families.[14] In Barysz (Barysh), in September 1939, the whole village watched the Soviet interior-ministry troops Narodnyy Komissariat Vnutrennikh Del (NKVD) leading a Polish landowner from his hideout in a peasant hut and transporting him into the unknown (his name will subsequently appear on the so-called Katyń list of approximately 21,000 Polish officers and civilians murdered by the NKVD in 1940).[15]

The residents of Galicia were also watching the deportation of Jews in 1941 and 1942. In towns that had a railway station, they saw their neighbors being crammed into cattle cars that would take them to extermination camps. At a certain point, both victims and onlookers became aware of where these trains were going. In smaller localities, Poles and Ukrainians saw Jews being hurried down the streets to ghettos in neighboring towns, or concentrated in the middle of the village, waiting for the Germans to decide where to kill them. In July 1941, in Dobropole, Nataliia Kul'chytska (b. 1933) left her house one day only to see her Jewish neighbor being dragged out of his house with his whole family and being rushed to join a column of other Dobropole Jews taken to the neighboring village of Wiśniowczyk (Vyshnivchyk), where most of them would be murdered.[16] In Wiśniowczyk, Yustyna Deretska (b. 1926) watched Dobropole and Wiśniowczyk Jews, crammed onto the former land-estate yard: "They sat there with their books and they prayed all the time and we, the children, ran to see them."[17] Poles and Ukrainians stood by the gates of their houses and watched. Kids, village outcasts and dogs followed the column of people.

---

[13] Dmytro Kup'iak, *Spohady ne rozstrilianoho* (Toronto: self-published, 1991), 103.

[14] Interview with Yosif Patetskyi, b. 1927, conducted in Bibrka in 2019 by Marta Havryshko. If not stated otherwise, the interviews were conducted in Ukraine and in Ukrainian.

[15] Archiwum Wschodnie Ośrodka KARTA (Eastern Archive of the KARTA Center, hereafter AW OK), AW OK II/98, Wanda Działoszyńska, 2–3; Interview with the daughter of Świdrygiełło-Świderski, Teresa Somkowicz, b. 1927, conducted in Pwllheli (Great Britain) in 2019 by Anna Wylegała. Interview conducted in Polish.

[16] Interview with Nataliia Kul'chytska, b. 1933, conducted in Dobropole in 2019 by Anna Wylegała.

[17] Interview with Yustyna Deretska, b. 1926, conducted in Osivtsi in 2018 by Wiktoria Kudela-Świątek.

The people hurried into the unknown were beaten and humiliated. When a landowner, Władysław Świderski from Barysz, was taken to a car, NKVD officers forced his employees to spit on him and beat him.[18] The humiliation of Jews—individuals or groups—was common. A woman-interviewee (b. 1927) from Hrymailiv (Grzymałów), remembers an old Jew who was abused by the Germans by the city pump; in Osowce (Osivtsi), a young Jew was placed at the head of a column of Jews, with a bouquet of thistles in his hands, and ordered to sing.[19] A woman who lived in Dobryniów (Dobryniv) at that time mentions that the Germans ordered the Jews to form a circle and dance: "I even saw [my neighbors], our Laika and her daughters, and everyone who was there. You should write it down, because I was there and saw everything, when they told them to dance."[20]

Deportation and humiliation announced what was about to happen. The residents of Galicia, above all, saw their neighbors die. They witnessed the deaths of individual people: in 1939 an interviewee from a village near Rohatyn watched a Polish landowner being forced to dig his own grave and then being shot by an NKVD officer.[21] Jerzy Klementowski, from the village of Psary (Pryozerne), was the son of a farm worker, first employed on the estate of Count Rey, and then on the same estate when it was administered by the Germans. The German administrator was strict and organized public tortures of his Polish and Ukrainian workers in the manor yard for minor offenses. As a child, Klementowski watched tortured people through cracks in the wall, and then, with his father, took away the bodies and cleaned the yard of blood.[22] A woman born in 1924 in Jaworów (Yavoriv) saw the Germans pulling out a Jewish boy her age from a house across the street and killing him on the spot, immediately after the German army had entered.[23]

---

[18] Interview with Anastasiia Ivantsiv, b. 1923, conducted in Barysh in 2019 by Marta Havryshko.

[19] United States Holocaust Memorial Museum (hereafter USHMM), RG-50.589*0244, Yahad-In Unum interview; Interview with Teodora Kanak, conducted in Osivtsi in 2019 by Marta Havryshko.

[20] Interview with a woman, b 1921, conducted in Stratyn in 2018 by Marta Havryshko. Some interviewees asked for anonymity and they are thus identified only by their gender and year of birth.

[21] Interview with a man, b. 1933, conducted in Rohatyn in 2017 by Anna Chebotarova.

[22] AW OK II/1323/2K Klementowski Jerzy, *Moje wspomnienia z lat dziecinnych z Sokołowa i Psar (1935–1943)*, 9.

[23] USHMM, RG-50.589*0193, Yahad-In Unum interview.

However, the landscape of mass war violence was dominated by killings of the Jewish population during Operation Reinhardt. Jews were shot with machine guns and buried in mass graves at a Jewish cemetery, in a nearby forest or in a field. The shootings were usually witnessed by children. Evheniia Zalutska, from Podhajce (Pidhaitis), born in 1929, followed a column of harried Jews, climbed a tree growing next to the mass grave dug in the middle of a field, and observed the murder of several hundred people.[24] Another interviewee (b. 1926) from Radłowice (Ralivka), observed the execution of local Jews from a distance, as he claims; however, he was able to determine who did the shooting, how people guarded the victims and how the bodies were laid in the dug ditches.[25] Even the younger children who were not allowed to run freely by themselves were not spared the view. Lubov Shelvakh was five years old when her mother sat her on a wall so that she could better see the murder of Jews in the cemetery in Podhajce. When people heard that the Jews were being killed, they left whatever they were doing, and rushed to the scene.[26] Another five-year-old, who spent the war in Skałat, observed the local "action" from the window; she saw Jews being murdered right on the street. What she remembered most was a young Jewish woman who threw her child out of the window and then jumped out herself.[27] In Galicia, as in other Eastern European countries, the Holocaust was a communal genocide (for the case of Slovakia, see Hana Kubátová's chapter in this volume); it was impossible to live where it happened and not have had direct contact with death.[28]

Violence against representatives of other groups was more intimate and happened quietly, but it was still noticeable. The residents of Galicia, even if they did not witness the very act of murder, saw dead bodies throughout the entire war. In June 1941, bodies of Soviet prisoners brutally murdered by the retreating NKVD units were exposed to public view. Seventeen

---

[24] Interview with Evheniia Zalutska, b. 1929, conducted in 2018 in Pidhaitsi by Marta Havryshko.

[25] USHMM, RG-50.589*0206, Yahad-In Unum Interview.

[26] Interview with Lubov Shel'vakh, b. 1938, conducted in Pidhaitsi in 2018 by Anna Wylegała.

[27] Interview with a woman, b. 1938, conducted in Hlibiv in 2019 by Marta Havryshko.

[28] Omer Bartov, "Communal genocide: Personal accounts of the destruction of Buczacz, Eastern Galicia, 1941–1944," in *Shatterzone of Empires: Coexistence and Violence in the German, Habsburg, Russian, and Ottoman Borderlands*, ed. by Omer Bartov and Eric D. Weitz (Bloomington: Indiana University Press, 2013), 399–420.

people were killed in Bóbrka. When we ask Yosif Mykytiv (b. 1923) about it, he describes how he and other boys ran to the courtyard of the local prison to see the corpses with their own eyes; the bodies lay naked, deformed, dreadful, and Mykytiv ran away screaming.[29] The parents of Nataliia Zaremba, only 11 years old in 1941, took her to a prison cellar covered with blood; when I asked her why her parents would take her to this horrific place, she answered: "All kids were taken there so that they knew what the Soviets had done to our people."[30] After the actions, dead bodies of Jews were commonly encountered. Józef Lesław Drecki, from Żółkiew (Zhovkva), remembers that when he went to work in December 1941, after the first deportation from the Żółkiew ghetto, he saw the body of Mrs. Taubowa, a Jewish woman he had worked for before the war, lying by a fence.[31]

Following the attacks of Ukrainian nationalists, people ran to see the bodies of Polish victims. In Hlebów (Hlibiv), several dozen people died overnight. An interviewee born in 1938 remembers the sight of the bodies of a Polish family murdered nearby: "I still remember us running there, little kids, in the morning, running to see them lying there, the father in the middle, and his little son by his side."[32] In Kurzany (Kuriany), Poles were killed individually, one family at a time. Mariia Koval'ska (b. 1930) remembers going to school one morning and almost tripping over the body of her dead neighbor, lying on the road completely naked.[33] The next morning, her neighbor and peer, Anna Khomiak, looked with a crowd of onlookers at the charred bodies of their neighbors, piled on the threshold of their own house. She remembers that the murdered young girl was naked from the waist up.[34] After 1945, there were bodies of other victims of Ukrainian partisans on the streets—for example, Russian female-teachers or chairmen of kolkhozes—and bodies of partisans who had been caught by the Soviet authorities and displayed for the public to see. In

[29] Interview with Yosif Mykytiv, b. 1923, conducted in Bibrka in 2019 by Marta Havryshko.

[30] Interview with Nataliia Zaremba, b. 1930, conducted in Lany in 2019 by Anna Wylegała.

[31] AW OK II/1272/2K Józef Lesław Drecki, 21.

[32] Interview with a woman, b. 1938, conducted in Hlibiv in 2019 by Marta Havryshko.

[33] Interview with Mariia Koval'ska, b. 1930, conducted in Kuriany in 2019 by Marta Havryshko.

[34] Interview with Anna Khomiak, b. 1930, conducted in Kuriany in 2019 by Anna Wylegała.

Hlibiv, one morning, on their way to school, children found the bodies of their teachers massacred, lying right on the street.[35]

Those who did not see bodies saw fresh graves. In Koropiec (Koropets), local Jews were murdered and buried in a deep ravine. After the shooting, Polish and Ukrainian children ran to see the newly dug graves.[36] A Pole from Bóbrka, eight-years-old in 1942, sneaked out without her parents' knowledge to the village of Wołowe (Volove), a few kilometers from town, where local Jews had just died. In her memory, the earth lying on her Jewish neighbors still moves and waves.[37]

Those who did not see the graves, smelled them. An interviewee born in 1934 remembers that when the last prisoners of the Jewish labor camp located near her hometown of Kamionki (Kam'ianky) were shot, the locals could smell the stench of bodies decaying in mass graves for a long time.[38] In Bogdanówka (Bohdanivka), bodies of murdered Jews had been burned and an awful odor of burned human bodies hovered over the village.[39] There were no funerals for Jews, and the victims of the assassinations that took place at the end of the war were buried in secret. However, almost 150 Poles, mainly women and children, murdered in Barysz in the winter of 1945 by Ukrainian nationalists (*Banderivtsi*), were openly buried in a cemetery. Ukrainians did not attend the funeral, but the Polish survivors did.[40] Entire communities participated in the public funerals of the victims of the Soviet prison massacres of 1941. Hundreds of mourners, adults as well as children, gathered at the cemeteries in Żółkiew, Bóbrka, Złoczów and in other Galician towns.

Everyone was close to violence, but some were much too close. Patrick Desbois, creator of the Yahad-In Unum archive, distinguishes three categories of witnesses to the Holocaust: indirect—those who only saw Jews led to their deaths; direct—those who saw the executions; and those requisitioned civilians who were forced by the Germans to help: to dig graves, carry bodies, sort clothes and so on. Desbois lists over 20 tasks performed

---

[35] Interview with Ol'ha Gerus, b. 1930 conducted in Hlibiv in 2019 by Anna Wylegała; interview with Teodosiia Diakiv, b. 1933, conducted in Hlibiv in 2019 by Marta Havryshko.

[36] Dmytro Boikiv, *Perezhyte osobysto abo Mitla* (Lviv: Kameniar, 2012).

[37] Interview with Helena Mazurs'ka, b. 1934, conducted in Bibrka in 2019 by Anna Wylegała.

[38] USHMM, RG-50.589*0219, Yahad-In Unum Interview.

[39] USHMM, RG-50.589*0224, Yahad-In Unum Interview.

[40] Interview with Władysław Skiba, b. 1932, conducted in 2020 in Kulin (Poland) by Anna Wylegała.

by locals by order of the Germans—from preparing food for torturers to pressing the bodies into graves.[41] Requisitioned civilians became the most entangled bystanders, involved not only by the very fact of seeing, smelling or hearing, but also by their—more or less willing—participation. Even before the murder, it had to be clarified as to who had to be killed. After the Poles in Barysz were killed, UPA moved to the neighboring village, where, unlike the situation in Barysz, Polish houses were widely scattered. To find the people they wanted to murder, they brought with them a Ukrainian resident of Barysz who had relatives in the village. His brother's wife (b. 1931) recalls the events in the following way:

> *Then they went into the valley, to the village, and took my husband's brother with them. It was so unfair, so terribly unfair! They took him to show the houses where Poles lived. There was his uncle, and his uncle's Ukrainian wife, and a Ukrainian daughter, they had a little girl, her name was Olya. [...] [Them too...?] Yes. [Even the Ukrainians?] Yes. [Didn't they know who was Ukrainian?] I don't know... They gathered them all in the shed and...*[42]

The Poles killed in Barysz had to be buried. There were almost 150 bodies, so the village council ordered kolkhoz workers employed as coachmen, to bury them. Thus, the bodies were transported by, for example, the 15-year-old brother of Mariia Kliotsko.[43] In Kurzany, Hanna Boiko (b. 1926) remembers that her father buried a Polish family murdered in the vicinity of their home. The victims were buried in their own yard, because the Catholic cemetery was far away and times were uncertain.[44] Civilians were employed to bury Jewish victims on a mass scale. Antoni Dereniowski from Narajów (Naraiiv) transported corpses from the ghetto to the Jewish cemetery and buried them in mass graves.[45] In Bóbrka, Ukrainian police led Jews to the place of murder, but they picked up men from randomly chosen houses and ordered them to dig huge ditches with shovels in the local brickyard. Yosif Patetskyi's father was absent, so they picked up his

---

[41] Patrick Desbois, "The Witnesses of Ukraine or Evidence from the Ground: The Research of Yahad-In Unum," in *The Holocaust in Ukraine: New Sources and Perspectives – Conference Presentations* (Washington: Center for Advanced Holocaust Studies, 2013), 91–100.

[42] Interview with a woman, b. 1931, conducted in Barysh in 2019 by Marta Havryshko.

[43] Interview with Mariia Kliotsko, b. 1929, conducted in Barysh in 2019 by Marta Havryshko.

[44] Interview with Hanna Boiko.

[45] AW OK II/1267/2K Antoni Dereniowski, Narajów.

teenage son instead. When the ditches were ready, the policemen chased the diggers away, murdered the Jews, and ordered people to fill in the ditches.[46] In Kamionki, the Germans surrounded the Jewish labor camp during liquidation in order to prevent prisoners from escaping, then they killed the prisoners and forced local Ukrainians to take care of the bodies. A man living nearby (b. 1928) remembers that his neighbors were forced to lay bodies on large grates and then set them on fire.[47]

At the Heart of Darkness: Towards Psychological Trauma

The consequences of the proximity of death can be traced at individual and group levels. The first reaction, especially among children, was often dread, shock and paralysis of sorts. Evheniia Sadivs'ka from Koropets (b. 1938) stood by the family's gate when local Jews were herded onto the street towards death. She was mesmerized and could not turn her gaze away, although, as she admits years later, it was a terrible sight. Her father forcefully pulled her away from the fence and took her home.[48] Anastasiia Ivantsiv from Barysh was 22 years old and had three children when local Poles were murdered in 1945. When the *Banderivtsi* raided the village, she locked herself up at home and shouted to her husband that it was the end of the world because she was being blinded by the red glow of burning houses. The following day, she was still afraid to go outside and barricaded herself at home.[49]

Many ran away and sought to distance themselves from what was happening. Yosif Mykytiv from Bóbrka (b. 1923) ran with other boys to see the massacred bodies of Soviet prisoners, but then ran away in horror. He could still see the Jews being led to the prison yard, but he would not watch them being ripped apart by an angry mob. When he came home, his mother yelled at him to stay away from everything, because it might end up badly for him.[50] The parents of Nataliia Havryshkevych from Bibrka (b. 1932) were to go to the funeral of Soviet victims in July 1941, attended

[46] Interview with Yosif Patets'kyi.

[47] USHMM, RG-50.589*0226, Yahad-In Unum.

[48] Interview with Evheniia Sadivs'ka, b. 1938, conducted in 2019 in Koropets by Anna Wylegała.

[49] Interview with Anastasiia Ivantsiv.

[50] Interview with Yosif Mykytiv.

by the entire town, but she herself insisted on staying home: "Of course I didn't go. As soon as I saw these people, I ran home and stayed there. It was awful."[51] Hanna Boiko from Kuriany (b. 1926), who was related to a Polish family murdered in the vicinity, recalls: "She was my aunt, I came, looked and ran home. I was so scared! After all, I used to visit her at home many times, and then I didn't ever go again, I was afraid to go there."[52]

For those who were more sensitive or who were forced to be closer to death than they wanted, the situation became unbearable at some point. While some children who observed mass executions were unmoved, others could not forget what they had seen. Lubov Shelvakh (b. 1938) watched from the cemetery wall the murder of the Podhajce Jews. However, when she saw children being thrown alive into a mass grave, she started screaming, lost consciousness, and had to be taken home by her mother. The girl would wake up at night and wet the bed for many weeks after this event. Her mother wanted to take her to see a doctor but that was not possible during the war.[53] Zygmunt Kubas from Bóbrka was 13 years old during the liquidation of the local ghetto. He wrote in his diary in the evening after the action: "I had a headache all day, I don't know if it's because of the shooting or because I had seen a lot of corpses and it affected me. I hadn't studied all day and couldn't even write in my diary."[54]

Not only children were deeply affected. Mariia Zamrozevych (b. 1927) from Kuriany recalls that when her father returned home from Brzeżany (Berezhany), where he witnessed the murder of local Jews, "he did not know what to do with himself."[55] He kept telling his family about what he saw. The father of another interviewee from the village of Radłowice (Ralivka), who was forced to assist in the murder of local Jews, experienced a nervous breakdown, stayed in bed for a long time and did not speak to anyone.[56] A resident of Chmieliska, who was forced by the Ukrainian police to bury about 50 local Jews alive during a wave of

[51] Interview with Nataliia Havryshkevych, b. 1932, conducted in Bibrka in 2019 by Anna Wylegała.
[52] Interview with Hanna Boiko.
[53] Interview with Lubov Shel'vakh.
[54] AW OK II/1347/2K, Zbigniew Kubas, *Dzienniczek od dnia 1 października 1942 r. do dnia 10 maja 1944 r.*
[55] Interview with Mariia Zamrozevych, b. 1927, conducted in Kuriany in 2019 by Marta Havryshko.
[56] USHMM, RG-50.589*0207, Yahad-In Unum interview.

anti-Jewish pogroms that swept through Galicia in July 1941, described
his experience in the following way:

> We all had trembling hands, and older men were as pale as ghosts. When we ran
> half a kilometer away from the crime scene, everyone made the sign of the cross
> but no one said a thing; we kept on running to get home as soon as possible. My
> neighbor had a heart attack and died the next day. He had participated in
> filling in the ditches with sand and his experiences caused his sudden death.[57]

While witnessing death became increasingly common with time, people
did not get used to the fear of one's own death and the death of one's
family. The situation of the residents of Galicia was unique because of a
constant change of roles—from witness to victim, from victim to perpetrator, and then back. At any time, Poles and Ukrainians could expect to lose
their shaky status as witnesses and (once more) become victims. In Delatyn
(Deliatyn),

> [...] at the beginning of July 1943 [t]hey dug out fresh pits at the Jewish cem-
> etery. People are nervous because there are no Jews left in the town, unless they
> catch someone who is in hiding. There are rumors that the pits are meant for
> beggars, old people and the weak.[58]

It also happened that being a victim did not exclude being a perpetrator
at the same time: as Marta Kurkowska-Budzan shows in her chapter in this
book on the executioners from the Polish underground, in occupied
Poland victims at times stood in the positions of victimizers, without losing their initial status of victims. In Galicia, every subsequent occupation
was making people anxiously look out for changes in the extermination
policy of the occupier. Who would be taken this time? Whom would they
kill? During the German occupation, Poles and Ukrainians became convinced that when the Germans were done with the Jews, they would turn
to the Slavs. Many interviewees cite Jews who were being led to die as
saying: "We are the leaven, you'll be the dough" (*Namy rozchyniat,' a
vamy zamisiat'*)—or other variants of the concept. Regardless of what the
Jews actually said in the final moments of their lives, these stories show the
scale of the fear of those times that can only be articulated in

---

[57] AW OK II/1223/2K.

[58] Vasyl' Yashan, *Pid brunatnym chobotom: Nimetska okupatsiia Stanyslavivshchyny v Druhii
svitivii viini, 1941–1944* (Toronto: New Pathway Publishers, 1989), 235.

religious-magical tropes or proverbs.[59] Individuals were also afraid of being mistaken for Jews. A woman-interviewee born in 1938, with olive skin and dark-hair, when stopped on the street by the Germans, had to explain that she was Ukrainian.[60]

In some cases, fear would become real and understandable, while in others, it was general, not specific but still intense. A Ukrainian woman from Koropets (b. 1935), who was a young child during the war, remembers this general fear. When talking about the murder of local Jews, she said: "We were scared, we were all so scared." When asked what they were so afraid of since they were Ukrainians, she hesitated before replying: "We were simply afraid. Well, we were not Jews, but it was so monstrous, what they did to people, it was so scary."[61] The situation did not improve when the Germans left and the Soviets returned. A woman-interviewee from Koropets (b. 1927), from a mixed family, recalls:

> *We were scared of the KGB officers, and of those from the forest, because there were Polish, Russian and Ukrainian guerrillas. [...] Everyone was scared, people were scared of one another. And they were even more scared in mixed families, because one group would beat up another and then those beaten would retaliate.*[62]

In some cases, fears would become more real. Anna Khomiak from Kuriany (b. 1930) says:

> *I remember them killing Poles, burning them, and how scared we were, how me and my mom were scared. We would run away to sleep in someone else's field, three houses away, so that they wouldn't... Because my mom was Polish, so that they would not kill us. [...] They will definitely kill us tonight, we thought. They'll set us on fire tonight...*[63]

Was an experience of the residents of Galicia during the war simply a series of unpleasant experiences, initially shocking and then something

---

[59] For analysis of the wartime folk tales and beliefs, see Olga Belova, "Legendy o voinie: arkhetipy v sovremmenykh folklornykh narrativakh," in *Problemy istorii Rosii*, 10, ed. by Aleksandr Redin (Ekaterinburg: NPMP "Volot," 2013), 227–35.

[60] Interview with a woman, b. 1938, conducted in Hlibiv in 2019 by Marta Havryshko.

[61] Interview with Eva Kulykovs'ka, b. 1935, conducted in Koropets in 2019 by Anna Wylegała.

[62] Interview with Olena Popiv, b. 1927, conducted in Koropets in 2019 by Anna Wylegała.

[63] Interview with Anna Khomiak.

everyone got used to, or was it an individual psychological trauma? Although there are many definitions of trauma at the individual level, most researchers agree that trauma is sudden and unexpected; it exceeds the limits of individual mental strength, and destroys the existing system of values, references and a sense of security. It is also an overwhelming experience for an individual.[64] It is difficult to diagnose the mental state of the wartime residents of Galicia using the sources from the war and even the contemporary interviews. All we have are rather subjective descriptions of its external symptoms observed in other people or a subjective assessment of one's own experiences, often carried out after many years.

In the USSR, for obvious reasons, there was no research conducted after the war on the impact of the brutality of war on civilians. However, in Poland, in the period of 1945–1947, over 6000 surveys were carried out among Polish youth, examining their mental state in relation to the war.[65] One cannot simply extrapolate the results of these studies to Galicia; however, attention should be paid to them for a number of reasons. First, the research covered a considerable number of young people displaced from the Eastern Broderlands, that means also from Eastern Galicia. Second, if the postwar mental state of Polish youth in general (most of whom experienced only the German occupation) was different from the mental state of Poles displaced from the Borderlands, then the group under study was likely to be in worse condition due to the multitude of occupational regimes subjected to and the experience of the Polish-Ukrainian conflict.

Seventy-five percent of respondents believed that they and their families suffered from a number of mental disorders—mostly their family members, but also about 20 percent of the young people themselves. The most common problems were depressive states, psychosomatic disorders (insomnia, difficulty concentrating, nervous tics), anxiety and neurotic

[64] Neil J. Smelser, "Psychological Trauma and Cultural Trauma," in Jeffrey C. Alexander, Piotr Sztompka, Ron Eyerman, Neil Smelser and Bernhard Giesen, *Cultural Trauma and Collective* Identity (Berkeley: University of California Press, 2004), 44; Robert Prince, "Historical Trauma: Psychohistorical Reflections on the Holocaust," in *Children Surviving Persecution: An International Study of Trauma and Healing*, ed. by Judith S. Kestenberg and Charlotte Kahn (Westport, CT: Praeger, 1998), 43–55.

[65] On this study, see Helena Radomska-Strzemecka, "Wpływ wojny na stosunek młodzieży do rodziny," *Przegląd Socjologiczny* 12 (1958).

states.[66] Although the majority of the issues described were rooted in direct experiences of death or mutilation of family members, a surprisingly large number of problems were related to situations when the respondents had only witnessed violence that did not affect their immediate family. Other studies show that Poles continued to dream about the war after it had ended—not only people who had been in concentration camps, had lost loved ones, had participated in combat operations—but also those who were "just" witnesses. Of the 1005 dreams collected just after the war, as many as 28.5 percent were associated with war violence.[67] Other studies carried out in Poland immediately after the war show that alcoholism had become a widespread phenomenon, also among children and young people: 27.9 percent of children aged between 7 and 15 regularly drank alcohol.[68] In other words, those who did not dream (or who dreamt too much) indulged in drinking to forget. According to Marcin Zaremba, author of one of the most insightful diagnoses of Polish society in the first postwar years, people drank vodka mainly because of its therapeutic value: "It was a tried and tested means of consolation in the moments of despair and defeat. [It] healed fear."[69]

The interviews being conducted today provide insight into the persistence of the trauma of witnessing mass violence and the sense of constant threat. The interviewees still lower their voices when talking about the Polish and Ukrainian victims of Ukrainian nationalists. They ask to go off the record when they reveal names; they stop in mid-sentence and make meaningful gestures. They cry, their voices tremble, they are unable to continue with the story when talking about the murders of Jews, especially if they saw death from up close. In some cases, they end the interview, claiming that they are unable to talk about the events that are interesting to the researcher. In some cases, after the first meeting, the family of an interviewee calls to cancel the next scheduled meeting because the interviewee had not slept all night and his/her heart ached from remembering the corpses. All of the above suggests that the war mentally wounded many residents of Eastern Galicia and does so still today.

---

[66] Biblioteka Jagiellońska (Jagiellonian Library, hereafter BJ), Przyb. 72/89, Helena Radomska Strzelecka, *Charakterystyka młodzieży okupacyjnej*, 53–4, 63, 65.

[67] Stefan Baley, "Psychiczne wpływy drugiej wojny światowej," *Psychologia wychowawcza* 1–2 (1948), 13.

[68] Marcin Zaremeba, *Wielka trwoga: Ludowa reakcja na kryzys* (Kraków: Wydawnictwo Znak, Instytut Studiów Politycznych PAN, 2012), 116.

[69] Zaremba (2012), 118.

LOSS AND DECAY: TOWARDS COLLECTIVE (COMMUNAL) TRAUMA

The witnesses of mass violence also experience less obvious traumas. One way to conceptualize trauma, although not from the psychological point of view, is to treat it as a trauma of loss. The residents of Galicia lose something with each disappearing or murdered human being. This process can be perceived on the individual level or from the perspective of an entire community. The most basic level of a trauma of losing is the loss of people who are important for the individual or the community. This was most painfully felt in many mixed rural communities existing before 1945, where marriages between Poles and Ukrainians were common, and the division into Polish and Ukrainian families was purely formal even up until the early 1930s.[70]

Inhabitants in Polish villages in Galicia, unlike in the neighboring Volhynia, were rarely slaughtered in entirety, but most probably there were no villages where no Poles were murdered. Those who did not die would have to leave—and, hence, they would still disappear from the community. In Hlibiv, where several dozen local Poles were killed during the war, out of several hundred, Ol'ha Gerus (b. 1930) testifies with hesitation: "It was so bad when they beat up those Poles. There were many mixed families. They left, and one had no family anymore."[71] Another interviewee from Rohatyn (b. 1933) refers directly to her experience: "Our entire family is gone. My mother's sister left [for Poland after the war] with her husband, and Stach, and Władzio, and Maniuśka, and the youngest, four children."[72]

The most severe loss is the loss of one's family, but residents also mourn their neighbors and friends. Stefania Shkvaryliak from Koropets (b. 1930) remembers her childhood best friend and neighbor, a Polish girl named Helka. After Helka left with her whole family after the war, Stefania did not make any new friends for a long time, and she corresponded with

---

[70] For more about the national relations in Galicia, see Olga Linkiewicz, *Lokalność i nacjonalizm: Społeczności wiejskie w Galicji Wschodniej w dwudziestoleciu międzywojennym* (Kraków: Universitas, 2018).

[71] Interview with Ol'ha Gerus.

[72] Interview with a woman, b. 1933, conducted in Rohatyn in 2017 by Wiktoria Kudela-Świątek.

Helka for many years.[73] The best friend of a Ukrainian woman (b. 1927) from the village of Usznia (Ushnia) was her Jewish neighbor; they went to school together, grazed cows together and grew up together. Like almost all Jews in Usznia, Tonia was murdered in the summer of 1942—probably with the participation of her Ukrainian neighbors.[74] Her Ukrainian friend has been crying over Tonia ever since. Teodora Kanak from Osivtsi (b. 1927) remembers that her father refused to hide their Jewish neighbor, but afterwards he cried and searched for the corpse in the plundered Jewish houses. We may only guess that while he did not find enough strength in himself to risk his own family and help his neighbor, he regretted it and felt he had failed the Jew, breaking long-lasting rules of neighborly loyalty.[75] One of the most shocking testimonies regarding the mourning of murdered neighbors is the conversation of two Ukrainian women from Kuriany, recalling the murder of their Polish neighbors:

It was summer... Yes, it was summer, what a summer that was. I still remember that Czesiek was at my place, they were at our place. After all, they were our friends, we sang songs until the evening, the girls were so cool... They were at our place on that day... What despair it was afterward! *We sang, we sat outside and sang. And they were murdered at night. In the morning...* My husband's father, he lived close to them, he dug a pit, put everyone inside, buried them, and that was it.[76]

Their memories show the uncertainty of life and death during the war: in the evening, your neighbor sits in your courtyard and sings songs, in the morning you go and see his dead body—and "that is it." Loss also takes place at a group level when communities lose members who had particular social or economic roles. In many communities, representatives of specific ethnic groups had dominated certain professions before the war. When Poles or Jews were killed, there was immediately a shortage of doctors, teachers, traders and shoemakers; the absence of doctors (and veterinarians) was perhaps the most severe outcome. At some point, the Germans lifted the ban on the treatment of Aryan patients by Jews because, after the

[73] Interview with Stefaniia Shkvaryliak, b. 1930, conducted in Koropets in 2019 by Anna Wylegała.
[74] USC Shoah Foundation, Visual History Archive, interview with Noyach Auerbach, no. 11568.
[75] Interview with Teodora Kanak.
[76] Interviews with Hanna Boiko and Mariia Kovals'ka.

deportation of most of the Polish intelligentsia to Siberia in 1939–1941, there was no one left who could treat patients. Baruch Milch, a Jewish doctor who was hiding in the vicinity of Tłuste (Tovste) throughout the war, recalled that as soon as he came out of hiding after the liberation, he was flooded with requests for medical help.[77] Vira Holinach (b. 1934), who lived in a village near Tovste after the war, remembers that her mother almost lost her injured leg because her family was unable to find a doctor to take care of the wound.[78]

There was a shortage of teachers after the war, which is not surprising since the Soviets predominantly targeted Polish and Ukrainian intelligentsia, and the Polish teachers who survived left Galicia as soon as possible when the Soviets returned. An interviewee from Rohatyn testifies that there were no "real" teachers after the war because they were killed by "one or the other."[79]

However, ethnic and political cleansing did not affect just the intelligentsia. In Galicia, during and immediately after the war, there was a shortage of traders, shopkeepers and craftsmen. In pre-war Stratyń, there was a bakery run by a Jew. When he was murdered by the Germans, the bakery remained closed, and it was never reopened. In Szczerzec (Shchyrets), the majority of Jewish-owned stores stood empty for several years.[80] Shortly after the war, Galician towns and villages were ghost-towns. Many of them irretrievably lost their town status and underwent secondary agrarianization. This was the case for many towns mentioned in this chapter—the populations of Koropets, from which Poles and Jews had disappeared, or Barysh, where a number of Poles had been murdered and the rest had left, decreased by more than half. Felsztyn, a small town before the war (the village of Skelivka in Lviv region after the war), was bitterly described in 1946 by a Ukrainian diarist as "once a town, today empty."[81]

[77] Baruch Milch, *Testament* (Warszawa: Ośrodek KARTA, 2001).

[78] Interview with Vira Holinach, b. 1934, conducted in Tovste in 2018 by Nataliia Otrishchenko.

[79] Interview with a man, b. 1922, conducted in Rohatyn in 2017 by Anna Chebotarova. On the shortage of staff in education, see Tamara Halaichak, ed., *Kul'turne zhyttia v Ukraini: Zakhidni zemli – Dokumenty i materialy*, Vol. I: 1939–53 (Kyiv: Naukova Dumka, 1995), 52–3.

[80] Interview with a woman, b. 1923, conducted in Stratyn in 2017 by Marta Havryshko; USHMM, RG-50.589*0173, Yahad-In Unum interview.

[81] Lev-Petro Savchyns'kyi, *Spohady* (Lviv: Krai, 2007), 103.

The residents of Galicia lost much more than significant people and their hometowns in the condition they had known them before the war. As the war went on, they lost their sense of security—they were waiting for the next occupier, a militia or a group of people aiming to destroy the ethnic or religious group they belonged to. They stopped trusting each other because it might turn out, at any time, that a neighbor wanted to take their life, or another neighbor was collaborating with the occupier and could show the latter who to arrest and kill. They lost what Piotr Sztompka calls a moral bond, understood as a special type of social bond that consists of loyalty, trust and solidarity.[82] Ol'ha Gerus from Hlibiv (b. 1930) mentions her father's cousin—a Pole who regularly eavesdropped on their conversations to find out which Poles the local *Banderivtsi* were planning to kill this time.[83]

The fact that a vast majority of acts of mass violence taking place in Galicia happened outside the state apparatus of violence had an extremely destructive effect on the integrity of local communities, a phenomenon that Natalia Aleksiun describes as "intimate violence."[84] The Germans were planning and controlling the Holocaust, but they engaged the Ukrainian police to perform auxiliary tasks that might involve shooting. And the pogroms that swept through Galicia in the summer of 1941 were the work of the neighbors of Jews: Ukrainians and Poles. The case of purges of Poles and retaliatory actions against Ukrainians was similar; in some cases, they were carried out by locally unknown guerrilla units, but much more often by locals, the victims' neighbors.

As a result, social order, understood as a system of norms and values that regulates social coexistence, also disappeared from Galicia. The more and less important norms became unstable. Consent of and growing indifference to violence emerged. More and more children and teenagers became perpetrators of atrocities. They not only witnessed executions, but also contributed to the deaths of their neighbors. Józef Anczarski, a Catholic priest who spent the war at the parish in Dobropole, describes in his diary how in October 1942 rural teenagers tortured and then murdered in front of the entire community an old Jewish woman who came to

---

[82] Piotr Sztompka, "Kulturowe imponderabilia szybkich zmian społecznych: zaufanie, lojalność, solidarność," in *Imponderabilia wielkiej zmiany: Mentalność, wartości i więzi społeczne czasów transformacji*, ed. by Piotr Sztompka (Warszawa: WN PWN, 1999), 265–82.

[83] Interview with Ol'ha Gerus.

[84] Natalia Aleksiun, "Intimate Violence: Jewish Testimonies on Victims and Perpetrators in Eastern Galicia," *Holocaust Studies: A Journal of Culture and History*, 23:1–2 (2016), 17–33.

the village.[85] Teenage Ukrainian boys participated in the murder of Polish residents of the village of Korościatyn (Korostiatyn), an act carried out in February 1944: Poles who survived the slaughter claimed that while the men murdered the inhabitants of one household after another, the boys robbed the victims and set fire to their houses.[86]

The act of watching monstrous public murders made further killings easier to commit and to watch.[87] Many researchers argue that the crimes committed by the UPA on Poles in Galicia and Volhynia happened because the perpetrators had had previous training with the Ukrainian police used by the Germans during the Holocaust.[88] The sources clearly provide an image of a society in a state of anomie, morally and socially instable, in economic chaos, while children's games of those times show how *á rebours* was the world of post-violent Galicia. Galician children—Polish, Ukrainian, and sometimes even Jewish, did not play "policemen" or "school." They played "round-ups," "shooting Jews" and "running away from Germans and Russians." The murdered "Jews," played by sparrows or mice, were buried in mass graves behind barns.[89]

All of the above, the loss of loved ones and neighbors, the loss of a sense of security, the collapse of a stable social structure, anomie and moral chaos, goes far beyond the definition of psychological trauma and should be defined rather as a kind of collective or communal trauma affecting not the individual but the entire community. According to Kai Erikson, collective trauma is "a blow to the basic tissues of social life that damages the bonds attaching people together and impairs the prevailing sense of

---

[85] AW OK II/1224/2K, ks. Józef Anczarski, *Kronikarskie zapisy z lat cierpień, grozy, zbrodni i ludobójstwa narodu, 1939–1946*, 215.

[86] Jan Zaleski, *Kronika życia*, ed. by Tadeusz Isakowicz-Zaleski (Kraków: Małe Wydawnictwo, 2010), 48–9; Motyka (2006), 383.

[87] This can be described as the normalization of violence. See e.g., Jared McBride, "Peasants into Perpetrators: The OUN–UPA and the Ethnic Cleansing of Volhynia, 1943–1944," *Slavic Review*, 75:3 (2016), 630–54.

[88] Cf. Grzegorz Rossoliński-Liebe, *Stepan Bandera: the life and afterlife of a Ukrainian nationalist: fascism, genocide, and cult* (Stuttgart: ibid. Verlag, 2014). Jan T. Gross rightly noticed that each act of plunder during the war made the next one easier: it appears that this statement can refer to any violence, see Jan T. Gross, "Social Consequences of War: Preliminaries to the Study of Imposition of Communist Regimes in East Central Europe," *East European Politics and Societies* 3:2 (1989), 198–214.

[89] AW OK II/1347/2K, Zbigniew Kubas, *Dzienniczek od dnia 1 października 1942 r. do dnia 10 maja 1944 r.*

communality."[90] Mass violence in Galicia certainly destroyed the social world. It took many years to restore and, in some respects, was never fully rebuilt. Framing this specific aspect of trauma as communal obviously refers to Omer Bartov's concept of communal genocide but goes beyond his definition. Communal trauma means both traumatic experience by the entire community and the destruction of the community as such. The community falls to pieces of entangled individual bystanders.

Living with the Dead: Long-Lasting Post-Traumatic Follow-Up

The third element of post-violence trauma consists of the necessity to live in places of mass death and, until very recently, to remain silent about it. Silence began during the war: people watching Jews being murdered did not speak, neighbors burying Polish victims in a rush did not speak, finally, parents of the UPA partisans looking at the bodies of their children, publicly displayed by the Soviets, did not speak (this was one of the methods used by the authorities to identify and repress the families of guerrilla members). Silence was safer than showing emotions, although it took a mental toll. Teodora Kanak from Osivtsi (b. 1927) recalls her feelings from the day when Jews were taken away from her hometown:

> *They cried a lot as they were hurried along. [...] And I cried a lot too, and then this soldier says to me: "Don't cry, or you'll go with them." So, I suppressed everything because I was scared. I was just a kid. This is what happened.*[91]

An interviewee from Kuriany (born 1927) answers the question of how people reacted to the fact that the Germans took Jews from the village: "What were they supposed to say? They turned their gaze away. We were scared to even look at them."[92]

After the war, the only (former) residents of Galicia who could openly and publicly speak about their war experiences were Jewish survivors who managed to emigrate to the West. Poles who were displaced to communist Poland and Ukrainians who remained in Soviet Ukraine were both

---

[90] Cited in Jeffrey C. Alexander, "Towards a Theory of Cultural Trauma," in Alexander et al. (2004), 5.

[91] Interview with Teodora Kanak.

[92] Interview with Mariia Zamrozevych.

deprived of that option. For obvious reasons, in both countries it was impossible to publicly discuss the topic of Soviet victims who were deported and then died in Siberia, were arrested and executed by the NKVD or were the UPA partisans who were murdered or died fighting Soviet troops. On the other hand, Polish victims of ethnic cleansing and Ukrainian victims of retaliatory actions could not be officially commemorated because the wartime Polish-Ukrainian conflict has been erased from official Polish and Soviet historiography. The case of the memory of the Holocaust was not so obvious. Neither in Poland nor in the USSR was the Holocaust denied as such; however, the official policy of the USSR was to treat the murdered Jews as civilian victims of the war, a position which contributed to downplaying the crimes perpetrated against this group.[93]

As a result, in the postwar years, the extremely difficult biographical memory of violence, often co-existing with individual psychological trauma, could not be translated into public commemorative practices, which might have had a therapeutic role. Both people who left Galicia and those who stayed behind had to deal with their traumatic experiences on their own. Nonetheless, local communities were not completely silent: people did not speak in public, but they could talk in a group of people they trusted. The fact that mass violence was discussed not only by mentioning "their" victims is evidenced by both the content of presently conducted interviews and the circumstances of the field studies. In the majority of towns where we conducted fieldwork, we heard detailed descriptions of local executions, not only from witnesses but also from people who were not present at the crime scene, namely, older as well as younger interviewees who were born after the war. Nataliia Havryshkevych (b. 1932) from Bibrka describes in detail the murder of Bibrka Jews in 1942 in the nearby village of Wołowe, but when asked if she saw it with her own eyes, she says indignantly that she did not, since she was a child. When I ask if her mother saw it, she again says no. Rather, the mother heard about it, and

---

[93] On the official memory of the Holocaust in the USSR, in particular in Western Ukraine, see Zvi Gitelman, "Soviet Reactions to the Holocaust, 1945–1991," in *The Holocaust in the Soviet Union: Studies and Sources on the Destruction of the Jews in the Nazi-Occupied Territories of the USSR, 1941–1945*, ed. by Lucjan Donroszycki and Jeffrey S. Gurock (Armonk: M.E. Sharpe, 1993), 3–28; Tarik Cyril Amar, "A Disturbed Silence: Discourse on the Holocaust in the Soviet West as an anti-Site of Memory," in *The Holocaust in the East: Local Perpetrators and Soviet Responses*, ed. by Michael David-Fox, Peter Holquist and Alexander M. Martin (Pittsburgh: University of Pittsburgh Press, 2014), 158–84.

told her ten-year-old daughter everything in detail.[94] The interviews recorded by the Yahad-In Unum team provide much corresponding data.

Very often, our interviewees are surprised by our question concerning the source of the precise information about events they had not witnessed, and answer that everyone saw everything, people talked about it in secret, how could we not know? The case of an interviewee from Hlibiv, where the local UPA partisans murdered several dozen local Poles in total, was very symptomatic. She was very reluctant to share her knowledge on this subject, but her granddaughter who was escorting us to the center of the village, told us about the crimes in detail: who died, who murdered whom and how, how the corpses were transported to the cemetery and how blood was dripping from the wagon.[95] It was obvious that she had heard it from her grandmother many times. After the war, knowledge of mass crimes against members of a local community—Ukrainians, Poles and Jews—was an "open secret," hidden from others for various reasons and absent from official discourse.[96]

Public silence also played a protective role in the mutilated Galician communities. As Hana Kubátová accurately notes in her chapter on Slovakia, after the war "former victims and perpetrators were expected to find a place as neighbors again." In Galicia, this necessity was even more acute. On the one hand, people co-responsible for crimes were protected from punishment, and, on the other, they could reintegrate into the local community in line with the principle that everyone knows, but because the victims are not here anymore, no one speaks up about it. In the majority of the communities under study, the oldest interviewees knew very well which local teenagers had been in the Ukrainian police and had participated in the shooting of Jews, and which later joined the guerrillas and killed Poles, and often these were the same people. In some cases, they were tried and convicted in postwar trials of collaborators or arrested as part of the fight against the Ukrainian underground, but most of the time they managed to avoid prosecution and continued to live in their hometowns.

For the community, the above mechanism enabled it to rebuild after the war, but for people from mixed families who stayed in Galicia after the

---

[94] Interview with Nataliia Havryshkevych.

[95] Interview with Ol'ha Gerus; informal conversation with her granddaughter.

[96] Marta Kurkowska-Budzan, "Imaging Jedwabne: The Symbolic and the Real," *Polish Sociological Review* 137:1 (2002), 113–7.

war, it deepened their war trauma. Apart from the memory of the sense of danger, the need to escape, and the loss of loved ones, they had to deal with the fact that, after the war, men who had wanted to kill them or had even murdered members of their family, could walk down the streets of their town. Anna Khomiak from Kuriany (b. 1930), who hid at the end of the war with her Polish mother and sisters (her father was a Ukrainian, so her brother was also considered a Ukrainian, unlike female members of the family) from her neighbors who had joined the UPA and hunted for local Poles, gave a symptomatic interview. When asked how she was able to look those neighbors in the eye after the war, she claimed that after the war everything calmed down and was normal. But when I ask for names, she says she has forgotten them (while she remembers other names without a problem).[97] Both Poles and Ukrainians from Galicia were not only entangled in what was happening there during the war, but also in memory of the violent past for many years after the war. Thus, the silence they experienced for so many years was a very complex phenomenon grounded in diverse reasons. Only in part did it emerge from the direct psychological trauma; another reason was politically and socially (communally) motivated repression from outside.

Unlike the Poles who were displaced from Galicia and took their sense of injustice with them, Ukrainians (and people from mixed families, such as Anna Khomiak) who stayed in Galicia, had to face many indirect and temporarily postponed traumas after the war. They had to learn to be silent; they had to learn to live alongside their perpetrators in order to allow their local community to survive; they had to live in crime scenes where the first murders of Polish landowners and the last executions of the UPA partisans had taken place. In many cases, they had to live in houses that belonged to a murdered person, or even literally live on someone's ashes.

The fact of taking over a house or an apartment after the war that had belonged to a Jew or a Pole no longer stirs emotions. It is not considered shameful and most interviewees openly call their own or their neighbors' houses "Jewish" or "Polish." This is due to two facts. First, in postwar Galicia, local authorities were responsible for distributing the non-destroyed houses that had belonged to the murdered or displaced via administrative orders. In very few cases had the new owner contributed in any way to the death or expulsion of the previous one. Second, the level of

---

[97] Interview with Anna Khomiak.

war destruction of residential buildings forced people to forget about their doubts in order to secure a roof over their heads.

The management of space around mass graves proved to be more problematic. In Galicia, as in the whole of the USSR, there were no mass exhumations of the murdered, but the majority of graves remained unmarked (often to this day). Under a mass campaign in the 1960s, many of the Jewish cemeteries in Galicia, where executions took place during the war, were removed to make space for public buildings.[98] In Shchyrets, a workers' hotel was erected on the site of a mass grave. At the Jewish cemetery in Barysh, where Jews were also murdered, the *matzevah* were razed to the ground and kolkhoz farm buildings were erected. A woman born in the 1940s testifies in dismay: "It's all done, there's not a sign there. They dismantled all grave markers and removed tombstones with inscriptions, when they were building the kolkhoz, the farm. This is now the foundation for the stables; we saw tombstones with Jewish inscriptions."[99]

In addition to public buildings, residential houses are also being built on mass graves. In a picturesque ravine not far from the center of Koropets, where Jews were shot, a local surgeon built his villa in the 1990s. Older residents shake their heads in disbelief, as if to say "how could he?" when discussing the matter. The house in Kuriany, on the doorstep of which a Polish family murdered in 1945 is buried, has changed owners several times and is currently home to a family that came from outside the village community. We were unable to talk to them, so we do not know if they are aware of the fact that the bodies of the hastily buried murdered family members are still there. In Zhovkva, a private owner built a house on the part of *kirkut* that had not been turned into a marketplace. Rumor has it that the house is cursed, that someone hanged himself there and that Jewish bones were found when the foundations were being dug. In other cases, mass graves had appeared under one's window. A woman-interviewee from the village of Pidhaichyky (Podhajczyki) did not choose to live next to the mass grave of her Jewish neighbors: Germans simply dug it within 100 meters from her house and she had to live with this fact ever after.[100]

---

[98] This was part of a wider campaign taking place in the USSR and the Soviet bloc. In Poland, for example, German cemeteries were removed under the 1964 decree of the Minister of Public Affairs, see Meng (2011), 141.

[99] Informal conversation with a woman, b. around 1945, conducted in Barysh in 2019 by Marta Havryshko.

[100] USHMM, RG-50.589*0213, Yahad-In Unum interview.

For many years after the war, the residents of Galicia were unable to forget about mass death, because they have literally lived on the bones of the victims—their own and others', and they have met the perpetrators on the streets—their own and others'.

CONCLUSIONS

To circle back to the main question of this chapter: what kind of trauma was experienced in Eastern Galicia by witnesses of mass violence, Poles and Ukrainians? First, some of them—more sensitive ones and/or those who have had particularly close contact with death and violence—experience *individual psychological* trauma with all its psychological and psychosomatic symptoms. It appears that the mental experiences of the witnesses had a gradation, and, while they did not always develop into a full traumatic experience on the scale from indifference to trauma, they were closer to the latter. Certainly, it should be emphasized that the psychological traumatization of one part of the group does not mean that another part of the group does not experience opposite emotions or is even guilty of perpetration.

The second aspect of post-violence trauma is *collective* trauma. The goal of this chapter has been to conceptualize it primarily as trauma of losing that affects the entire community, which loses its members (who have socially and economically important roles), a sense of security, the existing social structure, integrity and moral coherence. This trauma is less direct, and various members of the community experience it in varying degrees. Piotr Sztompka's theoretical concept of the trauma of social change helps to understand it.[101] Sztompka analyzes it most fully using the example of the Polish political and economic transformation after 1989, but his insights can be applied to any significant social change, such as the murder of several dozen percent of the Galician community over a few years. Sztompka unequivocally argues that major transformations and social crises are almost always accompanied by atrophy of social bonds and other elements of the social world including the structure and the system of values that define the shape of the community and society. It appears that in the long-term perspective, this aspect of post-violence trauma, although less obvious, was more significant for Galicia as a social organism than a

---

[101] In English, see Piotr Sztompka, "Cultural Trauma: The Other Face of Social Change," *European Journal of Social Theory* 3:4 (2000), 449–66.

number of individual psychological traumas experienced by its residents, because the trauma of losing affected everyone, not only the more sensitive ones. All this makes *collective* trauma in Galicia also *communal*.

Galician mass violence and death at the collective level might have been easier to work through if it had received the dimension of cultural trauma, as understood by Jeffrey C. Alexander. However, it did not, for a number of reasons. For collective trauma to become a cultural trauma it should be remembered, preferably also in the dimension of intergenerational transmission. The memory of it should acquire a culturally significant status, that is one that produces a powerful narrative of collective suffering, loss and tragedy that is recognizable to all members of the community. Finally, such memory should be associated with a strong negative affect such as pain, shame or guilt. According to Neil J. Smelser, "cultural traumas are for the most part historically made, not born."[102] In Galicia, the collective trauma of losing has not evolved into cultural trauma for two reasons. First, the totalitarian state does not provide conditions for an agent of memory. In a democratic state, it is the state or a structured social or ethnic group that finds it important to build a narrative about this particular trauma. Secondly, after the collapse of the USSR, when such opportunities arose, there were many other candidates for cultural trauma; the collapse of the USSR competes with Soviet repressions or the Chernobyl disaster, and the trauma of war violence stands no chance in this competition.

The third element of post-violent trauma is postwar silence on the one hand, and the necessity to continue living in places contaminated by violence on the other (*living with the dead*). In postwar Galicia there were almost no villages, towns or other sites without mass and individual graves; they were everywhere, just like the memory of those who were murdered and those who murdered—their own people and others.

These three elements of trauma, individual psychological trauma, collective and communal trauma of losing, and long-lasting trauma of silence and the necessity of "living with the dead," combine to form a multidimensional trauma of constant mass violence. Representatives of various groups of Galician residents, those who left after 1945 and those who remained, have experienced it to various degrees, but it has touched

---

[102] Smelser (2004), 36–7.

everyone. To turn to the words of one of the women-interviewees: "it has never been the same since they killed everyone."[103]

Acknowledgment The research for this chapter was funded within the project "Social anthropology of the void: Poland and Ukraine after World War II", financed by the National Program for the Development of the Humanities in Poland, no. 0101/NPRH3/H12/82/2014.

---

[103] Interview with Yosifa Fedorovych, b. 1927, conducted in Vyshnivchyk in 2018 by Anna Wylegała.

CHAPTER 6

Traumatized Children in Hungary After World War II

Tuomas Laine-Frigren

INTRODUCTION

The aftermath of World War II in Europe saw huge numbers of orphaned and dislocated children. Having been separated from their homes and families to escape the horrors of war, ethnic cleansing and genocide, they caught the attention of many around the world and concerns were raised about their mental health, and how they would readjust to postwar realities. Across these devastated European landscapes, psychologists, social workers and journalists encountered children who were at once physically fragile yet disturbingly unchildlike at the same time—"little old men and women," trying to learn how to play and go to school again after their

T. Laine-Frigren (✉)
Academy of Finland Centre of Excellence in the History of Experiences,
Tampere University, Tampere, Finland
e-mail: tuomas.laine-frigren@tuni.fi

© The Author(s) 2022   149
V. Kivimäki, P. Leese (eds.), *Trauma, Experience and Narrative in Europe after World War II*, Palgrave Studies in the History of Experience, https://doi.org/10.1007/978-3-030-84663-3_6

life-changing adventures.[1] These lost childhoods were not only a painful reminder of the experiences of wartime violence and upheaval, but were also brandished as symbols in discussions about the reconstruction of Europe. To counteract the psychological legacy of wartime violence, children (and their families) came to occupy a privileged position in many postwar societies. After the traumatic experiences of war, the children were seen both as vulnerable and in need of protection, but also as potentially dangerous and in need of control due to the "war inside" that they now suffered from. As a consequence, new psychological theories of healthy and harmonious childhoods and family life occupied the policymakers in postwar welfare states.[2]

This chapter examines how children's wartime suffering was culturally constructed in the particular time-bound context of victimhood and trauma in postwar Hungary. By analyzing a variety of source materials, such as published expert discourse, journalism and ego documents, I explore how children's suffering was interpreted in different contexts. I also examine how the processes of healing were understood, and what kind of social and political meanings were attributed to the children's traumas. My particular focus is the agency of people who did the actual practical work with children, such as psychologists, teachers and civil society activists, but I also refer to political and ideological constructions of childhood. Moreover, I make a tentative distinction between children as *victims* and children as *sufferers* in order to suggest (i) that not all war-related suffering found its manifestation in postwar public constructions of victimhood; and (ii) that there was in fact a wide range of war-related experiences among children.

After World War II, Hungary was economically and socially in ruins. The "last ally" of Hitler was now a defeated country, occupied by the Red

---

[1] Tara Zahra, *The Lost Children: Reconstructing Europe's Families after World War II* (Cambridge, MA: Harvard University Press, 2011), 90.

[2] Michal Shapira, *The War Inside: Psychoanalysis, Total War and the Making of the Democratic Self in Post-war Britain* (Cambridge: Cambridge University Press, 2013); Mathew Thomson, *Lost Freedom: The Landscape of the Child and the British Post-war Settlement* (Oxford: Oxford University Press, 2013); Stefania Bernini, "Mothers and children in post-war Europe: Martyrdom and national reconstruction in Italy and Poland," *European Review of History: Revue européenne d'histoire* 22:2 (2015), 242–58; Heide Fehrenbach, "War Orphans and Postfascist Families: Kinship and Belonging after 1945," in *Histories of the Aftermath: The Legacies of the Second World War in Europe*, ed. by Frank Biess and Robert G. Moeller (New York: Berghahn, 2010), 175–95.

Army and governed by the Soviet-led Allied Control Commission.[3] Hundreds of thousands of Hungarian Jewish citizens had died in Auschwitz, and the revisionist politics of the interwar period had reached a dead end.[4] Masses of half-orphaned, orphaned and homeless children were living in general poverty and destitution.[5] Social welfare institutions were hit hard by the war, and these already chaotic conditions were aggravated by the additional lack of schools, kindergartens and orphanages.[6] For thousands of children, hiding in shelters, bombing, devastation and death had been among their first experiences of life. In the midst of these generally miserable conditions, however, there was a certain political dynamism and optimism, particularly among left-wing psychologists and intellectuals whose position in the former regime had been insecure (due to antisemitism, for instance), but who now saw the postwar political constellation coalescing before their eyes as something altogether more promising. The psychological profession, for instance, was growing and it adopted a left-wing, progressive and public policy-oriented stance.[7] From 1945–1947, a national network of child psychology centers began to be set up by the state,[8] and the "Association of Mental Health Protection"

---

[3] Peter Kenez, *Hungary from the Nazis to the Soviets: The Establishment of the Communist Regime in Hungary*, 1944–1948 (New York: Cambridge University Press, 2006), 60–80.

[4] Raz Segal, "Beyond Holocaust Studies: Rethinking the Holocaust in Hungary," *Journal of Genocide Research* 16:1 (2014), 1–23.

[5] There is no exact information on the number of how many orphaned or homeless children lived in Hungary after World War II. Somewhat confusingly, the contemporary postwar estimates vary between hundreds of thousands and tens of thousands. UNESCO (1947) and the American Hungarian Aid Campaign (1945), for example, estimated that there were around 200,000 homeless children in postwar Hungary. In 1948, child psychologist Margit Hrabovszkyné Révész wrote that 20,000–25,000 children were "afflicted by war," but this figure is certainly too low. See *Children of Europe* (UNESCO, 1947); Margit Hrabovszkyné Révész, "Háborúsujtotta gyermekek," *Köznevelés* 4:22 (1948), 555.

[6] The postwar situation for children's health was also very bleak. In 1946, for example, over 40 percent of school-aged children were diagnosed with severe anemia, while diseases such as typhoid and tuberculosis were also very common. See Szabolc Varga, "A gyermekvédelem Magyarországon, különös tekintettel Sopron vármegyére (1945–1950)," *Universitatis Szegediensis: publicationes doctorandorum juridicorum* 6:1–8 (2004), 199.

[7] Melinda Kovai, *Lélektan és politika: Pszichotudományok a magyarországi államszocializmusban 1945–1970* (Budapest: L'Harmattan Kiadó, 2016), 143; Tuomas Laine-Frigren, *Searching for the Human Factor: Psychology, Power and Ideology in Hungary during the Early Kádár Period* (Jyväskylä: University of Jyväskylä Press, 2016), 206, http://urn.fi/URN:ISBN:978-951-39-6536-5

[8] Kovai (2016), 151–2.

was formed, grouping together progressive professionals from a number of fields and having the support of the Communist establishment and those in charge of science policy.[9] Following trends elsewhere in the world, and supported by the concrete aims of the country's top politicians, psychology professionals and educators in Hungary now began to plan new socialist policies for child welfare and education.[10]

Childhood during World War II has already been the subject of many important studies,[11] and there are also an increasing number that focus on postwar childhoods.[12] Many of the latter have focused on both the practical and theoretical work of civil activists, psychiatrists, teachers and social workers who dealt with these war children. Machteld Venken and Maren Röger, for instance, write about a Polish primary-school teacher in the provincial town of Submierzyce who in 1946 encouraged pupils to make drawings of what they had experienced in the war, drawing particular attention to the work of one boy who had experienced being a child forced laborer.[13] Meanwhile, the historian Ellen Schrumpf analyzes the essays of Norwegian schoolchildren asked to write stories about their life under the German occupation (1940–1945).[14] Ulrike Präger, in turn, investigates

---

[9] "Egy meg nem jelent folyóirat–a Jövő Embere," *Thalassa* 6 (1995), 1–2, 233–4, 248.

[10] Géza Sáska, "Alkalmazott lélektan és reformpedagógia 1945 után: Értelmezési kísérlet II rész," *Beszélő* 13:2 (2008), 6. Jewish left-wing psychologists and psychoanalysts in particular saw the general political conditions as promising; Kovai (2016), 137–52.

[11] See, for example Gabriel Moshenska, *Material Cultures of Childhood in Second World War Britain* (London: Routledge, 2019); Martin Parsons. *War Child: Children Caught in Conflict* (Cheltenham: The History Press, 2008).

[12] Machteld Venken and Maren Röger, "Growing up in the shadow of the Second World War: European perspectives," *European Review of History: Revue européenne d'histoire* 22:2 (2015), 199–220; Juliane Brauer, "Disciplining Young People's Emotions in the Soviet Occupation Zone and the Early German Democratic Republic," in *Childhood, Youth and Emotions in Modern History: National, Colonial and Global Perspectives*, ed. by Stephanie Olsen (Basingstoke: Palgrave Macmillan, 2015); Tuomas Laine-Frigren, "Children on the Move: Psychiatric Encounters with Child Evacuees Returning to Post-war Finland," in *Social Class and Mental Illness in Northern Europe*, ed. by Petteri Pietikäinen and Jesper Vaczy Kragh (London: Routledge, 2019); Nick Baron, ed., *Displaced Children in Russia and Eastern Europe, 1915–1953: Ideologies, Identities, Experiences* (Leiden: Brill 2016).

[13] Venken and Röger (2015), 199.

[14] Ellen Schrumpf, "Children and Their Stories of World War II: A Study of Essays by Norwegian School Children from 1945," in *Nordic Childhoods 1700–1960: From Folk Beliefs to Pippi Longstocking*, ed. by Reidar Aasgaard, Marcia Bunge and Merethe Roos (New York: Routledge, 2018), 205–19. Keeping in mind the multi-layered character of these narratives, Shrumpf detected many kinds of story types, from heroic adventures to tragic encounters

the "musical recollections" of German children expelled from the Sudetenland (as well as those who stayed there)—discussing the role of music in mitigating the traumas of war and loss of homelands;[15] while Viktória Bányai and Eszter Gombocz have noted that a similar therapeutic use of art was practiced in postwar Budapest, too.[16] In the Hungarian context, the outstanding work done by the social historian, Gergely Kunt, on wartime and postwar teenage diaries has been particularly valuable.[17]

The present study contributes to these wider historiographical trends by approaching the history of traumatized children in postwar Hungary from the two perspectives of discourse and encounter. In the first part of this chapter, I make use of Jeffrey C. Alexander's theories on trauma to examine how the discourse surrounding children's victimhood ensured that their suffering was interpreted as a painful "social wound," and consequently used to serve particular social and political ends.[18] In the second part of this chapter, I focus on the actual encounters between traumatized children and the adults who tried to help them. First, I look at one particularly interesting experiment in poem therapy that was carried out by a literature teacher in 1946 together with homeless children. After that, I look beyond the public "trauma drama" of children into a more personal account by examining the extraordinary wartime memoir and diary written by a volunteer nurse and Jewish survivor, Margit Tolnainé Kassai (1909–2000).

---

with death and loss, thus studying exactly how these stories stemmed from children's lived experience.

[15] Ulrike Präger, "'Musicking' Children From the Bohemian Lands: Nurtured and Hidden Musical Practices on Both Sides of the Iron Curtain," *European Review of History: Revue européenne d'histoire* 22:2 (2015), 310–30. See also Beata Halicka, "The Everyday Life of Children in Polish-German Borderlands During the Early Postwar Period," in *Borderland Studies Meets Child Studies: A European Encounter*, ed. by Machteld Venken (Frankfurt am Main: Peter Lang, 2017), 115–37.

[16] Viktória Bányai and Eszter Gombocz, "A traumafeldolgozás útjain: Holokauszt-túlélő gyerekek Magyarországon, 1945–49," *Regio* 24:2 (2016), 44.

[17] Gergely Kunt, *Kamasztükrök: A hosszú negyvenes évek társadalmi képzetei fiatalok naplóiban* (Budapest: Korall, 2017); Gergely Kunt, "The Psychological Coping Mechanisms of a Jewish Hungarian Teenager, Lilla Ecséry, as Reflected in Her Diary Written during the Holocaust," *Judaica et Holocaustica* 7 (2016), theme issue Women and World War II, 69–89.

[18] Jeffrey C. Alexander, *Trauma: A Social Theory* (Cambridge: Polity Press, 2012), Introduction, 101, 146.

CHILDREN AS VICTIMS

The end of the war in Europe saw many children whose mental well-being had been greatly affected by the violence they had experienced; and for whom there was now an increasing interest in their plight. Psychology experts and social workers, as well as state officials all around Europe, were very concerned that these children and adolescents might perhaps be too damaged to become active democratic citizens within postwar society. As Tara Zahra has shown, the sorry physical and mental state of the children caused many people at the time to fear for the future. Many worried, for example, that numerous children had been infected by the "foul education" provided by the fascists, while others were simply alarmed by the all-too-accurately dubbed "wolf children."[19] In Hungary, Gábor Sztehlo (1909–1974), Lutheran pastor and founder of the children's home *Pax*,[20] described how, in 1948, one of his children had spent one and a half years traveling across four countries fruitlessly looking for his father—all before the age of 12. The child eventually made it to the Austrian border where he fell into the hands of American soldiers, but only after having first wandered through Czechoslovakia and Romania. Sztehlo also described the feral appearance of another (13-year-old) boy who, upon arrival, was "almost naked and full of wounds," and "only carrying a flute [...]."[21] Meanwhile, in an account of what it was like working immediately after the war, a teacher from the village school of Uciechów in Lower Silesia, Poland, recalled the fate of those children who had arrived in the village after being transported all the way from the Ukraine. "These were big and small savages, almost all of whom had some psychological trauma, which was no wonder. After all, some of them had survived only by chance, hidden in some corner of the house in which some 'hajdamaks'[22] had slaughtered their closest relatives [...]."[23] Indeed, it would seem that a huge number of children in East-Central Europe had suffered traumas during

---

[19] Tara Zahra, "Lost Children: Displaced Children Between Nationalism and Internationalism after the Second World War," in Baron, ed. (2017), 198.

[20] This was a children's home and social facility for war orphans and other endangered children in Budapest.

[21] Andor Zsoldos, "Csoda a Budai Hegyek között," *Haladás* 3:27 (1947), 9.

[22] The word "Hajdamak" historically refers to a Ukrainian Cossack paramilitary fighter. In Poland, the term *Hajdamactwo* has very negative connotations, sometimes referring to Ukrainians as a whole.

[23] Halicka (2017), 131–2.

the 1940s caused by dislocation, hunger, violence and the loss of loved ones.

As also pointed out in Anna Wylegała's chapter in this book, the war experiences of these children were many and varied. In 1948, Hungarian journalist, Margit Izsáky (1899–1977), interviewed a number of underage conscripts who had been forcefully drafted during the last months and even weeks of war to fight an increasingly desperate struggle against the advancing Soviet Army. Izsáky was preparing a book about peoples' everyday lives during and after the Budapest siege. She was an experienced reporter and a specialist at investigating issues such as poverty and juvenile delinquency. In her book, which was soon to be published under the title, *Ország a Keresztfán* ("A Country on the Cross"), she reported on the day-to-day hunger and hardships of life in the bomb shelters during the last months of war, but her fundamental message was related to major issues of social and moral responsibility—and she started with the fate of children such as the ones mentioned below.[24]

The 15–16-year-old boys that Izsáky met all belonged, like most of their peers, to the nationalist paramilitary organization known as *Levente*—a nationwide youth organization (est. 1921) that provided military training for all Hungarian boys between the ages of 12 and 21. Throughout the war, *Levente* members had been actively involved in many kinds of military duties (e.g., as air-raid and fire wardens), but after the Arrow Cross coup in October 1944, they were increasingly used in combat situations.[25] Izsáky started her book with a description of these boys as having the appearance of "bitter old men," after the physical and mental stress they had clearly suffered at the hands of superior officers who had treated them very harshly.[26] This topic was also being discussed in the

---

[24] Margit Izsáky, *Ország a keresztfán* (Budapest: Müller Károly Könyvkiadó Vállalat, 1945). Izsáky's book was one of eight volumes in the Hungarian "Golgota" series (published in 1945). The openly expressed aim of *Magyar Golgota* was to stimulate discussion about the disaster of the recent past. See also Máté Zombory, "Magyar golgota: Politikai közösség és múltreprezentáció 1945 után," *Szociológiai Szemle* 25:1 (2015), 66–88.

[25] Attila Horvath, "War and Peace: The Effects of World War II on Hungarian Education," in *Education and the Second World War: Studies in Schooling and Social Change*, ed. by Roy Lowe (London: Routledge, 1992), 147–8; Caroline Mezger, *Forging Germans: Youth, Nation, and the National Socialist Mobilization of Ethnic Germans in Yugoslavia, 1918–1944* (Oxford: Oxford University Press, 2020), 188–9. *Levente* initially recruited only boys, but from 1942 onwards girls were also encouraged to join. This was voluntary at first but became obligatory after the takeover by Arrow Cross.

[26] Izsáky (1945), 13.

Hungarian Parliament at the time; as one MP pointed out in November 1945, many of these young *Levente* teenagers were now suffering in "unbearable circumstances" as prisoners in Allied-occupied Austria and Germany—it was high time to bring them back.[27] For Izsáky, these traumatized boys were not only victims of Arrow Cross and SS brutality, but also of a more generalized lack of moral responsibility and lack of courage on the part of adults to defend the children.[28]

Izsáky also met two teenage boys who had been given long prison sentences by the postwar Peoples' Court[29] for having taken part in the Arrow Cross's reign of terror—in particular, the infamous death march out of Budapest in which many Jews had been beaten to death. In one thought-provoking scene, the focus was thus turned towards the emotionally charged issue of children as potential *perpetrators*. Izsáky tried to describe how she felt in "the prison corridor" on her way to meet one of these boys. In spite of the fact that she had "already got used to the idea that the whole world was clearly one big mental asylum, full of evil imbeciles," she had to admit that it "was really scary" to think she was now going to meet convicted murderers who were barely teenagers.[30] But these were not psychopaths, she found, just kids from extremely poor backgrounds with little education—"typical Arrow Cross types," as she put it—who probably thought that messing around with submachine guns was a kind of game or "adventure." As twisted as these kids most certainly were, they were also clearly the victims of "poisonous, racist, and fascist propaganda" and the "worst kind of pulp fiction." Indeed, together with the misery they had "inherited," all these factors had combined to unleash their "murderous instincts." However, she was careful to play down the distinction between victim and perpetrator by also acknowledging that she, too, felt a certain responsibility (as indeed the whole country should have) for what had

---

[27] A nemzetgyűlés 2. ülése 1945. november hó 30-án, pénteken. The MP also referred to Hungarian Jewish children (although he did not explicitly call them Jews), who had somehow managed to survive being deported, but who were still in Austria and Germany. https:// library.hungaricana.hu/hu/collection/ogykdok_1945_1947/ (last accessed 23 January 2021).

[28] Izsáky (1945), 7–13.

[29] Between 1945 and 1950, more than 40,000 cases were heard in the Communist-led People's Tribunals, and over 22,000 defendants were found guilty. Tamás Bezsenyi and András Lénárt, "The Legacy of World War II and Belated Justice in the Hungarian Films of the Early Kádár Era," *Hungarian Historical Review* 6:2 (2017), 302.

[30] Izsáky (1945), 14–5.

happened: "I cannot feel pity – I only feel ashamed of myself. What kind of people did this to them? We are all guilty!"[31] In this way she not only claimed that adults should take real responsibility, but also raised the otherwise unspoken issue of collective guilt and perpetratorhood. The issue of children as potential perpetrators was thus used to illustrate broader cultural traumas in a country that had fought side-by-side with the Nazis.

In the immediate postwar years before the Communist takeover in 1948–1949, a large number of books and pamphlets were published, dealing with experiences of the recent past and the lessons that might be learned from them.[32] Among these were autobiographical narratives describing the Hungarian and Nazi German persecution of Jews, written by both Jewish and non-Jewish Hungarians.[33] Intellectuals raised questions about moral responsibility and soul-searching, while leftists especially blamed the "counter-revolutionary" regime of Miklós Horthy—at least in its last days, when the Arrow Cross members were given free reign—for having destroyed people's sense of morality. As the avant-garde writer, Lajos Kassák, put it—repairing these "poisoned minds" would not be something that could be done simply overnight.[34] Indeed, the problem was thought to be widespread; in 1945, the poet and politician, Dezső Keresztury, argued that the nation had been thrown into such a state of moral darkness by the terrible events of the recent past that "not even a lantern would help pick out a single person free of blame for what had happened in one way or another."[35] This was precisely the kind of discourse which used the symbol of the child as victim (and perpetrator) to highlight both a political community in crisis and the need for reconstruction and reform.

One rather typical way to articulate children's victimhood was to blame the "fascist" education they had been subjected to, and its dire consequences. This was a crucial subtext in Alice Hermann's arguments about the negative consequences of an authoritarian upbringing. Hermann (1895–1975) was one of the many left-leaning psychologists and child experts in postwar Hungary. An activist in the Social Democratic Women's movement, and a trained psychoanalyst, she represented the pre-war

---

[31] Izsáky (1945), 14–5.
[32] Zombory (2015).
[33] Ferenc Laczó, *Hungarian Jews in the age of Genocide: An Intellectual History, 1929–1948* (Leiden: Brill, 2015), 134.
[34] Lajos Kassák, "Vissza az életbe," *Világ*, 18 May 1948.
[35] See Dezső Keresztury, "Ember, ember, ember kívántatik," *Szabad Szó*, 15 June 1945.

heritage of the Budapest School of Psychoanalysis founded by Sándor Ferenczi (1873–1933). In 1946, Hermann published a popular guidebook entitled *Emberré Nevelés* ("Educating Humans"). Written against the backdrop of extreme violence in 1944–1945, the book at once advocated a liberal and humanist approach to education as the best means to avoid the dark past repeating itself and followed in the Hungarian psychoanalytic tradition. Indeed, the critique of conservative education—its hypocritical endeavor "to save the child's soul by severity"—had been at the core of Sándor Ferenczi's psychoanalytic work.[36] Most importantly, Ferenczi's conception of trauma being a consequence of broken social bonds was fundamentally based on his realist understanding of children's experience of parental violence and abuse.[37]

It was only logical that one of the major topics in Hermann's book would be authoritarian upbringing. She illustrated her ideas with a scene she had once witnessed in a Budapest marketplace when a mother hit her seven- or eight-year-old boy for running out after her as she left the house because he did not want to be left home alone. For Hermann, it was a clear illustration of how punishing children arbitrarily would breed submissive, fearful and timid human beings: well-behaved for sure, but ones whose "greatest satisfaction [would be] to follow the rules." Children so raised would never develop the capacity for making proactive and autonomous decisions. Instead, their sense of responsibility would extend "only to the point at which [...] the mission was completed and the command fulfilled."[38] What Fascism had revealed, Hermann argued, was not that the (German) people were themselves inherently cruel, but that since childhood they had been deeply ingrained with a "cult of obedience" which would explain why one day they might be organizing "Kraft durch Freude activities"[39] and on another "organizing pogroms."[40]

[36] Ferenc Erős, "Violence, Trauma and Hypocrisy," in *Psychology and Politics: Intersections of Science and Ideology in the History of Psy-Sciences*, ed. by Anna Borgos, Ferenc Erős and Anna Gyimesi (Budapest: CEU Press, 2019), 82–3, passim.

[37] Sándor Ferenczi, "Confusion of the Tongues Between the Adults and the Child (The Language of Tenderness and of Passion)," *International Journal of Psycho-Analysis* 30 (1945/1932), 225–230, translated by Michael Balint, https://icpla.edu/wp-content/uploads/2012/11/Ferenczi-S-Confusion-of-Tongues-Intl-J-Psychoa.-vol.30-p.225-1949.pdf (last accessed 23 January 2021).

[38] Hermann (1946), 34–5.

[39] Kraft durch Freude (Strength through Joy), or *KdF*, was a leisure organization for workers and their families in Nationalist Socialist Germany.

[40] Hermann (1946), 34–5.

On 12 November 1947, the topic of victimized children clearly became a vehicle for promoting a range of political agendas, when a parliamentary session[41] was called to debate a bill for establishing a new Juvenile Court in Budapest. Many of the speakers supported the rational and humanist idea that the Juvenile Court should use psychological expertise to help young delinquents readjust to society,[42] but many also used very pointed rhetoric to condemn the pre-war regime for what it had done to children.

Dénes Huszti, for instance, from the Smallholder's Party, talked about the "false patriotism" that had been peddled; he pointed out that children were universally very responsive to "all that was beautiful and noble," but since the old regime had failed to give them a proper humanist education, they had been easily marshaled in the wrong direction. The horrible events of the Jewish death march in 1944 were a testament to this. "Those of you who witnessed it," he argued, "will never forget the image of innocent people marching towards defamation and death," accompanied by 14–15-year-old bullies, who were beating and shooting dead anybody who faltered or tried to escape.[43] The Social Democrat MP, György Faragó, also referred to these "killing sprees"[44] in an attempt to make the listeners more responsive to child-related institutional reforms. Indeed, both Huszti and Faragó were keen to support the new proposals that psychology professionals work beside the judge in Juvenile Court to make sure that justice would be based on prevention, emphatic understanding and rational guidance—instead of punishment and nothing else.[45]

The Social Democrat, Fanny Auer (Ernőné Hajdú), gave one of the most powerful speeches of the day. She attacked an inherently conservative legislation which, because it had been "written by men," she argued, was blind to the occurrence of young girls being sexually abused (which was in turn a major cause of prostitution).[46] Auer also made positive remarks about new experiments in collective education and orphan care (e.g., *Pax* in Budapest), and demanded more psychology-based policies

---

[41] Az országgyűlés 18. ülése 1947. évi november hó 12-én, szerdán, https://library.hungaricana.hu/hu/collection/ogykdok_1945_1947/ (last accessed 23 January 2021).

[42] Az országgyűlés 18. ülése 1947. évi november hó 12-én, szerdán, 905–6, https://library.hungaricana.hu/hu/collection/ogykdok_1945_1947/ (last accessed 23 January 2021).

[43] Ibid., 904.

[44] Ibid., 888.

[45] Ibid., 888–9, 905–6.

[46] Ibid., 912.

for dealing with the menacing prospect of childhood crime in postwar Hungary. She believed the children would not easily forget the violence they had experienced, having internalized dangerous behavioral patterns during the war and the difficult times that followed it. "What should we expect," she asked, "from teenagers who saw and took part in so much killing themselves, who took part in looting homes and shops, and when the smartest kid in the family was the one who brought home as much of that loot as possible?"

THE PSYCHOLOGY OF CHILDHOOD TRAUMA

After the violent upheavals of World War II, social planners around Europe became more receptive to child psychiatry and psychology. As Michal Shapira and others have shown, the fate of children during the war and its aftermath provided a testing ground for psychological theories related to child development.[47] In Great Britain, Anna Freud and Dorothy Burlington famously voiced their concern over the evacuation of children from metropolitan areas to the British countryside. States and professionals were relying on findings made in the pre-war period, which had already seen a wide range of interventions in childhood issues,[48] and the emergence of the "child" as a key factor (and potential threat) for the future health and versatility of the nation.[49]

Hungary had an internationally significant tradition of child psychology, psychoanalysis and education, which now found fertile ground in the leftist (but still relatively pluralist) political context of the immediate postwar years before the Communist takeover. In light of the source material, however, the psychological consequences of war and genocide for children were rarely the main focus of expert discourses in postwar Hungary,[50] and

[47] Shapira (2013).

[48] See, for example, Dirk Schumann, ed., *Raising Citizens in the "Century of the Child": The United States and German Central Europe in Comparative Perspective* (New York: Berghahn, 2011); Nikolas Rose, *Governing the Soul: The Shaping of the Private Self* (New York: Cambridge University Press, 1999) 123–213.

[49] See, for example, Bengt Sandin, "Children and the Swedish Welfare State: From Different to Similar," in *Reinventing Childhood after World War II*, ed. by Paula S. Fass and Michael Grossberg (Philadelphia: University of Pennsylvania Press, 2011). Jutta Ahlbeck, "The Nervous Child and the Disease of Modernity," in *Childhood, Literature and Science*, ed. by Jutta Ahlbeck et al. (London: Routledge, 2018).

[50] The lack of explicit public attention of social and individual tragedies caused by war most clearly concerned the adult traumas. As observed by Melinda Kovai, this was particularly

when these matters were discussed by psychologists, that tended to happen in the future-oriented context of preventive strategies for mental health and democratic education. However, the professional opinions of psychologists were becoming increasingly visible and were often cited in the press. In October 1947, for example, a psychologist from the Budapest Institute for Child Psychology advised families not to send their small children to the countryside in winter. Referring to British wartime experiences, the psychologist argued that being separated from the mother was even more dangerous for a child than any poverty and deprivation they might experience at home.[51]

The wartime traumas of children were a direct cause of concern for Dr. Margit Hrabovszkyné Révész (1885–1956), who published an extensive study on "war-afflicted" children in 1948.[52] Between 1 May 1945 and 30 June 1948, Dr. Révész examined 226 children at the aforementioned *Pax* children's home (founded by Gábor Sztehlo), also known as *Gaudiopolis* ("the City of Joy") at the time.[53] *Gaudiopolis* was not only a child-welfare institution but also a large-scale collective experiment in civic education, a kind of city-state for children (that was also run by them).[54] Its roots were in the wartime rescue operations that Sztehlo had led, supported by the International Red Cross, using his Lutheran "Good Shepherd" orphanages to shelter around 1600 Jewish children and 400 adults during the Arrow Cross reign of terror and siege of Budapest in 1944–1945.[55] During its five years of existence (1945–1950), *Gaudiopolis* housed several

---

manifest during the first large psychiatric conference after the war in Hungary: only one of the speakers referred to mental problems caused by war. See Kovai (2016), 131. See also Ran Zwigenberg, "'Wounds of the Heart:' Psychiatric Trauma and Denial in Hiroshima," *History Workshop Journal* 84 (2017), 67–88. By now, many studies have argued that in many countries, war-related adult traumas (e.g., in soldiers) were not really understood or accepted by the mental health establishment after World War II.

[51] József Péter, "Gyermek-teleltetés," *Magyar Nemzet*, 19 October 1947, 4.

[52] Hrabovszkyné Révész (1948), 555–62.

[53] Zsoldos (1947).

[54] Stehlo's *Gaudiopolis* was a direct inspiration for Géza Radványi's classic film *Somewhere in Europe* (Valahol Európában, 1948), which depicts a gang of orphaned children building a new civilization out of the ruins of war. See Constantin Parvulescu, *Orphans of the East: Postwar Eastern European Cinema and the Revolutionary Subject* (Bloomington: Indiana University Press, 2015), 17–43.

[55] Éva Makai, "Háborús évek gyermekvédelmi közösségek utópiai," *Iskolakultúra* 6:2 (1996), 94–7.

hundred endangered children with different social backgrounds—although most had been either orphaned or half-orphaned by the war.

In her article, Révész presented a number of case studies, with her main intention being to show that children with different life histories, social backgrounds and ways of reacting to traumatizing events should be treated in different ways from each other. During the many moments she had spent with them over the years, she had noticed that many suffered from difficult inner conflicts, "persistent anxieties" and "fear of death." She believed the most important way to help these "mentally wounded" (*lelkileg sérült*) and "fearful" children was to give them moments of joy, beginning with a good regular diet and plenty of room to play and move around. Children's "natural curiosity," so often suppressed by the traumas they had suffered, should be revived by taking them on nature trips, giving them books or by taking them to see a film. Only after their basic emotional and "instinctive" needs were first met, could school assignments and other work tasks be set. In this way, it was hoped they could gradually shake off the debilitating sadness caused by the chronic lack of love and support they had suffered.[56] But as some of the children reacted aggressively and antisocially—needing to feel more active in actually controlling their environment—it was decided they should be given meaningful social roles in the community. In this way, Révész reasoned, their activity could be channeled to a "higher cultural level"—in which they could genuinely feel they were contributing to the children's community. Clearly, the civic and democratic upbringing offered by *Gaudiopolis* was one way to do this.

As noted by Constantin Parvulescu, orphans soon came to symbolize the allegedly superior social bonds represented by the socialist state in postwar Central and Eastern Europe. Révész, too, promoted the ideal of a benevolent institution, which, via individual teachers and other workers, would offer the kinds of psychological support that had previously only been entrusted to families (especially mothers). In her estimation, the orphans really longed for concrete support and help, and so when they got this, they tended to become the "very grateful" pedagogical subjects of those who truly took care of them, keen to identify the supportive

---

[56] Révész (1948), 561. Interestingly, Révész also related to physical symptoms. As she wrote, during the first months after the Budapest siege, the symptoms of mental trauma were primarily to be seen in "drastically reduced physical resistance," for example, prolonged gastrointestinal inflammation and various kinds of skin problems. In addition to them, very persistent "fear states" were the most striking phenomena during the first postwar months.

educator with the "missing parent" and the institution with a lost home. Révész recommended this humanistic institutional path particularly in those cases where the child's mother had died, as the mental wounds of these children often went unnoticed in family-care situations; especially when those families had themselves often been "mutilated" in so many ways.

The postwar momentum for psychology-based reforms was not solely driven by those in power and professionals in Budapest. There were also many teachers outside the capital with an interest in applied child psychology.[57] One of these teachers was Lívia Koralek, who had carried out psychological association tests with 55 orphaned Jewish children and detailed them in a report about her experiences in 1946.[58] The terms she used in the tests were "war," "home" and "mother," and the result she came away with was that all three were linked to "death and destruction" for these children. However, she argued that if teachers could develop ways of really listening to children's feelings, they could devise ways of alleviating their suffering and "make them smile again." In her opinion, it was the teacher's task to make the children realize that "nobody could ever again treat them in the way they had been treated a year ago." Only then could they, at some point, eventually realize there was in fact "a country waiting for them, and a country [Hungary] worth fighting for." Perhaps the children might gradually even forget their suffering. There was actually some reason for optimism, because several of her children "already knew how to laugh."[59]

One way of helping the children, Koralek suggested, would be for them to cultivate their own communities. Maybe the terrible things they had experienced in wartime could be something that provided the necessary impetus for building a "better future" together, insofar as they were events that they would absolutely want to avoid. She even went so far as to claim that their bad experiences had given them a certain "social awareness"[60] that their "Jewish brothers" had received more than their share of

---

[57] Kovai (2016), 150.

[58] Lívia Koralek, "A második világháború hatása a zsidó gyermek lelkivilágára," in *Tarbut Héber Kultúregyesület iskoláinak Évkönyve az 1945–46-os tanévről,* ed. by Aladár Spiegel (Budapest, 1946).

[59] Koralek (1946), 17.

[60] Koralek was clearly influenced here by the Hungarian pioneer of child studies, László Nagy (1857–1931), who had also detected war-induced "social sentiments" in his study of children's perceptions of war during World War I. See László Nagy, *A háború és a gyermek*

suffering,[61] thus also suggesting that the adults might also learn something from these children. The historian Gabriel Finder has also discovered somewhat similar images of children in his studies on Jewish child survivors in the Polish postwar collective memory. In a recent article, he focuses on how children were represented in the famous Yiddish film "Our Children" (*Undzere Kinder*, 1948).[62] The film dramatizes the encounter between two comedian actors and the residents of a Jewish children's home. The experience gives the children the chance to reflect on their wartime experiences and to criticize the artists' representations.[63] According to Finder, the children in the home (where most of the film's scenes are located) are portrayed as being terribly scarred by their experiences of the Holocaust, yet they are still able to build some kind of memory community for sharing these experiences together—especially when encouraged through artistic intervention. In this way, survivors of the Holocaust are for the most part depicted in the film as brave and future-oriented agents, rather than as passive victims. The film also suggests that adults can learn directly from children about the mental pain caused by war; about storytelling and music as potential ways of healing; and about how the future should be built.[64]

CHILDREN AS SUFFERERS

Where are you, mummy?
Here I am, my sweet son.
Although I won't see you long.
Come closer, my son.
And if I die.
Who's gonna look after you, my son?
I live on the pavement.
Someone will take me in.
Ernő Szecső[65] (1947)

---

lelke: Adatok a gyermek értelmi, érzelmi és erkölcsi fejlődéséhez (Budapest: A Magyar Gyermektanulmányi Tár, 1915), 141.

[61] Koralek (1946), 17.

[62] Gabriel N. Finder, "Child Survivors in Polish Jewish Collective Memory after the Holocaust: The Case of *Undzere Kinder*," in Baron, ed. (2017), 218–47.

[63] Finder (2017), 229–32. *Undzere Kinder* is also considered as one of the earliest critical filmic interventions to the problem of Holocaust representation.

[64] Finder (2017).

[65] The original Hungarian poem (translated by the author), written by the young orphan Ernő Szecső, goes as follows: "Hol vagy édesanyám? Itt vagyok édes fiam. Bár nem látlak

Orphaned children could be seen everywhere in the cities of Central and Eastern Europe by the end of 1945. As Constantin Parvulescu has suggested, their growing presence became a powerful reminder not only of the traumatic experience of war itself, but also the "grim deeds" of their parents' generation; symbolizing both the guilt of perpetratorhood and visions of a new civilization.[66] I, too, have argued in the first part of this chapter that children's victimhood was brandished ubiquitously in both professional and political discourses that envisioned a better society for postwar Hungary. The poem cited at the start of this section, however, was written as part of a "therapeutic" poetry experiment in a children's home by a teenager called Ernő Szecső whose mother had died. I will look specifically at this experiment next, as an example of a unique way of dealing with children's wartime traumas.

In 1947, teacher Zoltán Rákosi, renowned for his liberal educational ideas and great personality,[67] published an essay on teaching children about poetry.[68] Rákosi began by saying how in October 1946, "the learning went just fine," but that he sensed that there was a heavy feeling of resignation in the air that would just not go away. But in July of the following year, the famous poet Sándor Weöres (1913–1989) published a new collection of his poetry, *Elysium*, which included a children's poem called the "Dancing Song" (*Táncdal*), that played with nonsensical words, and Rákosi noticed how children would sometimes use a line from this poem they had heard (like "*panyigai, panyigai, panyigai* [...]"),[69] and use it for various purposes—as a joke, or expression of pity, for example. Inspired by this, he decided to "stir things up" a bit and challenged his class (mostly boys) by reading a poem he was "sure they wouldn't understand."

Rákosi's essay is a fascinating narrative of pedagogic discovery in the world of poetry; about how he and the kids started playing with rhymes, rhythms and sounds—"chewing" words and studying their emotional

sokáig. Gyere közelebb fiam. S ha meghalok. Ki fog gondozni, fiam? Az utca szélén lakom. Valaki csak befogad."

[66] Parvulescu (2015), 3.

[67] "'Erről a családról, amelynek oly sok nevezetes tagja volt' – Sárközi Mátyással beszélget Hegedűs B. András," *Beszélő*, 22 December 1994 (Karácsonyi melléklet), 14–5.

[68] Zoltán Rákosi, "Gyermekköltészet vagy a 'közönség' útja a művészethez: Részlet egy általános iskolai magyar tanár naplójából," *Válasz* 7:11 (1947), 414–26.

[69] Weöres' poem in English, see https://www.babelmatrix.org/works/hu/We%C3%B6res_S%C3%A1ndor-1913/T%C3%A1ncdal (last accessed 23 January 2021).

effects. Eventually, after several months of practice, the children were writing their own poems—and even got to meet the poet Weöres when he paid a visit to their class in person. In his essay, Rákosi clearly wants to convey the importance of a dialogic way of teaching; he was quite cleverly using children's existing ideas of poetry, but at the same time encouraging them to express even their strangest opinions and feelings. This method seems to have been successful: as one of the boys had revealed to Rákosi, "a peculiar feeling, difficult to grasp, grew inside me; it was mixed with pain [...] then I felt like I had grown wings and was now flying faster than the wind into the big world out there."[70]

Rákosi wrote in a self-reflective and gently ironic style, constantly weighing in on his role as a teacher, at the same time giving the impression that he, too, was participating in poetic discovery through playing. In 1994, one of his former students captured this playful aspect of his former teacher when remembering how they had gone on "strike against Mr. Rákosi's beard," refusing to participate in lessons again until the teacher shaved off his beard. This demonstration of the "will of the people" conveys something of the ideological sensibilities in postwar Hungary.[71] Not that Rákosi was a dogmatic ideologue; he wanted rather to inculcate a self-conscious and independent style of thinking among his pupils, as well as a love for the "music of poetry." This was not for any sublime nationalistic or collectivistic reason, but for the sake of art and life itself, even if it meant that the "statue of the Great Poet" would have to be toppled.[72]

Many of Rákosi's fifth grade elementary school students were badly traumatized Jewish children; and interestingly, the experiment itself took place in Sztehlo's aforementioned *Gaudiopolis*. As an educational institution, it combined early twentieth-century reform pedagogy, postwar socialist-democratic collectivism and Sztehlo's own experiences of the practice-oriented educational methods of the Finnish Folk High School movement, covering activities such as handicrafts, music, sports and hiking (Sztehlo had acquired a two-year fellowship to study theology and pastoral work in Finland at the turn of the 1930s).[73] For some reason, Rákosi did not mention in his essay that his students were from *Gaudiopolis*

---

[70] Rákosi (1947), 416.

[71] "Erről a családról" (1994), 14.

[72] Rákosi (1947), 420.

[73] Charles Fenyvesi, *When Angels Fooled the World: Rescuers of Jews in Wartime Hungary* (London: University of Wisconsin Press, 2003), 169; Makai (1996), 94–7. Based on his Finnish experiences, Sztehlo established a folk high school in Nagytarca (east from Budapest)

(maybe he wanted people to see his pedagogy as having more universal value). His primary aim was also not so much to disseminate a model of "art therapy" for traumatized children, but to recount the educational discoveries he had experienced together with his pupils.

Rákosi's article did, however, include both implicit and explicit references to the children's suffering. For example, in response to negative and sometimes rude feedback from children's relatives; claims from teachers and educational authorities that Rákosi's liberal methods were ruining the school's "prestige"; and letters accusing him of being "antisocial" and "inciting" hatred against the working class,[74] Rákosi made it very clear just how much his pupils had suffered during the war. He also pointed out how his critics had not noticed the importance of the poetry experience for the children—how it had truly affected their mental lives by, for instance, increasing their sense of belonging and inner purpose. In comparison, he noted that, after having been away for a couple of weeks over Christmas, the boys had become "orphans once more; pale and lifeless, they lingered around without a sense of purpose in their lives. It took several weeks of conscious caring to give them back peace of mind and the joy of poetic creation."[75]

Significantly, Rákosi was using poems that he must have known would have an emotional effect on homeless children: when the class studied a poem by János Arany (1817–1882), called *Family Circle* ("Családi kör"), he quickly recognized the emotions thrown into stark relief by the "light of the fireplace," which was "shining so invitingly" for these homeless children. At this point, he instantly began to suspect that the poem might easily lose its appeal if they tried to analyze it too closely. In any case, the poem certainly seemed to affect the children—they even used it to dramatize a *Commedia dell'arte* puppet play. Rákosi, in turn, was convinced that poetry and play could "expand the boundaries of life"[76] for these children, maybe even "relieve their souls of a great burden." The children also wrote and published their own poems (like the one at the start of this section) in their school newspaper, and 27 such poems were also published at

---

and directed it between 1937 and 1942. What especially intrigued him was the way Finland seemed to put resources on raising the cultural level of its agrarian population.

[74] Rákosi (1947), 418.

[75] Ibid.

[76] Rákosi (1947), 419.

the end of Rákosi's essay. Many of these poems were quite clearly reflecting upon the personal experiences of trauma and loss.

So, while his focus was more pedagogical than therapeutic, Rákosi was nevertheless acknowledging that poetry might serve as a means of psychological release for the traumatized children. This was reminiscent of the general approach proposed a year later by Révész in her 1948 article maintaining that all therapy and readjustment should be based on "increasing self-awareness." In other words, the children should each be encouraged to find the different elements needed for mental recovery from within themselves. But because this process of self-reflection was such a difficult path to take for these very conflicted children—not least because adults rarely had any idea about what these "secret mental paths" were—the presence of professionals was crucial to "holding their hands as symbolic mothers."[77]

Rákosi talked more openly about the therapeutic function of poetry in a newspaper article from 1948.[78] Understandably, many of his students had developed a state of mind that was "dark, strange, timid and distrustful"; almost all of his "sweet and unhappy children" had lost at least one of their parents in 1944–1945, and, after trying out many different methods, he felt he had failed to give them the comfort they needed. It was only when he introduced his "rhythm games" to the class that a completely new kind of psychological reality began to open up:

> At the point when a small 9-year-old orphan presented her deepest sorrows in four simple lines, describing the longing for her dead mother and father, she also felt relieved. She became something else. These children's poems are indeed strange, incredibly complicated, psychological mysteries.[79]

Rákosi described his pedagogical experiment as being born from the helplessness he felt when faced with the mental suffering of these pupils.

---

[77] Révész (1948), 560–1.
[78] Zsoldos (1947), 9. *Haladás* ("Progress"), was a radical anti-fascist (but not communist) newspaper established in 1945.
[79] Zsoldos (1947), 9.

A Child's-Eye View

In the last part of this chapter, I look at narrative representations of everyday wartime traumas in childhood by focusing on a particularly interesting memoir and diary written by Margit Tolnainé Kassai in the last year of the war. Kassai (1909–2000) was a Jewish woman who played a significant role in nursing Jewish children in temporary homes run by the International Red Cross in Budapest under the German occupation, during the Arrow Cross reign of terror and siege. The memoir, beginning in 1944, contains over 200 pages, dedicated to her faraway husband, and written in a matter of months between early March and early May 1945. On the day of Budapest's "liberation" by the Red Army (11 February 1945), she also started to keep a diary, where she described everyday life and conditions under the Soviet occupation.[80] Among many other things, Kassai's narrative portrays a number of children, which makes it an important document for studying their experiences. It also provides a fascinating hands-on view of what it might have been like to shelter children in such dangerous conditions. In what follows, I will look at how Kassai's "bottom up" narrative, and the interpretations of children it contains, possibly differed from the public discourse surrounding childhood in this era.

The memoir begins in April 1944, when Margit Kassai, an employee at the Hungarian General Credit Bank, gifted photographer and non-religious Jew, had to leave her house in Buda following the German occupation (19 March) and move to an apartment building especially designated for Jews in the inner city of Pest.[81] In this house, she lived together with many other families for a few months and organized day-care activities for the children there. However, after the Arrow Cross takeover (15 October), she found it too risky to stay in the house anymore, so she fled and stayed with friends for a couple of weeks, until managing to become a nurse for

---

[80] The original manuscript is kept in the Szabó Ervin Library in Budapest. The whole narrative (introductory letter, memoir and diary) has now been published: Margit Tolnainé Kassai, *Óvoda az óvóhelyen – Feljegyzések a Sztehlo-gyermekmentésről* (Budapest: Magvető Kiadó, 2020). The book also includes a thorough scientific introduction by Gergely Kunt.

[81] The authorities of Budapest decided in April 1944 that all the Jews had to move to the so-called Yellow Star Houses. In comparison to other cities in the East-Central European region, this was a rather unusual kind of ghetto and particular to the Budapest Jews (and their children) during the Holocaust. See Ágnes Nagy, *Harc a lakáshivatalban: Politikai átalakulás és mindennapi érdekérvényesítés a fővárosban, 1945–1953* (Budapest: Korall, 2013), 80–90; Zsuzsanna Ozsvath, *When the Danube Ran Red* (New York: Syracuse University Press, 2010), 97–9.

the International Red Cross with the help of Gábor Sztehlo, who was heading its child rescue program in Budapest at the time and looking for people to work in his previously mentioned Good Shepherd orphanages. As these shelters and their employees were (at least theoretically) under international protection, Kassai managed to survive both the Arrow Cross and Siege of Budapest, while taking care of the children she was also hiding with.

While Kassai's narrative is a potential source for many kinds of study, perhaps most obviously the life of Jews and others in Budapest in 1944–1945,[82] the everyday life she spent with children must certainly be one of its defining themes. One can see clearly how children made a deep impression on Kassai. Nursing gave meaning to the everyday struggles— for example, the dangerous trips for food and water, the lack of sleep and the terrible hygiene—thereby making them easier to bear. Ensuring that the children survived must have helped her build a sense of continuity for her own future too, as at many points in the narrative she admits that looking after the children and playing with them kept her sane amid the conflict of adults.[83]

At one point in the narrative, she illustrates these feelings with a small story called "Secrets of the Child's Heart." It takes place in a children's air raid shelter at some point towards the end of January 1945, when bombing and fighting were at their heaviest in Budapest. One day, however, when there was a relative lull in the violence, all the adults in the shelter went out into the courtyard to gather bricks from the rubble, and they built a protective wall to add protection. A few days later, while playfully chatting with the kids, she found herself asking them if only one nurse could look after them, who would it be? "Laughing, they looked at each other and answered right away that it would be either Aunt Margit (me) or Aunt Bozsi." The reason they gave for this, Kassai recounts, was because she and Bozsi were the adults who treated every child equally and without favoritism. It turned out that when the adults had gone out to gather bricks during the lull earlier that week, they had played a game about what to do if the courtyard suffered a direct hit, killing all the adults at once and

[82] For an overview of the many themes in Kassai's text, see Gergely Kunt, "Ironic Narrative Agency as a Method of Coping with Trauma in the Diary – Memoir of Margit K., a Female Holocaust Survivor," *Hungarian Cultural Studies* (e-Journal of the American Hungarian Educators Association) 7 (2014), https://doi.org/10.5195/ahea.2014.137

[83] Kassai (2020), 41.

leaving just the kids in the shelter. Then they played a variation, with the assumption that "either Aunt Bozsi or Aunt Margit" was the sole adult survivor. During this game, they imagined how they would organize the house and cellar, who would share with whom in each room, what they would do with the ham that still was left and who would do the cooking. The only problem was knowing what to do with the unbearable baby they called "Wald." So, they then played another variation, where the baby was also killed with the adults (save for either "Bozsi" or "Margit" of course). As Kassai writes to her husband, it was simply quite instructive to see how the minds of these children worked.[84]

The story is a fine example of the way Kassai generally wrote about the children—seeing them as active human beings rather than victims. She describes one 14-year-old "jeweler's assistant" from Józsefváros, for instance, as a "sharp-witted but lovable rogue" and "very good with his hands," in more ways than one: "one can't help forgiving his nimble fingers as they are great at fixing whatever goes wrong in the house too."[85] Then there was the 11-year-old son of a medical doctor, who had been forced to undergo plastic surgery to "rectify" his circumcision, and would often perform songs by Zoltán Kodály to the other kids. Then there was his cousin "Sutyi," who was constantly reading until eventually forced into the candlelit world of the basement. Some of the children, nevertheless, were clearly difficult, disorderly and messy; while some would bully other kids, others were refusing to eat, wetting their beds, or visibly miserable and clearly missing their parents.

But the latter sometimes developed their own strategies for dealing with the bullying—like "little Évike," a seven-year-old girl, who would often sing herself loudly to sleep in the dark.[86] She became especially close to a five-year-old boy called Palkó that Kassai wrote about more than once, probably because he was the first orphan she met. In these descriptions concerning Palkó, Kassai took stock of her overall relationship with the children, the feelings she attached to them and the challenges of keeping them calm in conditions of war and bombing. In doing so, though it is not explicit, a particular kind of "treatment ideology" seems to coalesce and take shape. At many times in the narrative, and particularly during the encounters with little Palkó, she confesses how difficult it was to maintain

[84] Ibid., 234–6.
[85] Ibid., 163.
[86] Ibid., 165, 259.

"proper standards of care," by which she meant keeping the correct emotional distance between herself and the children—almost certainly referring to what was known as the "Loczy method" in Hungary. According to this method, it was fine that children were not always missing their mothers, but at the same time it was wrong if the children became *too* emotionally attached to the replacement mother figure. Kassai claimed that she gradually learned to "remain calm" when faced with children's mental suffering ("in the same way a nurse gets used to blood"), but as her notes reveal, from time to time she found this impossible. When Palkó got sick, for instance, she wrote about how bad it felt to have to leave him for a couple of days (when she was forced to make a trip), and how she was afraid of losing him. As the sallow, withdrawn boy sitting in the corner said to her one day: "it's very bad for me to be here, because all the people are strangers." When Kassai then asked him if he felt she was a stranger, the boy answered: "only a half-stranger, but I love my mother the most."

As Gergely Kunt points out, Kassai's text can be approached as a special kind of trauma narrative—an attempt to process and reflect upon personal traumas through writing.[87] Kunt has studied the narrative strategies used by Kassai to construct meaningful experiences out of the traumatic events she faced. He convincingly suggests, for example, that Kassai's use of gentle irony and black humor was a coping mechanism to help her deal with stressful situations.[88] Kunt also points out differences in the tone and style of writing between her memoir and diary: the emotional atmosphere in the diary being somewhat less hopeful.[89] Kassai, herself, also shows a critical awareness of the "literary" qualities of her memoir when she writes in the introduction that she wishes she could have taken daily notes of her impressions and events until the very end of the siege, as she wanted to make "the whole thing more realistic and not so literary."[90]

One interesting dimension of this source relates to the way Kassai presents herself in the memoir. For example, she refers to many dangerous and frightening situations, in which she felt fear and even despair, but at no point does she want to give an impression of herself as a victim. Although she is very honest about the many anxieties she felt, and shares with her

---

[87] Kunt (2014).

[88] Ibid., 31.

[89] See, for example, the entry from 22 February 1945, which deals with plundering Soviet soldiers; Kassai (2020), 288–9.

[90] Kassai (2020), 17.

husband/reader even the most intimate physical problems (e.g., incontinence, menstrual issues and stomach troubles), it seems she also wants to convey how fearless she was. For instance, on one occasion when looking for water and candles, she saw some corpses "lying neatly next to one another [...] like a wagonload of goods waiting to be transported," and she describes how, "despite the thick snowfall," she felt like she was defying "the elements and a thousand dangers, just like the hero in a movie."[91]

If we compare this with a diary entry from 19 February 1945, however, the emotional landscape is somewhat bleaker, as Kassai tries to describe the difficult job of getting children into Sztehlo's new children's home on the hills of Buda. Though the siege and the fighting were already over, after months of physical and mental hardships, the long journey up the hill (with heavy loads to carry) was almost the last straw. At this point, the reactions of a ten-year-old girl gave her the chance to witness a child's-eye view of death. Kassai describes how the girl, who was "usually very smart, cheerful and balanced" suddenly started crying uncontrollably and refused to go any further when she saw corpses at the hospital gate in front of them. Getting increasingly hysterical (also because the other adult was yelling at her), the girl desperately asked if there wasn't another route they could take. But, because this was out of the question, Kassai decided to shield the sobbing girl under her coat so she would not have to see anything. As they passed the bodies, Kassai describes how "the girl's whole body shook," but how when they finally got to the children's home, she "bravely opened her eyes."

Conclusion

At this point, we return to Jeffrey Alexander, mentioned so far only briefly in the introduction to this chapter. His social-constructionist approach to trauma is based on the argument that people conceptualize pain and suffering in terms of collective stories. In this respect, his social theory of trauma offers a particularly useful framework for studying how different kinds of violent events have been publicly constructed as traumatic by specific institutions and carrier groups (according to their particular interests). Furthermore, as social psychologist Gilad Hirschberger has pointed out, collective traumas are not just social constructions of suffering, but

---

[91] Ibid., 187–8.

are often also used to build identities.[92] In this chapter, I have shown that children's victimhood was one such construction in post-war Hungary. In the devastating aftermath of the war, it was brandished as a sociopolitical metaphor for envisioning a better society of the future—as in many other countries (from Poland to Japan).[93]

However, Alexander's research design and his source material might not be so suitable for analyzing the real-life experiences of people who have faced everyday hardships during and immediately after a conflict. In this chapter, I have therefore tried to show how rare sources, such as Margit Kassai's wartime memoir and diary, can provide access to very personal experiences, and an alternative way to approach histories of trauma. What would be particularly interesting would be to systematically juxtapose such private narratives of suffering with public constructions of children's victimhood—especially if the private narratives were written in close proximity to the traumatic events they describe, and the public constructions were used for political and professional purposes. As we have seen, Kassai did not characterize the children she was in contact with as passive victims but as active ones, in spite of their suffering. What is also intriguing in her narrative is the unembellished and pragmatic picture she builds up of her everyday practice of nursing and helping children in the war. From Kassai's diary we get an immediate sense of the process she is going through to make sense of the traumatic events she is experiencing.

As Tara Zahra and others have rightly pointed out, the family and nation were widely regarded as central sources of emotional healing and individual strength for European children after World War II. In Hungary, the rather visible role of "war-afflicted" children might also have made them a suitable vehicle for articulating broader social, moral, and political issues of collective guilt and perpetratorhood. At the same time, the dynamics of traumatic memory were generally characterized by political and social taboos which meant that certain particularly painful issues for people and their families were not addressed, such as the rapes committed by Soviet soldiers, veteran

---

[92] Gilad Hirschberger, "Collective Trauma and the Social Construction of Meaning," *Frontiers in Psychology* 9:1441 (2018), 1–14; Alexander (2012), 125.

[93] See, for example, Owen Griffiths, "Japanese Children and the Culture of Death, January–August 1945," in *Children and War: A Historical* Anthology, ed. by James Marten and Robert Coles (New York: New York University Press, 2002), 167–8; Bernini (2015), 242–58. Griffiths studies the "culture of death" and sacrifice that was fed to children and teenagers in Japan during the Pacific War. According to Griffiths, this might have disappeared after Japan lost the war, but it was replaced with a "culture of life." Boys might not have been encouraged to die in battle anymore and girls were no longer encouraged to preserve their purity by killing themselves; but, instead, the new generation had to study hard and be brave in building a new culture.

traumas on the Eastern Front, and perhaps most notably the failure of Hungarian society to address the huge personal suffering of its Jewish citizens. For ideological and pragmatic reasons, the hegemonic Communist party did not want to differentiate between singular experiences of suffering, but, rather, treated all victimized groups as victims of "Fascism."[94]

The countries of Central and Eastern Europe emerged from World War II in a radically new political constellation. In Hungary, this change was characterized by historic land reforms and a general shift to the left, which also manifested itself in new psychological and educational discourses. Most importantly, as Hungary was now firmly in the Soviet sphere of influence, the Communists increasingly determined the substance of politics and public discourse.[95] In this chapter, I have referred to the popularity of including the issue of childhood trauma in the discourse arguing for a collective and future-oriented education at this time. This is also apparent in the public attention received by *Gaudiopolis*—the leftist political atmosphere at the time certainly supported these kinds of ideas and institutions.

However, the idea that a (children's) collective can be a potential site of healing should not be assessed solely against this backdrop of socialist nation-state-building, but also in the context of contemporary child psychology, not to mention the general socioeconomic and physical conditions that prevailed. One could argue that the institution appeared the most rational solution not so much because of the need to educate future socialist citizens, but because it was seen as the best (science-based) way to help orphans and other mentally distressed children readjust to a society ravaged by years of war and occupation.

In this chapter, I have paid attention to a range of voices and actors who either publicly discussed children's traumas or encountered them in their everyday lives. Indeed, the sources show a multiplicity of responses to childhood trauma, from abstract and future-oriented policy-talk to teachers and psychologists promoting specific ways of healing such as offering them moments of joy, taking them on nature trips and exploring poetry with them

---

[94] Hungarian historians have only recently started to unravel the social and psychological significance of these multiple silences. For sexual violence during and after the war, see Andrea Pető, *Elmondani az elmondhatatlant: A nemi erőszak története Magyarországon a II. Világháború alatt* (Budapest: Jaffa, 2018); Gergely Kunt, *Kipontozva: Nemi erőszak második világháborús naplókban* (Budapest: Osiris, 2019). See also Gábor Gyáni, *A Nation Divided by History and Memory: Hungary in the Twentieth Century and Beyond* (New York: Routledge, 2021), 67–87.

[95] See, for example Ignác Romsics, *Hungary in the Twentieth Century* (Budapest: Corvina, 1999), 245–64; Judit Meszáros, "Effect of Dictatorial Regimes on the Psychoanalytic Movement in Hungary before and after World War II," in *Psychoanalysis and Politics: Histories of Psychoanalysis under Conditions of Restricted Political Freedom*, ed. by Joy Damousi and Mariano Ben Plotkin (Oxford: Oxford University Press, 2012), 79–111.

in innovative ways. At the same time, we should keep in mind that while the postwar period did see an overall growth in child psychology, there were still many traumatized children who never got the chance to enter into a therapeutic relationship with a psychologist or progressive teacher, or to enjoy the warmth of an emotionally supportive institutional community. So, if we focus only on the role of psychology professionals, then we are ignoring the important role that many others played in helping children readjust—such as teachers, the civil society activists who were running different activities for children, and children's own communities. In the fledgling Socialist states of postwar Central and Eastern Europe, one way to approach children's readjustment was to actively engage them in a new future-oriented form of socialization, and perhaps there was also a "therapeutic" dimension to this. In postwar Hungary, for instance, the main ideological and political struggle "in the name of children" actually took place between the Hungarian *Kinderfreunde* movement, the Scouts, and the Communist Pioneers—the latter emerging victorious.[96] In this respect, contexts other than strictly professional therapeutic relationships were possibly more crucial for children's postwar readjustment than we have previously assumed. It could thus be rewarding for historians and others in the field of trauma studies to focus on studying these relationships more thoroughly in the future.

---

[96] András Kiss, "Gyermeksors a második világháború után–1946," *Archívnet* 9:1 (1999), https://www.archivnet.hu/hetkoznapok/gyermeksors_a_masodik_vilaghaboru_utan__1946.html (last accessed 23 January 2021).

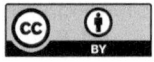

CHAPTER 7

"We will cry a little, but then we will forget": Narratives of Loss and Victory in Postwar Yugoslavia

Ana Antić

INTRODUCTION

In her seminal article on the notions of psychological trauma and shell shock in twentieth-century Russia, Catherine Merridale has argued that the Stalinist policy (and ideology) of stoicism, and its intolerance of psychological damage and weakness, resulted in fundamentally different attitudes to and discourses of psychological traumatization in the Soviet Union. While individual pain and victimhood were certainly experienced by exceptionally large numbers of Soviet citizens throughout the 1930s and 1940s in particular, there existed no public cultural or political framework in which such suffering could be expressed or discussed—and survivors, both civilians and military veterans, were unlikely to benefit in any way from insisting on their own victimhood narratives. According to Merridale, the end of World War II saw a politically orchestrated

A. Antić (✉)
Department of English, Germanic and Romance Studies, University of Copenhagen, Copenhagen, Denmark

© The Author(s), under exclusive license to Springer Nature Switzerland AG 2022
V. Kivimäki, P. Leese (eds.), *Trauma, Experience and Narrative in Europe after World War II*, Palgrave Studies in the History of Experience, https://doi.org/10.1007/978-3-030-84663-3_7

emergence of "a myth of endurance and stoicism which did not allow for victimhood or personal weakness." This myth in turn radically shaped the collective as well as personal memory of the war violence, and profoundly affected Soviet citizens' experiences and discourses of hardship, suffering and survival.[1] In her innovative analysis of children's experiences of the Leningrad siege, Lisa Kirschenbaum suggested that it might be useful to replace the dominant framework of trauma with the concept of (psychological) resilience when discussing experiences and memories of Soviet child survivors of the Leningrad siege and the Great Patriotic War. This approach, Kirschenbaum argues, can shed more light on those children's own understandings and memories of their wartime experiences and hardships, and can provide a productive analytical framework for interpreting Soviet discourses of heroicism, strength and endurance.[2] Rather than dismissing survivors' narratives of endurance, strength and resilience as inauthentic products of a coercive regime's political propaganda, both Merridale and Kirschenbaum argue, we might need to explore how such official discursive denials of traumatization affected individual expressions and experiences of extreme pain, loss and suffering.

The absence of the language of traumatization, weakness and suffering from the Soviet postwar narratives of the war raises further questions about possible meanings and limitations of the framework of psychological trauma outside the modern Western world. While a significant number of researchers have recently explored psychological legacies and effects of World War II, most of these works have been focused on Western Europe and the United States. In particular, there has been almost no research into different cultural, political and psychiatric conceptualizations of psychological trauma in Eastern and Central Europe beyond the Soviet Union. This chapter aims to address this gap, asking whether narratives of collective endurance and resilience were more widespread across the region, and to what extent the socialist ideology and socialist regimes in Eastern Europe affected the conceptualizations of psychological suffering and healing. Focusing on socialist Yugoslavia, the chapter argues that, given the absence of developed postwar psychiatric and political discourses of trauma and wartime suffering, we need to explore how narratives of

---

[1] Catherine Merridale, "The collective mind: Trauma and Shell shock in twentieth-century Russia," *Journal of Contemporary History* 35:1 (2000), 39–55.

[2] Lisa Kirschenbaum, "The meaning of resilience: Soviet children in World War II," *Journal of Interdisciplinary History* (Spring 2017), 521–35.

psychological loss and pain were articulated indirectly—in broader cultural and public spheres.[3] If psychological trauma was not the dominant paradigm used to understand and describe psychological suffering in socialist Yugoslavia, how were the effects of extreme wartime violence and loss addressed, discussed and represented in postwar artistic productions? How did psychiatrists, writers, artists and filmmakers understand the concept of a damaged psyche and how did they envision its recovery? Were the psychological experiences of war and violence seen as potentially undermining the efforts at postwar reconstruction?

In the aftermath of World War II, Yugoslavia was a ravaged country: its human and material losses at the end of the war were higher than in any of the warring countries except for Poland and the USSR. Years of brutal occupation and an even more brutal civil war, fought on ethnic and ideological grounds, left the economy in ruins, so that the immediate postwar period was marred by a scarcity of basic foods, materials and housing options. Even more devastating than material destruction was the tremendous psychological impact of the war: there was hardly a family untouched by the mass murder and incarceration of civilians, and, well into the postwar years, many were still waiting for information on their loved ones. Tens of thousands witnessed unprecedented crimes and cruelty.[4] And yet, the country's flourishing psychiatric—and psychoanalytic—profession had

---

[3] I refrain from using "trauma" as an analytical framework for the chapter—instead, I only refer to the concepts (or narratives) of psychological trauma and traumatization as parts of medical, psychiatric or broader cultural discourses, and I don't employ those notions as general terms to describe the reality of psychological suffering. I believe the concept of trauma to be historically, politically and culturally specific, and agree with scholars such as Didier Fassin and Derek Summerfield, who think critically about its transhistorical and transcultural/transnational applicability. As a result, I don't assume that "trauma" would necessarily be the most appropriate framework for understanding and describing World War II's psychological consequences in Yugoslavia (or Eastern Europe)—the chapter thus makes a distinction between experiences of psychological suffering and trauma as an interpretive framework. The latter is arguably one of many paradigms that could be employed to analyze the psychological aftermath of war and violence.

[4] Jozo Tomasevich, *War and Revolution in Yugoslavia, 1941–1945: Occupation and Collaboration* (Stanford, CA: Stanford University Press, 2001), 744. Although figures remain contested, total human losses are taken to exceed 1.5 million in the entire country (Bogoljub Kocovic, *Zrtve Drugog svetskog rata u Jugoslaviji* [London: Naše delo, 1985], 172–80). The Yugoslav Reparations Commission estimated material losses at over 9 billion US dollars, which included over 20 percent of residential housing destroyed or heavily damaged, around 60 percent of livestock killed or plundered and over 19 million tons of grain and other crops taken out of the country between 1941 and 1945 (Tomasevich [2001], 715).

very little to say about possible long-term psychological effects of such extreme violence, personal loss and dislocation. At the first postwar Yugoslav neuropsychiatric congress in 1946, leading Croatian psychiatrist Bosko Niketic briefly acknowledged the immense psychological suffering ("much sadness, worry, uncertainty and fear") to which the country's population had been exposed, and enumerated the unspeakable atrocities many had witnessed—"mass shootings, hangings, slaughters... loss of almost all family members, and waging a resistance war in the most difficult circumstances imaginable." Nevertheless, Niketic concluded his discussion of such harmful psychological disturbances and their possible consequences in the very next sentence, stating that, fortunately, the Yugoslav peoples had "persevered in their struggle" despite this, and that all their mental anguish had been "crowned"—and presumably cured—by the ultimate triumph of the anti-fascist forces.[5] Niketic and the other congress speakers then proceeded to discuss Yugoslavia's peacetime psychiatry and its future tasks.

To my knowledge, only two trauma-related issues were discussed for a brief period after the end of the war. Dr. Nikola Nikolic, a survivor of the infamous Jasenovac concentration camp ran by the Croatian fascist Ustasha organization, published a book on the psychological and medical aspects of camp experiences based on his observations of his fellow inmates and coined the term "horrorosis" (*hororoze*) to indicate that a completely new diagnosis was needed to describe and understand the effects of such brutal torture and incarceration.[6] Nikolic's concept of unique Yugoslav psychoses and neuroses did not catch on, and its discussion largely remained limited to his manuscript. On the other hand, another specifically Yugoslav illness did receive more sustained public, political and psychiatric attention, because it affected the military. "Partisan hysteria," a form of war neurosis only diagnosed in Yugoslav anti-fascist guerrilla soldiers (partisans), was defined as a unique psychological disorder, unknown in the rest of the world and fundamentally different from the battle fatigue or shell shock noted in Western armies. But the case of "partisan hysteria" demonstrated just how politically sensitive such discussions could be, especially at a time when the victorious partisans were becoming the bearers of the new state's foundational narrative of resistance. While partisan neurosis caused quite a stir in the immediate postwar years, primarily because of its

---

[5] Bosko Niketic, "Otvaranje konferencije," *Narodno zdravlje* 2:3 (1946), 4–5.
[6] Nikola Nikolic, *Jasenovacki logor smrti* (Zagreb: Nakladni Zavod Hrvatske, 1948).

theatrical and disruptive character, a leading Yugoslav psychiatrist pronounced it completely cured soon after, and there was no further political or psychiatric discussion of this problem after the mid-1950s.[7]

But if references to trauma dropped out of psychiatric discussions, this did not necessarily mean that war-related psychological distress disappeared from the emotional worlds of Yugoslav (and other East European) citizens. In his article for this volume, Robert Dale has demonstrated that narratives of psychological traumatization were by no means absent from Soviet psychiatrists' daily practice and considerations, nor from former Red Army soldiers' own "vernacular languages" of suffering after World War II. In a similar vein, Ville Kivimäki has argued that "traumatic memories" persisted in Finnish soldiers' dreams and permeated their experiences and recollections of wartime violence long before Finnish psychiatric discourses integrated such concepts. To some extent, similar trends marked Yugoslavia's postwar period. At the Third Congress of Yugoslav medical doctors in 1971, Slovene psychiatrist Janko Kostnapfel made a passing reference to the lingering psychological effects of World War II among his patients: "Memories of the horrors of the last war are still very fresh. From our patients of younger and middle generations we often hear horrible stories about the war every day." Kostnapfel concluded that this was not at all surprising, given that Yugoslavia lost about ten percent of its prewar population, or about 1.7 million people: "just that number tells us about the emotional difficulties of their surviving family members."[8] Kostnapfel's intervention offered an important (and unprecedented) insight into the workings of Yugoslavia's postwar psychiatric clinics: they were reportedly inundated with traumatic narratives of World War II, and by patients who were still experiencing severe war-related psychological distress. It was not unexpected, then, that such narratives, expelled from medical or political forums, would find their way into socialist Yugoslavia's artistic and literary production.

This chapter, thus, explores how the theme of damaged psyche and individual psychological pain was explored outside psychiatric and official political discourses. Due to space restrictions within one chapter, the analysis will be largely limited to Yugoslav film production in the 1950s, 1960s

---

[7] See Ana Antić, "Heroes and hysterics: Partisan hysteria and Communist state-building in Yugoslavia after 1945," *Social History of Medicine* 27:2 (2014), 349–71.

[8] Janko Kostnapfel, "Rat I mir sa stanovista psihijatrije," *Zbornik III. Kongresa lekara Jugoslavije* (Ljubljana: Savez lekarskih društava Jugoslavije, 1971), 281–2.

and 1970s, with occasional reference to important literary works that developed the topic of wartime suffering and its postwar psychological consequences. The chapter argues that it was Yugoslavia's renowned Black Wave cinema which broached this subject most systematically and consistently. It will, therefore, offer the first analysis of the role that some of the most significant Black Wave films played in exploring the psychological consequences of World War II, and in demonstrating how Yugoslav citizens' immense (publicly unacknowledged) pain and suffering shaped postwar reconstruction. The Black Wave in Yugoslav cinematography primarily marked the 1960s, the period of political, economic and cultural liberalization in the country, and received significant international esteem and attention. Researchers have extensively analyzed these films' complex, innovative and multi-layered critique of the socialist regime, but they have never explored their powerful engagement with the notion of war trauma and with the war's emotional and psychological effects on all individuals and groups within society. In fact, a significant aspect of the films' political critical edge was their undogmatic, poignant and often controversial portrayal of the multiple clashes between individuals scarred by the war and postwar revolutionary realities.[9] These films' themes, as well as their reception, can shed much needed light on the complex processes through which individual pain and suffering were translated into the public cultural and political discourses of a socialist country.

Broken Soldiers on Film

In 1945, the Yugoslav People's Army was plagued by a virtual epidemic of war neurosis, which affected thousands of partisan soldiers. The end of the war seemed to only exacerbate the spread of the illness.[10] This was a disorder that bore no resemblance to the war traumas in the other nations that had participated in the conflict: it did not manifest itself in the form of an

---

[9] Gal Kirrn, *Surfing the Black: The Yugoslav Black Wave Cinema* (Maastricht: Academienplein, 2001); Daniel Goulding, *Liberated Cinema: The Yugoslav Experience* (Bloomington: Indiana University Press, 1985); Pavle Levi, *Disintegration in Frames: Aesthetics and Ideology in the Yugoslav and post-Yugoslav Cinema* (Stanford, CA: Stanford University Press, 2007); Constantin Parvalescu, "Gleaming Faces, Dark Realities: Dušan Makavejev's Man is not a Bird and the Representation of the Working Class after Socialist Realism," *Senses of Cinema* 49 (2009), 47–56; Milan Nikodijevic, *Zabranjeni bez zabrane: Zona sumraka jugoslovenskog filma* (Belgrade: Jugoslovenska Kinoteka, 1997).

[10] Arhiv Sanitetske sluzbe Ministarstva odbrane, R-19, "Neuropatija (slicna histeriji)," 1–2.

urge to withdraw from the frontlines, as was the case in the British and US armies, where battle exhaustion, anxiety and demoralization emerged as the most popular diagnoses by 1944. Rather, Yugoslav war neurotics demonstrated a heightened willingness to fight, as their new disorder consisted of violent and potentially harmful epileptiform seizures which simulated wartime battles and attacks. The seizures could occur at any moment and under any circumstances, usually when there was an audience—in the middle of a conversation, at lectures or meetings, while driving or riding in a car, in front of superiors, for example. According to Dr. Hugo Klajn, Vienna-educated Belgrade psychoanalyst and psychiatrist who treated a number of the partisan patients in the immediate aftermath of the war, these involuntary seizures started when soldiers fell into a state of trance of sorts, during which they subjectively re-experienced intense feelings related to fighting.

Even more importantly, only certain ranks of partisan soldiers seemed to be affected by the illness. By 1945, the partisan neurotic appeared to be a precisely defined type from a very distinct (low) socio-economic position, the serious psychiatric repercussions of which seemed to clearly demonstrate the dark side and subversive potential of increased social mobility. The Yugoslav form of war neurosis apparently most frequently affected the uneducated, socially immature and emotionally less sophisticated—in some reports even "primitive"—members of the partisan troops, who were given important political responsibilities but experienced severe trauma and anxiety due to their own inadequacy and unpreparedness. Partisan neurosis was virtually only diagnosed in extremely young, uneducated (frequently illiterate) and immature soldiers, whose limited intellectual capacities frequently clashed with the highly responsible assignments that they had been given (or to which they aspired) towards the end of the war.

Yugoslav psychiatrists, therefore, explained "partisan neurosis" almost exclusively in terms of ambition, social mobility and intellectual inadequacy rather than that of psychological suffering. According to this interpretation, the specter of military ranks, awards and hierarchies explained the mysterious outbreak of hysteria at the very end of the war: the decision to dispense with guerrilla formations and build a traditional military organization in 1943 was the reason why virtually no partisan neuroses had been recorded before that year. The distribution of officer ranks, distinctions and status rewards within the victorious army in the spring of 1943 was held to be responsible for the hysterical seizures experienced by many

of the "incompetent" and overly ambitious partisans who found themselves in lowly positions within the hierarchy: these changes "incited envy
and awoke ambition and desire for rewards among the partisans, especially
in uneducated, young and psychologically immature soldiers." When
advancement was denied or jeopardized, "the wish emerged in immature
and vain partisans to vent their anger and receive what they thought was a
deserved award."[11] In fact, Klajn highlighted the "wish for being recognized" as the single most important psychological factor in the development of partisan neurosis. While this wish could easily be satisfied during
the war in battles (through self-sacrifice and consequent admiration by
comrades, commanders, and the local population), the circumstances after
the end of the war offered fewer opportunities for immediate acquisition
of rewards and praise while at the same time made such acquisition ever
more important in the context of a newly hierarchical army. Consequently,
"neurosis represented a promissory note for that type of recognition, seizures – a dramatic display of one's claims, of one's (under-appreciated and
unrewarded) achievements and sacrifices, much more effective than mere
talking about them would have been."[12]

It is indeed very telling that the motive of social advancement came to
dominate psychiatric discussions, especially since patient case files offered
a wealth of evidence that numerous other extreme social and psychological
factors and pressures might have had an exceptionally adverse effect on the
partisans' mental health. Most "hysterics" hospitalized in Kovin had
extremely tragic and violent life stories to share with Klajn. In their narratives, the sheer magnitude of wartime suffering, trauma and losses emerged
with crystal clarity, and testified to the unprecedented catastrophe endured
by the Yugoslav population. Many of these soldiers were barely teenagers
when the war started, and most of those examined by postwar psychiatrists
had lost some of their closest family members in the course of the war. Ivo
C. only decided to join the partisans after the Ustasha slaughtered his
father, mother and younger brother. His sister survived, but he did not
have time to check on her after years of fighting when he passed through
his village with his unit at the end of the war—and this is when he started
having his first seizures.[13] Conversely, Stevo T. found out that his entire
family had been slaughtered by the Ustasha after he had already become a

---

[11] Hugo Klajn, *Ratna Neuroza Jugoslovena* (Belgrade: Tersit, 1995 [1955]), 17–8.
[12] Klajn (1995), 42.
[13] Klajn (1995), 76.

partisan soldier.[14] Velizar P. admitted that he experienced the first symptoms of his mental illness at the very end of the war, in March 1945, after he "remembered that his sister had been shot, his father was in prison, and he himself had no education to speak of." Moreover, earlier in the war, Velizar had escaped from in front of a firing squad at a Hungarian concentration camp.[15] Many partisan hysterics had experienced Croatian, German or Hungarian concentration and detention camps or prisons: Zivadin P. told Klajn that he had escaped a Croat camp "where he was beaten and tortured so brutally that he asked to be executed." Following the escape, Zivadin decided to take revenge for his murdered father and brother, and took part in shootings of the partisans' POWs, mostly Ustasha soldiers. In his seizures, Zivadin was likely plagued by the fact that he himself took other people's lives and yelled: "I was tortured as well, they did deserve it!"[16] Still, even in the face of such a mountain of evidence of the intensity of the partisans' psychological traumatization, Klajn was the only psychiatrist to acknowledge the importance of the wartime exertions and suffering of the "hysterics" to the development of their neurosis. But even within Klajn's explanatory framework, this was at most a secondary factor: wartime horrors and hardships were not the main cause of the seizures, and could not, on their own, have provoked the Yugoslavs' war neurosis.

In 1957, a group of Zagreb-based psychiatrists, led by Stjepan Betlheim, conducted a follow-up study of wartime neurotic patients, aiming to inquire into their adaptation to civilian life in the course of ten or so years after the end of the war. After interviewing 34 former patients, who had all received treatment in military hospitals after the end of the war, the psychiatrists concluded that in the majority of cases the former partisans had suffered from "superficial neurosis" that did not harm deeper layers of their personality, and consequently they faced no larger problems reintegrating into postwar society. This was true particularly for those interviewees who were younger than 18 at the time of their seizures: according to the study, they overcame their neurotic disorders very easily, since those appeared to be just a phase in the maturation and development of their personality.[17] The authors recommended superficial psychotherapy, with

---

[14] Klajn (1995), 109.
[15] Klajn (1995), 69–70.
[16] Klajn (1995), 79–80.
[17] Stjepan Betlheim et al., "Adaptacija ratnih neurotika," *Vojno-sanitetski Pregled* 9 (1957), 508–9.

particular attention to mental hygiene measures and prevention. In their conclusion, this group of eminent military psychiatrists argued that the outbreak of "partisan hysteria" did not seem to have left any deeper wounds in the Yugoslav society: the former neurotics apparently shed their neurotic condition fairly quickly and were able to adapt to the peacetime circumstances without major disturbances. They were cured: they out-grew their "hysteria," leaving it behind in the course of their personal development, education and perhaps also their social ascent.

Except for this final piece of psychiatric analysis, which confirmed the complete disappearance of Yugoslav soldiers' war trauma from the socialist state, there were no further psychiatric, political or cultural references to "partisan hysteria" following the heated discussions of the immediate postwar months and years. The diagnosis itself seemed to have vanished from Yugoslavia's public discourse, and the first (and only) time this com-plex neurosis re-appeared was in Mica Popovic's highly controversial 1968 film *Delije* ("Heroes").[18] Even though this film refrained from any explicit criticism of the regime, its close examination of two young partisans' dif-ficult re-adjustment to peacetime circumstances in 1945 proved too sub-versive to the authorities, and *Delije* was withdrawn from cinema distribution before it ever had a chance to premiere.[19] It remains (to my knowledge) the only piece of visual art which directly depicted bouts of partisan neurosis—in the form of a young partisan woman, whose unsta-ble psychological state turns her into a truly tragic figure. Her two seizures followed the descriptions in Klajn's and Betlheim's psychiatric treatises—they were violent, gave expression to her own traumatic experiences in the war, and consisted of re-enactments of wartime situations and language; they were shown as highly public, as the woman had to be restrained by her comrades or random passers-by, but after each seizure, the woman was simply abandoned by everyone and left to her own devices, if occasionally pitied, even though it was clear that her psychological state was rapidly deteriorating (in a memorable scene, she tries to board a train together with her comrades but is a few seconds late and is therefore left behind, running desperately after them, crying and gradually losing any hope that

[18] *Delije*, dir. Mica Popovic (1968).
[19] Milan Nikodijevic, *Zabranjeni bez zabrane: Zona aumraka jugoslovenskog filma* (Belgrade: Jugoslovenska kinoteka, 1995).

she might be able to continue her return journey to her village).[20] In contrast to the postwar psychiatrists' interpretations, moreover, in Popovic's film "partisan hysteria" is understood solely in the context of war-related psychological suffering—exposure to as well as perpetration of extreme violence. While in Klajn's and Betlheim's treatises and case histories such hysterical seizures often served as tools for the partisans' self-promotion or as protest if they did not receive awards and recognitions, the young woman in *Delije* only relives her own unprocessed wartime distress and does not seem to have any ulterior careerist motives: "if only you knew how they shot at us…," she screams.

But Popovic's engagement with partisan neurosis was not limited to a minor character: more importantly, the two brothers themselves represent some of the most important emotional and psychological traits of the feared postwar partisan hysteric. Unfortunately, the brothers remained unable to overcome or grow out of their psychological predicament, and their hopeless, desperate and ultimately tragic attempts at reintegrating belied the idea that soldiers' neurosis and traumatic memories could be left behind easily, or that the war only damaged superficial layers of their psyche.

The brothers, Gvozden and Isidor, fit the ill soldiers described on the pages of Klajn's book a bit too neatly for this resemblance to have been a mere coincidence: they are deeply immature (both socially and sexually), extremely politically confused and uninformed, and disturbingly unaware (and incapable) of any postwar revolutionary tasks. In addition, they are both peasants and barely literate, with no formal education and, coming from an extremely underdeveloped region, they would most certainly be described as "primitive" in the psychiatric and medical culture of postwar Yugoslavia.

Just as in the historical cases of partisan hysteria, Isidor and Gvozden are most unsettled at the prospect of demobilization—they are both certain that the end of the war means the end of their lives. Gvozden takes the news of demobilization with resigned calm: "I understand, we are not needed anymore, we had served our duty," while their female comrade gives voice to their true feelings, screaming "I can't live!" These reactions echoed those of many of Klajn's patients, whose profound disorientation

[20] After the young woman had a seizure in the street, one of the brothers, himself deeply damaged by the war, says dismissively "as if we don't know what women's nerves are, and what they are for!"

at the end of the war left them angry that their capabilities as soldiers were suddenly less important and seemingly underestimated. For instance, 20-year-old peasant Niko N., demonstrated this sentiment very clearly: as Klajn reported, Niko stated that he first started getting seizures because he was "'unnerved that the war had ended,' because now soldiers were facing tasks which he, as an illiterate person, could not and would not accomplish. He wished the war was still going on."[21] Like Niko and Klajn's other patients, Isidor and Gvozden were constantly reliving the war and war situations, which irretrievably transformed their lives and psyche; their dreams were exclusively of the war.

The sentence "it's over" became a leitmotif of sorts throughout this film. Repeated over and over again by various protagonists, mainly by Gvozden himself, it referred to the end of the war, the death of the brothers' family, the tragic obliteration of their village by the Germans, but also to the end of any life possibilities for the two brothers in the aftermath of the war and the subsequent revolution. As Gvozden concludes upon their return to their destroyed village, "we fought for other people's lives." Or, as another one of Klajn's patients, Nikola P. put it, "this was not what I fought for." While in wartime he had been "fierce, throwing bombs, shooting [...] yelling and breaking," now Nikola complained of injustice, his own poverty and living conditions. In that sense, the postwar as a concept becomes impossible and inconceivable from Gvozden's and Isidor's perspectives: as their commander lectures about postwar, civilian battles awaiting them—"battles for a new man... continue in your homes, families, workplaces"—they look extremely unsettled and clearly fail to take in the meaning of those important words. In contrast, the one moment when the brothers' faces shine with happiness and renewed confidence is when they hear distant shots in their village and run in their direction hoping that the war has started again ("God willing," whispers Gvozden as they approach)—unfortunately for them, they only encounter a hunting party, the members of which inevitably laugh at them, while the scowling head of a killed bear appears to mock their naiveté.[22]

But while in the psychiatric interpretations, the trauma of demobilization was almost always tightly linked to soldiers' concerns about their

---

[21] Klajn (1995), 78.

[22] Marko Krstic, "Apsurd podela, pobede I slobode: 'Covek iz hrastove sume' I 'Delije' Mice Popovica," in *Novi kadrovi: Skrajnute vrednosti srpskog filma*, ed. by Dejan Ognjanovic and Ivan Velisavljevic (Belgrade: Clio, 2008), 289.

status and their inability to rise through the ranks, Isidor's and Gvozden's simple-mindedness and ingenuousness left no space for ambition or careerism: it was the wooden chests which they carried around—a not so subtle metaphor for the heavy psychological and emotional baggage of their violent war-waging days—that made it impossible for them to move on. The chests were filled with weapons, and the brothers' constant ominous references to them throughout the film indicated how deeply and irretrievably their personalities had been transformed by the orgy of violence which had surrounded them for four years.

The film depicts the volatility of the postwar situation, which was clearly described in Klajn's patient case files; the brothers' pent-up aggression remains a constant threat to the people (and children) whom they encounter on their way and who might inadvertently trigger their violent impulses and painful memories. Throughout the film, the brothers repeat how they are itching to use their rifles again, and how "sweet" it would be to fire them. Once they take their weapons out of the boxes, towards the end of the film, the spiraling of violence out of control seems inexorable: Isidor in particular behaves uncontrollably and cannot stop shooting, apparently oblivious to any external stimuli. The brothers' death is tragic precisely because it is inevitable. In fact, the entire final sequence of the film, when Isidor is chasing the one remaining German soldier in the village, could be read as a protracted seizure of a typical partisan hysteric. The "mad Kraut" (*ludi Svaba*) reportedly lost his mind when his unit was ordered to kill and burn the entire village: he shot and murdered his comrades instead and stayed on in the area hiding in the mountains and occasionally throwing small stones at passers-by. In the final scenes, Isidor slowly descends into a psychotic state and starts chasing the German in the barren, lunar landscape of his destroyed village, reliving, and relishing in, the wartime memories and experiences, which he and his brother pined for throughout the film. After he kills the German, Isidor runs and laughs uncontrollably, and continues shooting and singing—possible further references to the behavior of those suffering from "partisan neurosis."

Suffering and Revolution

The brothers' family had been obliterated—as was their house and the entire village—while death, loss and misery now permeate the postwar reality of their home region. Isidor's and Gvozden's reaction to this news was ambivalent and understated: even though they appear indifferent

throughout most of the film—singing, joking and laughing quite frequently—their grief and incredulity in the face of a tragedy of such pro-
portions occasionally comes to the fore. Isidor in particular seems to have
a difficult time coping with the losses—asking over and over again "who
killed Manojlo, I wish I knew" (in addition, the film repeatedly cuts to a
shot with this sentence written on the wall, which then becomes one of
the core motives throughout the story, even though we never learn who
Manojlo was and why his death was troubling Isidor so much), and trying,
with heartbreaking urgency, to get an eyewitness to tell him more about
the perishing of their family. In a crucial scene, Gvozden scolds his brother:
"You can't sing and not think. You can't forget. It doesn't work. No
father, no mother. No house. It's over." Gvozden's words point out, in a
simple and straightforward manner, the painful paradox of Yugoslavia's
war victory and postwar reconstruction: in the midst of revolutionary celebrations and victorious enthusiasm for building a new and better society,
the all-pervasive grief and mourning sat uncomfortably, incongruously,
and masses of those whose lives were irretrievably scarred by the war's
tragedies did not always find easy ways to express their sorrow while
responding to the state's postwar expectations.

In the film, the brothers appear gloomy and awkward as they mingle
with street celebrations and merriment, failing to take in the carnivalesque
atmosphere of the very end of the war. They are as profoundly uncomfortable with such public parties as when they are themselves celebrated as
postwar heroes or forced into any ordinary social contacts and relationships. The psychological wounds of the war are everywhere, marring the
joyful surface of the postwar days: the brothers come across a variety of
deeply tragic figures whose return to society seems impossible—men crying and cursing furiously on the railway tracks while waiting to board a
train loaded with caskets carrying their dead family members; a mother
crazed with grief and anxiety, begging them to help release her imprisoned
daughter (the narrator's voice tells us that the woman "was worn down
[*pohabala se*] in one night" when her daughter was arrested by the new
authorities, and that "she remembers that people used to say that she had
laughed in the past.") Gvozden's "it's over" certainly applies to all of
them. Their pain and misery regularly act as an awkward, almost embar-
rassing reminder of the war's long dark shadow.

The figure of a dark, psychologically troubled person against the background of public end-of-the-war festivities became a common one in
Yugoslav films of the late 1950s and 1960s, and particularly in Black Wave

cinema. In Branko Bauer's *Tri Ane* ("Three girls named Ana"), the main protagonist is a retired tram driver whose young daughter disappeared after a Chetnik massacre during the war, but who is suddenly informed, years after 1945, that she might have survived.[23] The father's grief and desperate determination to find his child still cause benevolent bemusement among his neighbors and friends who appear permanently astonished by Red Cross statistics indicating very high numbers of missing persons in postwar Yugoslavia, as if this information did not correspond to their own experiences and memories, as if the war had happened to someone else. Clad in black, the father pushes through crowds of jubilant people, in whose joy he could never partake. This motive is taken even farther in Purisa Djordjevic's widely acclaimed 1967 film *Jutro* ("Morning"), which narrates, in a beautifully poetic as well as an often ironic manner, the very last day of the war in a small Serbian town.[24] *Jutro* juxtaposes the sheer joy of victory and survival and a deep, inspired commitment to the revolution with the unspeakable anguish of those who lost their loved ones in the previous four years (or might still lose them in the course of Communist reprisals). As one film critic noted, while *Jutro* symbolizes the dawn of the new era and the "gun fire has stopped, struggles still continue within ourselves. In the film, we see both blossoming fruits and dead people hanging from the trees. Flowers and corpses denote a moment in which the end of the war and the beginning of peace merge into one."[25]

But Djordjevic's film sought to demonstrate more than the mere coexistence of such contradictory emotions and psychological states: it emphasized the incongruousness of these two motives in often provocative ways, and partly because of this, *Jutro* caused major political controversies and debates among Yugoslavia's cultural public.[26] One of the most colorful and provocative characters, partisan Mali, attracted particularly severe disapproval from more conservative sections of the audience, and in particular of those who saw themselves as the guardians of the memory of the revolution. Mali was accused of disrespecting the victims of the war, when, at one of his comrades' funerals, he announced that he was simply too elated to have survived to weep and feel true sorrow: "I can't feel

---

[23] *Tri Ane*, dir. Branko Bauer (1959).
[24] *Jutro*, dir. Purisa Djordjevic (1967).
[25] Abel Desi, "Poetska istina 'Jutra'," *Borba*, November 17, 1967.
[26] Radina Vucetic, *Koka-kola Socijalizam* (Belgrade: Sluzbeni glasnik, 2012); Bogdan Tirnanic, *Crni Talas* (Belgrade: Filmski centar Srbije, 2008), 49–65.

sorry for anyone anymore, [...] I can't lie anymore when everything in me rejoices that I managed to stay alive, my ears, eyes, feet." Mali's response, often dismissed as too cynical by contemporary critics and commentators, still captured very well the complex, apparently irresolvable contradictions of that liminal postwar moment: as the film zooms in on his dead friend's obituary ("our beloved son and brother, shot in December 1944..."), Mali invites his female comrade to go dancing. In Djordjevic's (and Mali's) defense, film critic Zivko Milic argued that Mali was hardly a monster but an authentic representative of Yugoslavia's postwar "morning of the victory," which, despite the massacres, death and mass grieving, was marked by "outbursts of delight": "on that day, in our streets as well as in the souls of our people, were there lights of joy, were there round dances everywhere, or did everything look like a funeral?"[27] But Djordjevic likely did aim to do more than simply describe the elated atmosphere of the immediate postwar: the very outrageousness of Mali's words was meant to challenge and provoke, and it indicated that happiness, celebrations and enjoyment might have come at the expense of grieving, that they made the articulation and expression of sorrow and mourning impossible. As a young female partisan says to a Soviet officer who jokingly asks her what she would do if he dies during the upcoming battle for Berlin, "We will cry a little, but then we will forget."

Jutro begins with a memorable sentence, uttered by one of its leading female characters: "peace resounded like a bomb," which emphasizes multiple psychological continuities between wartime and peacetime. The film's cheerful and breezy tone is, however, often intercut with deeply disturbing scenes of grieving or dead people and with narratives of wartime brutalities. Juxtaposed with Mali's *joie de vivre* are the drawn, haggard faces of elderly women and men who march around the town carrying photographs of their dead or missing family members, attempting to find out how they died. An arrested Chetnik soldier is walked through the town before his execution, chanting "I killed seventy-two of your comrades," while a crowd of desperate locals follows him around, showing him their sons', daughters', fathers' or neighbors' photographs as he explains with chilling calmness and indifference how and where he slaughtered each one of them.

The song which runs through the film further symbolizes the complex emotional moment of this extraordinary last day of war and first day of

[27] Zivko Milic, "'Jutro' ne laze," *Borba*, November 10, 1967.

peace. The melody and the female singer's voice are cheerful, light and buoyant, but this cheerfulness is undermined by the song's unnerving lyrics, which narrate the seemingly endless list of names of all those who were killed or slaughtered in the course of the war, by the "Germans, Bulgarians, Hungarians." As we watch the town prepare for a mass funeral, and family members and neighbors gather in somber silence, the song warns that "the Germans have killed the face" of the town, and wonders how to tell all the mothers, sisters, girlfriends about so many deaths of their dearest, doubting whether they might be able to recover. "It is peace, but Jovan is dead," laments the song further, asking what to do with all the pain and absences once the morning arrives and the war is finally and formally over. When the morning of the revolution dawns, will true peace be possible, or has, as the song cryptically concludes, this "new-born freedom shot peace in the heart?"[28]

In 1961, young film director Zivojin Pavlovic condemned Yugoslavia's film industry as a whole, accusing it of no less than "falsifying" the history of World War II and the revolution. "Recalling memories burnt by the war, poring through authentic documents and photographs, and carrying the scars of heavy traumas which that time left on our childhoods," the generations growing up in the aftermath of the war, concluded Pavlovic, had to notice that a true and complete artistic representation of this "bloody and fateful history" was completely missing from Yugoslav filmography, even though numerous World War II films had been produced.[29] In these acclaimed war movies, the soldiers and activists who created the venerated legacy of the revolution seemingly "did not truly waste away in dungeons, did not die and did not kill." Pavlovic protested vehemently against the Yugoslav film artists' tendency to sanitize and beautify the enormous tragedies and psychological suffering of wartime and cover them with "idealized romanticism," producing the "kitsch of the revolution instead of revolutionary art." Juxtaposing a photograph of an actual partisan soldier—ragged, emaciated but with a supremely determined look in his eyes—with a still from an early Yugoslav war film, depicting polished, made-up and well-dressed partisans, Pavlovic asked whether it was not "shameless for 'art' to give [real resistance soldiers] such doubles" as in the second picture. Instead of dealing honestly with "tragic deaths," Yugoslav war films offered "dilettante performances." In Pavlovic's view,

---

[28] Goulding (1985), 91–3.
[29] Zivojin Pavlovic, "Laz o revoluciji," *Danas*, July 5, 1961.

this sustained artistic "lie about the revolution" in fact offended those whose lives were permanently scarred by the tragedy of the German occupation, civil war and ideological infighting, denying them authentic (and poetic) representation and an opportunity to grapple with the difficult social and psychological legacies of the all-pervasive death and violence.[30]

Pavlovic's angry article did not pass unnoticed. Unsurprisingly, it was Vjeko Afric, the director of the very first World War II film *Slavica* (also hailed as Yugoslavia's first sound film), who took issue with Pavlovic's (rather harsh) interpretations. In Afric's response, it became clear that any artistic insistence on suffering, trauma and psychological pain experienced in the course of the war was seen as incompatible with narratives of struggle, proud resistance and victory: "does [Pavlovic] think that our fighters for freedom died tragically? That they suffered in silence? That they went down under the blows of fate? [...] Our fighters fought and died. Under the gallows they still fought. This is what the raised fist of Stevan Filipovic [a partisan about to be hanged] tells us, not about 'tragic deaths.'"[31] In this narrative, therefore, Pavlovic's suggestion that World War II visited tragic deaths and individual suffering upon citizens of Yugoslavia (and its resistance soldiers in particular) worked to undermine the history of struggle, fighting and resistance: those who fought and felt no fear in the face of occupiers did not die tragically, and those who resisted could not have suffered, even though they might have experienced unspeakable hardships and torture. In this sense, for Afric, a former partisan himself and one of Yugoslavia's foremost directors at the time, the very fact of revolutionary resistance and heroic anti-fascist struggle denied the possibility of suffering and tragedy; the latter were reserved for those who "took it in in silence."[32]

Afric's response was quite representative of the official take on this debate. Petar Volk, one of Yugoslavia's most influential film and theatre critics, scholars and decision-makers, referred to Mica Popovic's *Delije* as a "strange and difficult film," and dismissed its complex engagement with the war's damning psychological legacies as an attempt to "make waging wars senseless and turn victory and freedom into sources of new misery

---

[30] Ibid., 17.
[31] Vjeko Afric, "'Laz o revoluciji'," *Danas*, July 5, 1961.
[32] Ibid., 2.

and absurdity."[33] Moreover, in Volk's interpretation, the film's overbearing cynicism denied the very meaning of life. Popovic's exploration of the emotional turmoil and internal struggles faced by those who lost everything in the war was thus deemed subversive in and of itself, as it might undermine the Yugoslav audience's confidence in the overall meaning of the revolution and anti-fascist resistance.[34] As Volk noted in relation to another one of Popovic's controversial films, such close examinations of people's descent into destructiveness and criminality might "kill faith in man" and "threaten our humanity."[35]

It is striking that in Yugoslavia, whose population suffered one of the most brutal occupation systems in World War II Europe and witnessed (and took part in) a merciless civil war, discussing the tragic nature of the 1940s and their possible psychological legacies proved to be controversial. In his contribution to the public debate about Purisa Djordjevic's *Jutro*, film critic Zivko Milic felt it appropriate to remind his collocutors that "war is an awful human tragedy and the fact that our revolution had a progressive role did not mean that it was not a war as well, that it did not have its sinister side of horrors."[36] Here, Milic seemed to object to the idea that revolution and suffering were incompatible, and that narratives of tragic wartime losses and psychological sacrifices somehow undermined the achievements, legacies and progress of the revolution. Moreover, Milic continued, "hating the war does not mean hating the revolution, it does not even mean hating those who took part in the war, its flags, its victories." In other words, an honest appraisal and remembrance of war-related psychological wounds and war's emotional toll did not tarnish the heroic memory of resistance, anti-fascism and socialist victory. However, Milic's article might also offer a glimpse into why postwar discussions of "war traumas" were so difficult and controversial: writing of the war's horrors, he urged the public to understand and accept the film director's decision to show even those "individuals who, as victims of war psychosis, behaved

---

[33] Petar Volk, *Svedocenje: Hronika jugoslovenskog filma 1945–1970,* 2. deo (Belgrade: NIP Knjizevne Novine, 1975), 144.

[34] Volk followed the Party line: subsequent to the release of *Delije*, the Yugoslav Communist Party's Commission for Culture condemned the film's attempt to "soil the revolution and all its legacies, putting a question mark over everything that was good and positive in that revolution." Quoted in: Radina Vucetic, *Monopol na istinu: Partija, kultura I cenzura u Srbiji sezdesetih I sedamdesetih godina XX veka* (Belgrade: Clio, 2016), 274.

[35] Volk (1975), 144.

[36] Zivko Milic, "'Jutro' ne laze," *Borba*, November 10, 1967.

in ways which might be unexpected in a civilization aspiring to be humanistic." It would appear that Milic's understanding of "war psychosis" and
its victims only extended to those members of the victorious army who
acted in objectionable and inhumane ways, who might have compromised
the revolution and the purity of the Communist Party's victory through
their troubled and unreasonable actions. Importantly, this narrow reading
of war trauma seemingly excludes all other (military and civilian) victims
who may have struggled to cope with their unspeakable wartime experiences, and makes it easier to understand why Yugoslav officials, leaders of
veteran organizations and more traditional film makers preferred to avoid
any detailed discussions of the issue.[37]

Given Zivojin Pavlovic's strong opinions about cinematic representations of the war in Yugoslavia, it is unsurprising that his 1969 film *Zaseda*
("Ambush") proved to be so politically (and even artistically) controversial.[38] Pavlovic himself described the film as a product of his own childhood trauma, and his troubled memories of the immediate postwar
violence and disappointments: "something stormed out of me there – my
experience, my spasm over history, which included my childhood and
youth, my spasm over divisions, dilemmas, differences... over the fate of a
community which was created then and whose roots dated to that time."[39]
The film follows yet another complex lead character, Vrana, whose tragic
wartime losses only seem to increase his pure faith in the revolution and in
building a better world. But the events and trends he witnesses in a small
town in the immediate aftermath of the war cause him increasing distress,
and his enthusiasm steadily turns into depression, anxiety and bitterness.
Just as in Milic's observation, the deceitful and intolerant behavior of
some of Vrana's comrades seems to be linked to traumatic experiences: for
instance, following the show trial of one of the town's distinguished figures, a group of young Communists proceeds to vandalize his house in a
bout of aggression and zealousness which indicates their unstable psychological state. As one film critic complained when the film was released, it
was the partisans' "instincts"—political, sexual, psychological—which
were portrayed as pathological, irretrievably perverting the revolutionary

---

[37] For some of their very critical responses to the "black-wave" cinema, see also Dusan
Miljanic, "Velika laz o jednom vremenu," *Borba*, November 14, 1967; Radoje Radojevic,
"Poricanje smisla revolucionarne borbe," *Borba*, November 7, 1967.

[38] *Zaseda*, dir. Zivojin Pavlovic (1969).

[39] Tirnanic (2008), 94.

dream.[40] In addition, the film depicts the psychological and emotional price of multiple conflicts and divisions—social, political, ideological— which played out in the postwar months and years. In the heady days of Yugoslav Stalinism, according to Pavlovic, the revolution showed its brutal face, drawing the population in while playing on their psychological or moral weaknesses.[41] Avdo Humo, a prominent member of the Communist Party's Commission for Culture, condemned *Zaseda*'s narrative line, which, in his opinion, portrayed the partisans literally "losing their minds" after years of fighting and infighting.[42] Pavlovic's film was additionally politically disruptive in its portrayal of Vrana as the only true, honest revolutionary, whose death at the Communists' own hands signified that, already in 1945, such ideals were dead as well.

In *Zaseda*, more than in any other film focusing on psychological trauma, the political disruptiveness of narratives about the personal suffering of war participants came to the fore, while Pavlovic linked his harsh critique of the foundations of the Yugoslav regime with an exploration of dire psychological effects of the immediate postwar era.[43] As one critic of the film exclaimed, "where are the joys and passions, where is the laughter and exaltation, the brightness and self-confidence, where is the life of a revolution!"[44] Unlike some of the most popular war films of the time, *Zaseda* did nothing to maintain the "revolutionary enthusiasm" of the Yugoslav population, digging instead into the origins of the communist state and shedding unforgiving light on the wounds which the revolution inflicted upon its own most valuable heroes. A jury member of Yugoslavia's most prestigious film festival in Pula, Croatia, noted that *Zaseda* should be given a prize because it "distressed viewers the most," while another believed that the film was "a great truth." Still, despite winning a large number of jury votes, *Zaseda* was not honored with any of the most

---

[40] "Ostaje nam da cutimo I da patimo," *Knjizevne novine*, August 16, 1969 (minutes of the special jury meeting of the Fifteenth Yugoslav Film Festival in Pula, July 26–August 2, 1969).

[41] Zivojin Pavlovic, *Djavolji film: Ogledi I razgovori* (Belgrade: Institut za film, 1969), 202.

[42] Quoted in Vucetic (2012), 288.

[43] For a more detailed account of the regime's harsh criticism of the film, see Vucetic (2016), 285–9.

[44] Veljko Micunovic, "Tematika domaceg filma," in Fedor Hanzekovic and Stevo Ostojic, eds, *Knjiga o filmu*, (Zagreb: Spektar, 1979), 393.

important awards, having been deemed too ideologically and politically "flawed" and an "angry negation of history."[45]

Perpetrators

While these cinematic narratives directly addressed the complex conse-quences of witnessing or experiencing extreme violence, one of the core themes of Black Wave war films was the trauma of perpetrating violence, of becoming a murderer. This was clearly an issue that would have affected large numbers of Yugoslavs who lived through the war: soldiers from the Yugoslav lands who fought on all sides were a primary concern, but another important and common trope developed in relation to civilians who might have engaged in different forms of violent collaboration while the country experienced an exceptionally brutal occupation system. This was far from a uniquely Yugoslav phenomenon: in Britain as well, for instance, postwar authorities and "psy" professionals grew increasingly anxious about the volatility of violent, destructive impulses which might have been triggered by the external violence of World War II. Some of the most important Black Wave films (as well as pieces of literature) expressed this anxiety about the future of a society which now consisted of possibly experienced perpetrators, whose impulses, reactions and psychological structures might have been irretrievably altered through their involvement in murders and executions. Frequently, the same people would be both—victims and perpetrators of violence—which further complicated postwar challenges and dangers.

In *Delije*, it was the extreme immersion in violence as perpetrators which made it impossible for the brothers to resume their peacetime social roles ever again. In a flashback, Isidor remembers how difficult it was for him to perpetrate his first wartime execution (of a German soldier): after the shooting, which he performed together with his brother, he froze and vomited, while Gvozden encouraged (or consoled) him—"you'll get used to it." The problem was, this film suggested, that Isidor and Gvozden did get used to shooting—and murder—as a normal, even necessary aspect of life, and were apparently hardly able to control themselves once demobi-lized: their obsession with violence meant that they found no other way to release their fears, frustrations and psychological pain. Through their con-versations about the existence of God and from flashbacks, it becomes

---

[45] "Ostaje nam da cutimo I da patimo," *Knjizevne novine*, August 16, 1969.

clear that they were religious before the war but lost that faith through their participation in numerous executions. In *Jutro*, the lightness and carelessness of some of the postwar executions of civilians is shocking, and the partisans who perform them appear unable to feel any empathy for fellow human beings in those moments (even though those same partisans are by no means depicted as monsters): when, at a party, a local piano player, for instance, admits that he served as a German translator during the occupation, he is shot immediately, on the spot, without any prevarication or further inquiry.

One of the most deeply unsettling scenes in this respect comes from yet another film which offered an anguished personal (rather than heroic epic) narrative of the war from the point of view of a partisan soldier turned tragic hero. Stole Jankovic's 1978 *Tren* ("Moment"), based on another war-veteran Antonije Isakovic's acclaimed novel, follows Arsen's internal ethical struggles throughout his challenging wartime experiences. His arrival in his home village at the end of the war deals the worst blow to the partisan's psychological stability: upon his return, he finds his house destroyed and his entire family killed.[46] But it is the realization that his family was the only one targeted by the Nazis in this way that sets Arsen off on a quest to understand how this might have occurred. When it becomes clear that the entire village betrayed his family in order to save themselves, Arsen faces his neighbors in long and torturous conversations, in which the villagers are portrayed as, at the same time, victims of extreme violence, silent witnesses of suffering and complicit in murder and destruction. The villagers explain that, after the body of a German soldier appeared in the water, they were required by the occupation authorities to surrender a certain number of hostages from their midst to be shot in reprisals. They directed the Germans to Arsen's family and told them he was in the Communist resistance.

When Arsen confronts the villagers, they gather in a circle around him: the dividing line between them could not be clearer, Arsen is completely alone, a moral hero of pure conscience but carrying unbearable pain; he could never again be part of the village community, which held responsibility for the death of the innocent. The village elders seem to be undecided regarding the value of re-telling this difficult story, and of revealing the truth: they do want to commemorate the tragedy of Arsen's family through formal rites and monuments, but reject any continuous

---

[46] *Tren*, dir. Stole Jankovic (1978).

reminders of the pain they helped inflict (as it transpires, they killed the family's dog following the execution, because its barking and whimpers made it impossible to forget what had happened, and also indicated the dog's hope that someone—Arsen—might return and exact revenge). This scene still ultimately plays out like group therapy, in which the villagers relive their own complicity and other wartime experiences, recount what they did and ask for forgiveness. The villagers are themselves deeply ambivalent about their own role in the executions, however, and they never take full responsibility: "war is always dirty, it tumbles everything," one of them says; another one adds that "people must defend themselves in war," and the line between victims and perpetrators is blurred even further when the village elders start recounting their own suffering and extreme fear at the hands of multiple occupation armies which passed through their community in Arsen's absence. The very participation in the betrayal of Arsen's family seemed to have caused exceptional grief as well, and one village elder breaks down in tears remembering the moment when he was tasked with choosing ten hostages from the village: "counting the tribute in blood – it's horrific business."

The villagers recognize this war as fundamentally different from any other conflict in their memory, precisely because of its totality, which both targeted civilians and demanded their involvement in massacres and hostilities. "It was your war," one of the village elders tells Arsen, in a strangely accusatory tone, "a different war, internal, without borders." Arsen's former neighbors do not believe in "his" wars and revolutions, but, as penance for their deeds, they are willing to obey his decisions: "we want to come with you, to your socialism. We will elect you as president, nobody else, the one and only authority, rule over us, we will endure." From the point of view of postwar reconstruction and recovery of communities and individuals, this was perhaps the film's most unsettling message: psychologically compromised and deeply morally damaged by their fateful and murderous choices in the war, the villagers are not capable of evolving into independent political citizens and full-fledged members of the new socialist society. They cannot contribute to the revolutionary makeover in any meaningful way. At best, they can offer to be obedient, docile, and "endure" the socialist government in order to escape any fundamental moral reckoning. Moreover, both the village community and Arsen appear to be irretrievably broken by the roles which the war and the occupation forced them to take on, and the act of confession does not seem to ease the pain of either party in any way: Arsen leaves the village in disgust, having turned gray within only a few hours, and never recovers from his loss (and his own sense of responsibility and guilt), while the villagers strive to perform their repentance and move on, but remain anxious and worried that Arsen might curse them. The film as a whole, and this final scene in particular, raise the question of the war's *longue durée* psychological and political effects, and offer a rather pessimistic interpretation of possible attempts to overcome such traumas through commemoration, political change or reconciliation.

PERSONAL AND NATIONAL TRAUMAS

By the 1980s, the political situation had changed radically, and this had a decisive effect on the public presentation and discussions of the notions of trauma and violence. For the first time, a Yugoslav film adopted a broadly psychoanalytic approach to the issue of war-related psychological suffering: Aleksandar Fotez's *Lazar* was made in 1984 and dealt with traumatic memory and repression by zooming in on a particularly troubled village family in postwar Serbia.[47] The film follows a mother and her son—Lazar—who eke out a miserable existence about twenty years after the war. The mother is deeply and permanently mentally disabled, while Lazar, born during the war, is mute and appears developmentally stunted; their lives seem to be frozen in the tragic events of the war, from which they could never move on. One day, the mother tells Lazar the full story of the experience which transformed their lives—a Chetnik attack at the very end of the war. The story of the war's escalating tragedies takes up the entire film and Lazar undergoes immense pain, at times trying to force his mother to stop talking, but once everything is told and relived, he grows out of his mutism and infantilism, and the sinister, lurking presence of the war's evil moves away from the house. It is necessary, the film seems to suggest, to relive and "work through" the most difficult of memories in order to break the traumatic event's hold on one's psyche. Once the "original trauma" is remembered, retold and shared, its effects become manageable.

Despite its prevailingly dark and labored atmosphere, the film ends on a surprisingly optimistic note. But by the mid-1980s there was little reason for political optimism, especially in relation to commemorating the war's most difficult events: in the public discourse, the issue of recovering "repressed" wartime memories came to the fore, but it was not personal

---

[47] *Lazar*, dir. Aleksandar Fotez (1984).

memories that political elites were addressing—the discussion moved to the plane of "national trauma" and the collective suffering of individual ethnic communities in Yugoslavia. In fact, the 1980s in Yugoslavia witnessed what Jasna Dragovic-Soso referred to as an "outburst of history": a period of intense reconsiderations of some of the most sensitive themes in Yugoslav communist historiography.[48] These discussions escalated—and became extremely popular well outside academic and intellectual circles—in the decade following Tito's death, when political, constitutional and economic crises were confounded by rising nationalist tensions in the multi-ethnic state. Unsurprisingly, they were dominated by nationalist revisionist reinterpretations of World War II and the establishment of socialist Yugoslavia. Such revisionist narratives were almost always couched in terms of repression: the supposed political repression of particular national or opposition groups, as well as the repression of traumatic memories of wartime massacres and crimes in the official socialist historiography. While the Yugoslav historiography of World War II and the attendant civil war by no means suppressed the historical knowledge and memory of fascist and collaborationist violence against civilians, it often aimed to "de-ethnicize" it, de-emphasizing the national belonging of both perpetrators and victims, and subsuming them under the overarching narrative of the Yugoslav peoples' common struggle against fascist occupation and bourgeois collaborators.

The most important and wide-ranging debates along these lines occurred in Serbia. From the early 1980s on, some of the most prominent Serbian intellectuals insisted that, in socialist Yugoslavia, Serbs, as the largest constitutive nation, suffered numerous injustices, while their enormous victimization at the hands of the Croatian Ustasha in the course of World War II remained a taboo. These historians, writers, poets saw the current political crisis as a result of the Serbian nation's subordinated position, and its alleged inability to mourn and get justice for its own wartime victims. In that sense, the Serbian people took the role of Lazar in the above-mentioned film—just like Lazar's illness could not be cured until the full horror of his wartime experience was openly recounted and relived, the Serbs had to have their own suffering acknowledged and aired in public

[48] Jasna Dragovic-Soso, *Saviours of the Nation: Serbia's Intellectual Opposition and the Revival of Nationalism* (Montreal: McGill-Queen's University Press, 2002), 64.

before their political community could heal and move on.[49] It is striking that this motive of the repression of traumatic memories played such an important role in the deterioration of relations between different national groups in Yugoslavia in the 1980s: the narrative of a victimized and suppressed nation, whose wartime suffering was further exacerbated by postwar humiliation and political weakening, was central to the Serbian national mobilization and the violent escalation of ethnic conflicts.[50] Towards the end of Yugoslavia, when complex psychological effects of difficult and violent wartime (and postwar) experiences could finally be discussed more openly in the public sphere, the attention of Serbian public opinion shifted away from personal suffering to commemorating collective, "national traumas."

These narratives of national injustice and victimization were developed primarily in literary works and theatre plays. Some of the most popular and widely read Yugoslav novels of the 1980s addressed the brutal crimes of the collaborationist Ustasha regime against Serbian and Jewish citizens of the wartime Independent State of Croatia; these novels abounded in gory details of the Ustasha violence, and often depicted socialist Yugoslavia as an artificial, forced political creation, built upon silence about the genocide against Serbs. Such works also sent a problematic message about the future of Yugoslavia's multi-ethnic structures: they often described lingering postwar tensions between different ethnic communities, primarily in Bosnia and Croatia, which, according to this interpretation, stemmed from their inability to talk about their wartime conflicts (and the role of Croat and Muslim populations in crimes against Serb civilians). Such is Jovan Radulovic's 1983 play *Golubnjaca* ("Pigeon Pit"), which poignantly painted the hopelessness and misery of a mixed Serb and Croat village of the 1960s.[51] The long shadow of the wartime massacre against Serbian villagers (whose bodies were thrown into a nearby ravine—the Pigeon Pit) made it impossible for either community to overcome such experiences, precisely because, according to the play, the socialist authorities prevented any serious discussion of those massacres, its victims and its perpetrators and their responsibility. The abyss which thus opened between the two

---

[49] David Bruce MacDonald, *Balkan Holocausts? Serbian and Croatian Victim-Centered Propaganda and the War in Yugoslavia* (Manchester: Manchester University Press, 2002); Đorđe Stanković, "Srpska medijalna kultura sećanja," *Tokovi istorije* 3 (2006), 274–5.

[50] Bette Denich, "Dismembering Yugoslavia: Nationalist ideologies and the symbolic revival of genocide," *American Ethnologist* 21:2 (1994).

[51] Jovan Radulovic, *Golubnjaca* (Belgrade: BIGZ, 1983).

communities could not be papered over in any way, and the play demonstrated how inter-ethnic hostility and lack of understanding were perpetuated in the behavior of the local children. The official ideology of communist "brotherhood and unity" was thus depicted as a hollow and at times cynical attempt to prevent entire families from seeking closure and justice for their unspeakable pain. The bleak reality of postwar multi-ethnic communities, filled with threats, fear and recriminations, could not be further from the communist aim of building a supranational state. The staging of the play was, unsurprisingly, very problematic, and it was repeatedly banned as it was deemed that "its treatment of relations between nations is unacceptable."[52] In spite of this, the narrative which the play promoted became the leitmotif of the 1980s. These were the roots of the subsequent (and widely accepted yet highly problematic) narrative of the 1990s' wars as an eruption of stifled ethnic conflicts, which had been brewing under the surface of the seemingly harmonious socialist Yugoslavia.

According to 1980s' Serbian public opinion, therefore, the fundamental conflict, which was at the core of Yugoslavia's political crisis and undermined the very possibility of multi-ethnic solidarity, was one between personal or family war memories of Serbs, and the official (repressive) state memory. The revival of those personal memories, however, was not to serve the purpose of psychological healing and emancipation of affected individuals: it was orchestrated by a variety of elites to foment fear of future crimes and massacres. The existence of supposedly unacknowledged past genocides against Serbs, and of the communist state's "conspiracy of silence," which Serbian intellectuals argued protected perpetrators in the name of political stability, was used to suggest that such crimes might happen again. The narrative of repressed traumatic memories promoted the idea that the Serbian nation was in existential danger yet again; for instance, a leading Serbian historian attempted to prove that the Croatian elites harbored centuries-long "genocidal intentions" towards Croatian Serbs.[53]

While the Serbian intellectual revisionist debates were the most wide-ranging and prominent, the late Yugoslav period saw a revival of a number of other painful historical memories, whose discussion was difficult and sensitive in the preceding decades. Alongside books and plays about Serbian victimhood, new memoirs and fictional works about inmates'

[52] Dragovic-Soso (2002), 106.
[53] Dragovic-Soso (2002), 111.

experiences at the Goli Otok camp—an exceptionally brutal prison where the Yugoslav regimes sent those suspected of pro-Stalinist sympathies following the 1948 break with the Soviet Union—flooded the Yugoslav market from the mid-1980s on.[54] At the same time, right-wing Croatian intellectuals, mirroring the Serbian debates, sought to portray Croats as the greatest victims of World War II, and raised the issue of the victorious communist army's reprisals against (collaborationist) Croat soldiers as well as large numbers of civilians in the final weeks of the war. Public commemorations of these victims in the Bleiburg Field (in Austria, near the Slovenian border, where thousands of retreating collaborationist military units, the Ustasha political leadership and many civilians surrendered to the British troops but were then sent back to Yugoslavia and captured by Tito's forces) continued throughout most of the socialist period but were heavily monitored by the Yugoslav intelligence services. The Bleiburg tragedy functioned as the core symbol of the communist repression of the Croat nation, and it quickly took center stage in the cultural politics of the newly independent Croatian state.[55] In that sense, the 1980s saw an exceptionally successful and widespread construction of mirroring narratives of repressed wartime traumas, violence and victimization, which were all linked to intensifying demands for a radical reconsideration of the history of World War II. Moreover, the wars of the 1990s were directly related to experiences of World War II precisely through such narratives of repressed memory and unarticulated trauma. At the end of Yugoslavia, in stark contrast to its early period, discussions about wartime "trauma" dominated the public sphere and political relations, but they served explicitly national(ist) rather than personal psychological aims.

---

[54] Dragovic-Soso (2002), 83.

[55] Vjeran Pavlakovic and Davor Paukovic, eds, *Framing the Nation and Collective Identities: Political Rituals and Cultural Memory of the Twentieth-Century Traumas in Croatia* (London: Routledge, 2019).

CHAPTER 8

Guilt, Responsibility and Trauma: Restoring the Moral Self-Image in Postwar Slovakia

Hana Kubátová

INTRODUCTION

Elegantly crafted, with subtle yet powerful acting, "The Shop on Main Street" (*Obchod na korze*, 1965) is one of the most praised Czechoslovak movies of all times. Based on a short story authored by Ladislav Grosman, a Holocaust survivor, the Oscar-winning drama unfolds as World War II is raging.[1] Situated in a small town of eastern Slovakia in the early 1940s, the

---

[1] The movie was inspired by a short story, "The Trap" (*Past*), which Ladislav Grosman adapted into a script and a novel by 1965, already bearing the name *Obchod na korze*. The movie was produced by directors Ján Kadár and Elmar Klos. In Great Britain, it appeared under the title *The Shop on High Street* but was screened as *The Shop on Main Street* for the North American audience. The movie starred Ida Kamińska as Rozália Lauptmannová, and Jozef Kroner as Tono Brtko. For a wider context, see for example, Jiří Holý, "The Six Versions of The Shop on Main Street," in *Aspects of Genres in the Holocaust Literatures in Central Europe*, ed. by Jiří Holý (Praha: Akropolis, 2015), 97–113.

H. Kubátová (✉)
Faculty of Social Sciences, Charles University, Prague, Czechia
e-mail: hana.kubatova@fsv.cuni.cz

© The Author(s), under exclusive license to Springer Nature Switzerland AG 2022
V. Kivimäki, P. Leese (eds.), *Trauma, Experience and Narrative in Europe after World War II*, Palgrave Studies in the History of Experience, https://doi.org/10.1007/978-3-030-84663-3_8

movie follows the unusual bond between Rozália Lauptmannová and Tono Brtko. Mrs. Lauptmannová, as she is typically referred to in the movie, is an old widow and hard of hearing. Immersed in a world that is long gone, she has only little understanding of things around her, let alone of the mounting anti-Jewish legislation in one of Nazi Germany's closest allies. For the clerical fascist regime of wartime Slovakia (1939–45),[2] Mrs. Lauptmannová is first and foremost a Jew and the owner of a small button shop located on the town's main street. While making little to no revenue, the shop, just like much else owned by the Jews, is now subject to "Aryanization," a euphemism for widespread robbery that made large sections of the society complicit in the Holocaust.[3] Tono Brtko is a middle-aged carpenter with little ambition in his life, an ordinary man on many accounts. Spurred on by his wife Evelína and assisted by his brother-in-law and member of the paramilitary Hlinka Guard (*Hlinkova garda*) Markuš Kolkotský, Tono, called in the movie by his first name most of the time, acquires Mrs. Lauptmannová's button shop. Where the movie seems to border on farce, Tono is softened by Mrs. Lauptmannová's vulnerability, remaining torn between his conscience and societal pressure. Unable to find the courage to disclose himself as the Aryanizer (*arizátor*), Tono assumes the role of a distant cousin. The movie climaxes in a tragic finale. Distressed about whose life to protect, Tono aggressively pressures Mrs. Lauptmannová to go into hiding and avoid being deported. Mrs. Lauptmannová, still unaware of what is happening but increasingly suspicious, suffers a fatal heart attack. Upon finding her dead, Tono commits suicide.

It was its focus on the "little" people, on the many like Tono and Mrs. Lauptmannová themselves, on the choices and experiences of "ordinary" men and women in the Holocaust, both Jews and Gentiles, that turned the movie into a "masterpiece, a flawless examination of the toll of indecision and the penalty of passive decency."[4] Reviewers from North America, where the movie was screened early on, seemed fascinated by the "deep

---

[2] Hana Kubátová and Michal Kubát, "The Priest and the State: Clerical Fascism in Slovakia and Theory," *Nations and Nationalism*, online first (November 30, 2020), https://doi.org/10.1111/nana.12664

[3] Hana Kubátová, *Nepokradeš! Nálady a postoje slovenské společnosti k židovské otázce, 1938–1945* (Praha: Academia, 2013).

[4] Eleanor Perry, "A Haunting Masterpiece of Unrequited Hate: The Shop on Main Street," *Life*, April 2, 1966, 8. See also Ján Kadár, "Not the Six Million but the One," *New York Herald Tribune*, 23 January 1966, https://www.criterion.com/current/posts/139-the-shop-on-main-street-not-the-six-million-but-the-one

affection" between Tono and Mrs. Lauptmannová, a couple that could be considered odd in peaceful times, let alone in the setting of a genocide.[5] They praised the "film's lasting power" in posing questions that were only rarely asked in public then: "If it had been you, what would you have done?"[6]

The response the movie received in then Communist Czechoslovakia was more complex. The unflattering portrayal of the majority society during World War II, seen as bearing its share of responsibility for the Holocaust, was difficult to digest for many. Alexander Dubček, the leader of the Slovak branch of the Communist Party of Czechoslovakia, apparently sent a letter to President Antonín Novotný, criticizing the movie for insulting the people of Slovakia and the memory of the Slovak National Uprising.[7] The argument Dubček was making is that with one of the largest resistance actions against Nazi Germany, lasting from 29 August until late October 1944, and involving more than 60,000 army personnel and 18,000 partisans on the side of the rebellion, Slovakia had no reason to be self-flagellating about its past. If there was any guilt for allying the country with Germany, it lay with an undefined and largely anonymous category of fascists. Resistance supposedly cleared the name of the people. The widespread participation in robbing the Jews was explained by resorting to the ideological language of the era. Emil Lehuta, a renowned film critic, for instance, dismissed what he understood as a schematic interpretation of the seizure of Jewish property in the movie. For Lehuta, public involvement in Aryanization needed to be understood as a consequence of class struggle.[8]

Taking the debate triggered by the movie as a point of departure, my chapter examines attempts at restoring the moral self-image in postwar Slovakia. For its history as a model Nazi ally during World War II, but

[5] Ben Kern, "'The Shop on Main Street' Told with Cinematic Skill," *Star Tribune*, 1966, 42. See also, e.g., Bosley Crowther, "The Shop on Main Street," *New York Times*, January 25, 1966.

[6] Perry (1966), 8.

[7] Arnošt Lustig and František Cinger, *3 x 18 (portréty a postřehy)* (Praha: Mladá fronta, 2007); *Obchod na korze, 1965: Interview with Elmar Klos jr.*, DVD (Praha: Bontonfilm, 2005); Radoslav Passia, "Ladislav Grosman—muž jedného scenára?" *Pravda*, December 11, 2015,   https://zurnal.pravda.sk/esej/clanok/376584-ladislav-grosman-muz-jedneho-scenara. Accessed April 20, 2020.

[8] Emil Lehuta, "Obchod na korze," *Slovenské pohľady* 82:1 (1966), 144.

equally so for its anti-fascist rebellion and the role the 1944 uprising played in official narratives of the past, I am interested in how complicity and collaboration were publicly processed, most often rejected but also acknowledged, in the period leading to the political "thaw" of the 1960s. I build on two arguments here. First, and in line with social identity theory, I understand that individuals are inclined to perceive their in-group, as well as in-group's actions in the past, favorably.[9] When the moral self-image of the in-group is threatened, individuals typically resort to what are called avoidance strategies. It is only when these fail that experiences of collective guilt may, but also may not, arise. While presenting a negative emotion, experiences of collective guilt are crucial for reducing bias and elevating intergroup relations.[10] Historians of the aftermath often equate avoidance strategies, be it in deflecting guilt onto others, minimizing the harm committed, or shifting attention to heroic accounts of World War II, such as resistance and rescue, with silence, with an absence of emotions. My chapter offers a different perspective. It treats avoidance strategies as a response to the voicing of experiences that conflicted with the official discourse, as a reaction to them being brought into sayability, to paraphrase Peter Leese's introduction to this volume.[11]

Second, understanding national identities as "built around symbolic commemorations of the past,"[12] nations as communities of "common memory and common destiny"[13] and nation-states as being both "new" and "historical,"[14] I bring further attention to the role of guilt, responsibility, and trauma in community formation and erosion. Referring to

[9] Henri Tajfel and John Turner, "The Social Identity Theory of Intergroup Behaviour," in *Psychology of Intergroup Relations*, ed. by Stephen Worchel and William G. Austin (Chicago, IL: Nelson-Hall, 1986), 7–24.

[10] See e.g., Michal Bilewicz, "History as an Obstacle: Impact of Temporal-Based Social Categorizations on Polish-Jewish Intergroup Contact," *Group Processes and Intergroup Relations* 10:4 (2007), 551–63.

[11] Peter Leese is referring here to the work of Targol Meshab, "Why Does the Other Suffer? War, Trauma and the Everyday," Ph.D. thesis (University of California, Santa Cruz, 2006), 44.

[12] Johanna Ray Vollhardt and Michal Bilewicz, "After the Genocide: Psychological Perspectives on Victim, Bystander, and Perpetrator Groups," *Journal of Social Issues* 69:1 (2013), 2.

[13] Mary Fulbrook, *German National Identity After the Holocaust* (Cambridge: Polity, 1999), 21.

[14] Benedict Anderson, *Imagined Communities: Reflections on the Origin and Spread of Nationalism* (London: Verso, 1991), 11.

works of Omer Bartov and Natalia Aleksiun on the everyday, even inti-mate nature of the Holocaust in Eastern Europe, I understand the Holocaust as communal genocide.[15] With neighbors seeing brutal round-ups, writes Bartov, hearing shots from nearby forests and, hence, having first-hand knowledge of the Holocaust, "it left a deep and lasting imprint on all surviving inhabitants of these localities."[16] Going beyond the notion of communal genocide, Anna Wylegała introduces the concept of com-munal trauma in her chapter on the memory of ethnic cleansing and mass violence in Eastern Galicia during World War II. For Wylegała, communal trauma encompasses "both traumatic experience by the entire community and the destruction of the community as such." Of course, there are important distinctions to draw between the wartime situation in Slovakia and that of Eastern Galicia. Yet, the Jewish-Gentile experience in the Holocaust was a tangled one in Slovakia, too, as the choices made by Tono and Mrs. Lauptmannová's chances of survival demonstrate in the movie.[17] Similarly entangled, even if conflicting, were also the responses to the events of the past.

As shown here, the immediate postwar decade was transformative for the memory of the Holocaust in Slovakia, and the public articulation of previously omitted themes in the cultural production of the 1960s, such as "The Shop on Main Street," was a culmination of a tension between the public remembering of the past and the experiences of Jews in wartime Slovakia. As former victims and perpetrators were expected to find a place as neighbors again, the category of the Slovak as a heroic victim was cemented with the help of a resistance mythology. This said, complicity in the Holocaust may have been avoided in the official discourse of World War II but the traumatic past, the experience of exclusion, violence, and

[15] On communal genocide, see Omer Bartov, "Communal Genocide: Personal Accounts of the Destruction of Buczacz, Eastern Galicia, 1941–44," in *Shatterzone of Empires: Coexistence and Violence in the German, Habsburg, Russian, and Ottoman Borderlands*, ed. by Omer Bartov and Eric D. Weitz (Bloomington: Indiana University Press, 2013), 399–420; Omer Bartov, *Anatomy of a Genocide: The Life and Death of a Town Called Buczacz* (New York: Simon & Schuster, 2018); Natalia Aleksiun, "Intimate Violence: Jewish Testimonies on Victims and Perpetrators in Eastern Galicia," *Holocaust Studies: A Journal of Culture and History* 23:1–2 (2017), 17–33.

[16] Bartov (2013), 44.

[17] Wulf Kansteiner, "Hidden in Plain View: Remembering and Forgetting the Bystander of the Holocaust on (West) German Television," in *Probing the Limits of Categorization: The Bystander in Holocaust History*, ed. by Christina Morina and Krijn Thijs (New York: Berghahn Books, 2018), 266–90.

murder was certainly not forgotten by Jewish witnesses. In this sense, to reiterate my argument, avoidance strategies should not to be mistaken for erased memories; they signify the very destruction of a commonality.

My theoretically driven chapter rests on historical documentation in the form of institutional written accounts, official newspapers but also ego-documents, such as testimonies. A category that lies somewhere in between institutional and personal sources are the letters and petitions addressed to official bureaus by individuals in charge of bodies that represented Jewish victims, many of them being survivors themselves. In this chapter, I am particularly interested in how the concept of harm or wrongdoing (*krivda*) was defined and utilized by a range of memory actors and vehicles.

Given the fact that my chapter places the restoring of the moral self-image at its center, I use terms "in-group" and "majority society" largely interchangeably here. This said, I find it important to distinguish between the terms "collective guilt" and "responsibility." Philosopher Hannah Arendt, debating the question of German collective guilt with psychiatrist and philosopher Karl Jaspers, among others, rejected the notion of collective guilt, setting it aside from what she called political responsibility. For Arendt, the concept of guilt, and hence also the concept of innocence, applies to individual actions only. Guilt is a moral and legal category, and "Where all are guilty, nobody is. Guilt, unlike responsibility, always singles out; it is strictly personal."[18] Distinguishing between guilt and responsibility is also useful for my chapter. Here, I follow political scholar Marion Young's interpretation of responsibility that "does entail *doing* things (and perhaps not doing things) but doing things that indirectly contribute to the enactment of crimes or wrongs."[19] In short, in what follows, I understand guilt as a legal category, collective guilt as an inward negative emotion that results from accepting in-group's responsibility for the committed harm—whether one was directly or indirectly, personally or not, implicated in the events.

My chapter proceeds as follows. I start by outlining the Slovak role in World War II and the Holocaust, clarifying how the country aligned itself with Nazi Germany and expanding on local complicity and collaboration in the destruction of historically multiethnic communities. I then expand

[18] Hannah Arendt, "Organized Guilt and Universal Responsibility," in idem, *Essays in Understanding, 1930–1954*, ed. by Jereme Kohn (New York: Harcourt-Brace, 1994 [1945]), 121–32.

[19] Iris Marion Young, *Responsibility for Justice* (Oxford: Oxford University Press, 2011), 81.

on the long shadows of the Holocaust, pointing to the different effects guilt, responsibility, and trauma had on the societies of Europe. I make a case for why Slovakia in particular and Eastern Europe in general needs to be more tightly integrated into scholarship on Holocaust memory and its restoration. I then expand on the different avoidance strategies that countries took to avoid facing responsibility for the harm committed. What follows is an empirical investigation into the parallel, and, at times, conflicting processing of the past by the postwar establishment, and by the Jewish witnesses in postwar Slovakia. From this perspective, the intertwined lives of Tono and Mrs. Lauptmannová, in "The Shop on Main Street," epitomize the tension between the heroic resistance-focused official narratives of World War II and the personal accounts of the Holocaust on the part of the Jewish witnesses.

THE COMPLICITY OF SLOVAKIA

Slovakia has enough reasons to reflect on its role in World War II and the Holocaust. The wartime Slovak Republic was established on 14 March 1939, a day before Nazi Germany occupied the Bohemian lands, installing Protectorate Bohemia and Moravia. Propaganda presented the historically first Slovak state as the fulfillment of a centuries-long quest for self-determination on the part of the people, and the regime as independent, liberated from alleged oppression in the first Czechoslovak republic (1918–39). In reality, the country's establishment was a mere side effect of a "deep political and moral crisis in Europe, German aggression and the break-up of pre-Munich Czechoslovakia."[20] While enjoying substantial self-rule until the suppression of the Slovak National Uprising and the subsequent German occupation of Slovakia in 1944, the country's independence was curtailed as early as on 23 March 1939 when a Treaty of Protection with the Third Reich entered into being. In return for guaranteeing its territorial integrity, a particularly sensitive point for newly established Slovakia following the Hungarian occupation of southern and southeastern parts of the country, the actions of the local administration with respect to military, foreign policy affairs and economy were to be

---

[20] Ivan Kamenec, "The Slovak State, 1939–1945," in *Slovakia in History*, ed. by Mikuláš Teich, Dušan Kováč and Martin D. Brown (New York: Cambridge University Press, 2011), 175.

taken in "close agreement" with Nazi Germany.[21] The Slovak government, led by President-Priest Jozef Tiso, obeyed the German master, sometimes going to great lengths to prove its loyalty. Slovakia was the only country that joined the German attack on Poland on 1 September 1939, which led to the outbreak of World War II. In November 1940, Slovakia joined the Axis powers and followed Germany and Italy in declaring war on the Soviet Union in June 1941 and on the Western powers, Great Britain and the United States, in December of that year. Slovakia's participation in Germany's war efforts was minimal in the larger picture of things, yet substantive, given its limited military, whose key officials had been trained in the Czechoslovak army and were hence reluctant to support the war effort in the first place. Nevertheless, the Slovak Army sent almost 60,000 men to the Eastern Front and while many were withdrawn and others deserted in the face of great losses, it fought the Soviet forces until August 1944.[22]

Slovakia's complicity was structural, in terms of allying with Nazi Germany, but also ideological, through pursuing an aggressive policy against its proclaimed enemies, the Czechs, Hungarians, Roma and especially the Jews. Before the outbreak of World War II, the country was home to approximately 89,000 Jews, two-thirds of whom were murdered in the Holocaust. While Nazi Germany held significant sway over Slovakia, the national establishment not only followed the Nazi lead in approaching the so-called Jewish question, but at times also initiated more draconian policies. Competition within different wings of the official Hlinka Slovak People's Party led to a further radicalization of the already harsh anti-Jewish measures. Given the fact that a majority of the population here identified with one of the Christian churches, most notably the Roman Catholic Church, Tiso and multiple other clergymen used their religious standing to sanction the persecution of the Jews, explaining the various discriminatory steps as being in accordance with Christian teaching. Propaganda encouraged the vision of a state that was finally "Slovak,"

---

[21] John Grenville and Bernard Wasserstein, eds, *The Major International Treaties of the Twentieth Century: A History and Guide with Texts* (London: Routledge, 2013), 219.

[22] Jozef Pecina and Michael Tkacik, "Eastern Front Operational Constraints on Slovak Artillery, 1941–1943," *The Journal of Slavic Military Studies* 18:1 (2005), 75–107. See also Igor Baka, *Slovenská armáda vo vojne proti Sovietskemu zväzu a slovensko-nemecké vzťahy 1941–1945* (Bratislava: Vojenský historický ústav, 2019); "Padlí, zomrelí a zabití slovenskí vojaci v priebehu protisovietskeho ťaženia (jún 1941—august 1944)," Ústav pamäti národa, accessed 25 April 2020, https://www.upn.gov.sk/sk/padli-zomreli-a-zabiti-sl-vojaci

liberated from the oppressive Jews, but also from the Czechs and the Hungarians. Official bureaus invited complicity by making the argument that the theft of Jewish belongings was intended to elevate the living conditions of the majority society. Many locals participated in robbing their former friends and neighbors. Auctions of properties often coincided with Jews being loaded onto carriages and deported to almost imminent death. Testimonies from non-Jewish witnesses not only provide evidence of them observing the deportations, seeing the removal of Jews firsthand, but demonstrate how locals informed the authorities on Jews in hiding.[23] Religious arguments lent further legitimacy to the fable about Aryanization as the rightful return of property to Gentiles. The promise that people would benefit from the state-sponsored theft of Jewish belongings resulted in the fact that, for the most part, Slovak politicians could count on support from below. Popular backing of the regime started to crack only in late 1943, around the fall of Italy, at a time when it was also becoming clear that Nazi Germany would not win the war.[24]

Resistance activities, carried out by both Communist and civic groups, culminated in August 1944 in, as it became known, the Slovak National Uprising. In point of fact, the uprising was largely international, with about 30 different nationalities taking part.[25] Between 800 and 1200 Slovak Jews joined the resistance as well.[26] A number of Slovak Roma participated in the rebellion, paying a heavy price: according to estimates, about 1400 Slovak Roma were murdered in the course of the uprising.[27]

[23] Hana Kubátová and Monika Vrzgulová, Being "Local" in Eastern Slovakia: Belonging in a Multiethnic Periphery, manuscript accepted with *East European Politics and Societies*.

[24] For Slovak-Jewish relations during World War II and popular responses to the Holocaust, see, for example, Kubátová (2013); Hana Kubátová, "Accusing and Demanding: Denunciations in Wartime Slovakia," in *Lessons and Legacies: New Approaches to an Integrated History of the Holocaust: Social History, Representation, Theory*, ed. by Alexandra Garbarini and Paul B. Jaskot, Vol. XIII (Evanston, IL: Northwestern University Press, 2018), 92–111; Kubátová and Láníček (2018).

[25] Dušan Halaj, "SNP a európska rezistencia," in *SNP v pamäti národa: Materiály z vedeckej konferencie k 50. výročiu SNP, Donovaly 26.–28. apríla 1994* (Bratislava: NKV International, 1994), 249–71.

[26] Yeshayahu Jelinek, "The Role of the Jews in Slovakian Resistance," *Jahrbücher für Geschichte Osteuropas* 15:3 (1967), 415–22.

[27] See e.g., Arne B. Mann and Zuzana Kumanová, *Ma bisteren! Nové poznatky o holocauste Rómov na Slovensku* (Bratislava: Občianske združenie IN MINORITA, 2015), https://www.databazeknih.cz/knihy/ma-bisteren-nove-poznatky-o-holocauste-romov-na-slovensku-332941. Accessed 10 May 2020.

After some heavy fighting, especially on the Slovak-Polish border, the German Wehrmacht, accompanied by Einsatzgruppe H of the Security Police and the SS, crushed the rebellion in late October of that year. The end of the war was particularly brutal for Slovakia. As historian Lenka Šindelářová has established, between September 1944 and March 1945 approximately 4000 people were murdered, often in a cruel way: hanged, strangled, burnt, or buried alive. Among the victims were mostly Jews caught in hiding or when fighting with the partisans, but also Roma and other real or alleged partisans and their supporters. Approximately 90 villages and towns were burned down in revenge.[28] Propaganda organs of the wartime state quickly denounced the uprising as the act of a handful of domestic traitors, Bolsheviks, Czechs, and Jews. A more radical Slovak government was introduced, and new Emergency Units of the Hlinka Guard were employed to help suppress the rebellion. Again, locals were engaged to help locate and hunt down everyone who had or could have supported the uprising, first and foremost the Jews. To show the Germans that the Slovak government had not abandoned them, on 30 October 1944, Tiso celebrated a mass of gratitude and decorated German soldiers who had helped crush the insurgency. Following the suppression of the resistance, German units, assisted by Slovak radicals, renewed deportations of Slovak Jews. In the last months of the war, approximately 12,600 Slovak Jews were deported from Slovakia, most of them to Auschwitz or Theresienstadt, with most of them not surviving.

Subsequent to the collapse of the fascist regime, legal continuity with the prewar Czechoslovak republic was emphasized. Slovakia not only joined the victorious powers as part of the renewed Czechoslovakia after World War II, but what is more, placed its troubled past within a parenthesis. As will be shown and problematized, while avoiding reference to the crimes committed, the postwar establishment highlighted the 1944 uprising, claiming that resistance, not collaboration, epitomized Slovak actions in the war. After all, as historian Tony Judt noted when writing on similar efforts across postwar Europe, for a country to be innocent "a nation had to have resisted and to have done so in its overwhelming majority."[29]

---

[28] Lenka Šindelářová, *Einsatzgruppe H: působení operační skupiny H na Slovensku 1944/1945 a poválečné trestní stíhání jejích příslušníků* (Praha: Academia / Múzeum Slovenského národného povstania, 2015), 101–16.

[29] Tony Judt, "The Past Is Another Country: Myth and Memory in Postwar Europe," *Daedalus* 121:4 (1992), 90–1.

The Long Shadows of World War II

There is a wide scholarly consensus concerning the long shadows of violence, and the deep emotional effects genocides have on individuals and societies at large. Negative feelings, fear, anxiety, and grief do not cease with an armistice or liberation. On the contrary, "[o]bservers of interethnic conflict report that people speak of atrocities committed against their group without necessarily differentiating between events that occurred yesterday, a decade ago or a hundred years ago."[30]

"Trauma," as a medical term, is reserved for an acute organic or physical wound. As a term within the social sciences and humanities, its meaning has gradually "expanded to incorporate the emotional insult or shock to the mind resulting from physical and/or emotional injury."[31] Within Holocaust studies itself, research into trauma has been closely intertwined with questions of memory and repression, silence and voice. Ever since the 1970s, scholars have striven to understand the "significance of the Holocaust inheritance for those who come after."[32] The interlocutors in the works that have appeared on Holocaust trauma were mostly survivor families, a group that came to be called the "second generation."[33] Memoirs, commemorative books, ego materials at large, as well as intimate conversations, actual or imagined, that family members had with their loved ones who survived or perished in the Holocaust, have given impetus to investigations of the intergenerational transmission of trauma.[34] Around the same period we can also witness the emergence of first works,

[30] Michael J. A. Wohl and Nyla R. Branscombe, "Forgiveness and Collective Guilt Assignment to Historical Perpetrator Groups Depend on Level of Social Category Inclusiveness," *Journal of Personality and Social Psychology* 88:2 (2005), 288–303; Michael Ignatieff, "The Elusive Goal of War Trials," *Harper's Magazine*, March 1, 1997; Elazar Barkan, *The Guilt of Nations: Restitution and Negotiating Historical Injustices* (New York: Norton, 2000).

[31] Aaron R. Denham, "Rethinking Historical Trauma: Narratives of Resilience," *Transcultural Psychiatry* 45:3 (2008), 395.

[32] Eva Hoffman, *After Such Knowledge: Memory, History, and the Legacy of the Holocaust* (New York: PublicAffairs, 2011), xi.

[33] Helen Epstein, *Children of the Holocaust: Conversations with Sons and Daughters of Survivors* (New York: Putnam, 1979).

[34] See, for example, Gabriele Schwab, *Haunting Legacies: Violent Histories and Transgenerational Trauma* (New York: Columbia University Press, 2010).

many of them autobiographical, that examine the emotional effect the Holocaust also had on perpetrators' children and grandchildren.[35]

Even more recently, scholars have pointed their attention to the processing of past injuries in different national contexts. Researchers have largely focused on Germany, France and Italy. Germany is often given as an example of a country that managed to process its past, and where emotions of collective guilt have been experienced. As sociologist Bernhard Giesen has reminded us, however, the German *Vergangenheitsbewältigung* needs to be understood as gradual and twisted. In early postwar years, an exculpatory narrative was introduced that highlighted "the opposition between oppressors and the people," between Hitler and the Germans.[36] The highest echelons of the Nazi party, and Adolf Hitler especially, were defined "as satanic seducers who had approached the good and innocent German people from outside and deprived it of its common sense like a drug, a disease, or a diabolic obsession."[37] This avoidance strategy, the shifting of blame intertwined with victimhood, was not unique for post-1945 Germany. Scholars working on postwar France and Italy, among them historian Rebecca Clifford, noticed that, for a long period, these countries avoided questions of complicity in the Holocaust by fostering an image of the good-hearted people who had stood in opposition, if not resistance, to the fascists, representing the outer fringes of their national communities. As Clifford demonstrates, "the notions of the *bons Français/italiani brava gente* played important roles in postwar-national identity, and the power and persistence of these myths held in check public discussion of the extent of French and Italian cooperation with and participation in the persecution of Jews."[38] Indeed, France is cited as an example of a larger trend in how the Holocaust has been ousted from public recollections. Historian Henry Rousso termed the cutting away of

[35] See, for example, Anne Fuchs, Mary Cosgrove and Georg Grote, eds, *German Memory Contests: The Quest for Identity in Literature, Film, and Discourse since 1990* (Rochester, NY: Camden House, 2006); Laurel Cohen-Pfister and Susanne Vees-Gulani, eds, *Generational Shifts in Contemporary German Culture* (Rochester, NY: Camden House, 2011).

[36] Bernhard Giesen, "The Trauma of Perpetrators: The Holocaust as the Traumatic Reference of German National Identity," in Jeffrey C. Alexander, Piotr Sztompka, Ron Eyerman, Neil Smelser and Bernhard Giesen, *Cultural Trauma and Collective Identity* (Berkeley, CA: University of California Press, 2004), 119.

[37] Giesen (2004), 119–20.

[38] Rebecca Clifford, *Commemorating the Holocaust: The Dilemmas of Remembrance in France and Italy* (Oxford: Oxford University Press, 2013), 6.

the uncomfortable past the "Vichy syndrome," a disorder which seemed to have spread throughout the Old Continent like an epidemic, hardly sparing any country.[39]

If the 1960s and 1970s are seen as allowing a breakthrough into a more honest engagement with wartime history for the West, an often-repeated assumption is that for the East, the processing of the Holocaust started only in 1989, when the countries of the former Soviet bloc were released "from the burden of officially mandated Communist interpretations of World War Two."[40] While the political liberation of the late 1950s and 1960s in Communist Europe resulted in a social and cultural transformation as well, this was seen as temporary and short-lived, an interruption rather than a shift in the overall trend. Scholars working on the role of history in Slovak nationalism, like the political scientist Shari J. Cohen, claimed that "the word holocaust did not enter the Slovak debate until 1989 (though small groups of nationalists and democrats discussed it). On the territory of that small country whose leaders traded nominal independence for collaboration in one of the country's greatest crimes, this history was never made meaningful."[41] In line with these views, the handling of the past in postwar Slovakia and Eastern Europe in general has often been reduced to the attempted "erasure of the Jewish memory" in public and vernacular culture, and the avoidance of "ethnic and religious tags" when approaching the topic of World War II in official narratives of the past, including Marxist historiography.[42] Historian Mary Fulbrook, when comparing the impact of the Nazi past on the Federal Republic of Germany and on the German Democratic Republic, has offered scholars a way out of this dichotomy. By studying how "West Germans continued to be obsessed with an unresolved past" in connection, and not outside of, "more immediate problems with a divided present" on the part of the East Germans, Fulbrook also made a convincing case as to why we need to

---

[39] See Henry Rousso, *The Vichy Syndrome: History and Memory in France since 1944* (Cambridge, MA: Harvard University Press, 1994).

[40] Tony Judt, *Postwar: A History of Europe Since 1945* (New York: Penguin Books, 2006), 821.

[41] Shari J. Cohen, *Politics Without a Past: The Absence of History in Postcommunist Nationalism* (Durham, NC: Duke University Press, 1999), 11.

[42] Sławomir Kapralski, "The Impact of Post-1989 Changes on Polish-Jewish Relations and Perceptions: Memories and Debates," in *The Religious Roots of Contemporary European Identity*, ed. by Lucia Faltin and Melanie J. Wright (London: Continuum, 2007), 90; Judt (2006), 823.

move past a blind appraisal of the West (for its supposedly objective and courageous facing of the past) and a harsh criticism of the East (for its ideologically coded narration of events) when scrutinizing the attempts to come to terms with the Holocaust.[43]

While recollections of what had happened in Slovakia during World War II were ethnically determined, while Communist-mandated official narratives significantly distorted the history of both World War II and the Holocaust, while only a few in the postwar era were open and willing to listen to Jewish voices, these voices were certainly not absent. On the contrary, however slow, reluctant, and limited the articulation of past harms was in the early postwar decades, Jewish experiences served as counter narratives to the official discourse on heroism, their narratives confronting the moral self-image of Slovakia.

Restoring the Moral Self-Image

The processing of local participation in the Holocaust in different, Eastern and Western European national contexts has shown that the reckoning with one group's wrongs is a multilayered process, one that evolves in time and space. Reactions to past wrongdoings are far from mutually exclusive, and different attempts to restore the moral image of the in-group are picked up by different actors and vehicles. This observation is in line with psychological research, which takes note of a wide range of group-protective and avoidance strategies in the aftermaths of violence.[44] These strategies are not limited to the examples identified earlier, especially the deflecting of guilt onto others, but also include an outright denial of facts or an in-group's flattering interpretation of past injuries.[45] Where historians and nationalism scholars are in agreement with social psychology scholarship is in the role that history, and socially shared representations of the past, play in fostering and maintaining the idea of a nation.[46] Confronted with a negative aspect of their past, individuals may,

---

[43] Fulbrook (1999), 177.

[44] Stanley Cohen, *States of Denial: Knowing about Atrocities and Suffering* (Cambridge: Polity, 2001).

[45] Roy F. Baumeister and Stephen Hastings, "Distortions of Collective Memory: How Groups Flatter and Deceive Themselves," in *Collective Memory of Political Events: Social Psychological Perspectives*, ed. by James W. Pennebaker, Dario Paez and Bernard Rimé (Hillsdale, NJ: Lawrence Erlbaum Associates, 1997), 277–93.

[46] Anderson (1991); James Liu and Denis Hilton, "How the Past Weighs on the Present: Social Representations of History and Their Role in Identity Politics," *British Journal of Social Psychology* 44 (2006), 537–56.

for instance, try to "avoid the negative position implied by their group's history" by seeking a higher, for instance, European, or lower, local or personal, identification.[47] These and other responses support the claim that what actually stands in the way of social-change processes is the trauma of victims, an organic or physical wound, but primarily a psychological condition, as well as the unprocessed communal trauma of the societies at large. In this sense, reluctance to face the past on a part of the in-group is a symptom of communal bonds being broken.

Avoidance strategies have one additional role. In an attempt to restore the moral self-image of an in-group, social psychologists Michael J. A. Wohl, Nyla R. Branscombe and Yechiel Klar tell us that people "engage in a variety of group-protective strategies which are aimed at alleviating the adversarial experience of guilt that stems from a shared group membership with the harm-doers."[48] In other words, blaming the Germans, the radicals, such as members of the paramilitary Hlinka Guard in the Slovak case, rationalizing past actions and even presenting the in-group as the actual victim of the story, is a group-protective mechanism, one that is nevertheless inward driven. Avoidance strategies protect the in-group from experiencing collective guilt, and they also foster an ethnically exclusive understanding of community or group.

Compared to any form of retribution, which always takes the form of an outside-imposed ruling, collective guilt is a form of self-judgment. Being a self-conscious negative emotion, as already outlined, "positive consequences for the harmed others may follow" from experiences of collective guilt.[49] These may include actions intended to alleviate the wrongdoing, including apologies and reparations. As mentioned, in the long run, collective guilt experiences may have positive effects on out-group attitudes and, as such, reduce bias in intergroup and intragroup contact.[50]

---

[47] Bilewicz (2007), 552; Liu and Hilton (2006); Nyla B. Branscombe, Ben Slugoski and Diane M. Kappen, "The Measurement of Collective Guilt: What It Is and What It Is Not," in *Collective Guilt: International Perspectives*, ed. by Nyla B. Branscombe and Bertjan Doosje (Cambridge: Cambridge University Press, 2004), 16–34.

[48] Michael Wohl, Nyla Branscombe and Yechiel Klar, "Collective Guilt: Emotional Reactions When One's Group Has Done Wrong or Been Wronged," *European Review of Social Psychology* 17 (2006), 1–37.

[49] Wohl, Branscombe and Klar (2006), 3.

[50] Wohl, Branscombe and Klar (2006), 9.

Collective guilt is conceptualized as a self-conscious emotion that "stems from the distress that group members experience when they accept that their in-group is responsible for immoral actions that harmed another group."[51] Collective guilt is a psychological experience and does not "involve actually being guilty in any sense of the word. This is an important distinction."[52] What is equally important to stress is that collective guilt can only be experienced when avoidance strategies fail.

Available research agrees on several necessary factors that facilitate the experience of collective guilt, these being self-categorization as a member of the group that committed harm, understanding that it was the in-group that was responsible for the harmful actions and agreeing that the harm committed was "illegitimate or immoral." The actual degree of "collective guilt experienced will depend on the perceived difficulty and costs to the in-group of correcting the wrongs committed."[53] With communal bonds broken in the Holocaust through complicity and collaboration, the stakes for correcting past wrongs were too high, especially as this would, in the Slovak case, entail the restitution of Jewish property.

THE HEROIC AND TRAUMATIC PAST
OF A COMMUNAL GENOCIDE

The screening of "The Shop on Main Street" in Czechoslovakia coincided with the culmination of what has been referred to in literature as the ritualization of resistance remembrance.[54] Preparing for the 20th anniversary of the uprising, plans were drawn up for a grandiose museum to be built in the town of Banská Bystrica, the former center of the anti-Nazi rebellion (the museum eventually opened in 1969). Memorials and monuments

---

[51] Nyla B. Branscombe and Bertjan Doosje, "International Perspectives on the Experience of Collective Guilt," in Branscombe and Doosje, eds (2004), 3.

[52] Ibid., 3–4.

[53] Wohl, Branscombe and Klar (2006), 9.

[54] Miroslav Michela and Michal Kšiňan, "The Slovak National Uprising," in *Komunisti a povstania: ritualizácia pripomínania si protifašistických povstaní v strednej Európe (1945–1960) = Communists and Uprisings: Ritualization of Remembrance of the Anti-Nazi Uprisings in Central Europe (1945–1960)* (Kraków: Towarzystwo Słowaków w Polsce, 2012), 36–66.

dedicated to the uprising started to be built as soon as the war was over, first as part of local initiatives.[55] Raised away from main crossroads, "on the sites where fallen warriors were put to eternal rest, plain crosses, stone memorials, but also massive pylons emerged, made by former co-warriors, families and other engaged inhabitants." New memorials were constructed in centers of towns and on the orders of official government bureaus following the 1948 Communist takeover. Carved inscriptions, giving thanks to the partisans and anti-fascist fighters, were now supplemented with a red star, turning it into "the central theme of the Uprising's iconography."[56]

The Slovak participation in World War II was, in the official discourse, reduced to the anti-fascist rebellion. Two things are worth pointing out when examining how the 1944 rebellion was presented to the public, and what role it played in the further exclusion of the Jews from the community. First, in contrast to the plaques dedicated to the fallen soldiers of World War I, for instance, tributes built to honor those who died while in uniform in World War II were largely anonymous. If names were included, they typically belonged to those who fell in the last months of the war at the hands of the Germans, hence sidestepping Slovak soldiers who fought and died alongside the Wehrmacht. Whether identified or anonymized, victims of the 1944 uprising were very much nationalized. This was also the case with the 1949 Memorial to the Victims of Fascism at Kremnička, today one of the boroughs of Banská Bystrica. As the German forces were progressing in crushing the rebellion, many Jews who joined the uprising fled to that partisan stronghold. As the town fell, 747 alleged and actual partisans were murdered in Kremnička. Whereas at least half of them would be considered Jewish according to the racial legislation then in place, and they were also hunted down and shot to death as Jews, the impressive monument with a relief made of three crosses and a red star was simply dedicated "to the tortured partisans."[57] The nationalization of victims in Kremnička (and in general) is best seen when placed in contrast to

[55] See, for instance, Ľubomír Lipták, "Pamätníky a pamäť povstania roku 1944 na Slovensku," *Historický časopis* 43:2 (1995), 363–69.

[56] Michela and Kšiňan (2012), 42.

[57] See, for instance, Gila Fatran, "Holocaust and Collaboration in Slovakia in the Postwar Discourse," in *Collaboration with the Nazis: Public Discourse after the Holocaust*, ed. by Roni Stauber (London: Routledge, 2010), 186–211.

the overall number of Czechoslovak victims of the "various battlefronts in the fight against fascism," which is usually estimated at 360,000. The number of "Czechoslovak victims" here includes the approximately 277,000 Jews from the Bohemian lands, Slovakia but also Subcarpathian Rus who perished in the Holocaust.[58]

Second, despite the violent suppression of the uprising and the terror that followed, and notwithstanding the number of memorials dedicated to the victims, there was a visible absence of mourning in postwar Slovakia. The uprising was celebrated and looked up to, and fallen partisans were termed "martyrs," as if sacrificed for the whole. Through the renaming of towns and villages, institutions and army units; the installation of memorials and commemorative plaques as well as the introduction of awards; and through annual anniversaries aimed to "anchor the meaning of the Uprising,"[59] a road to a heroic national narrative was paved in postwar Slovakia. As mentioned above, the undoubtedly heroic deeds of the insurgents were used to acquit the majority of all wrongdoings. According to this tale of the nation, the majority society played the role of an innocent and heroic victim, the clerical fascist regime was an "imposed and artificial result of Nazism and fascism,"[60] and the complicity in anti-Jewish persecution, violence and murder was determinedly avoided.

If guilt, responsibility and trauma revolve around harm and wrongdoing, it is interesting to read how these concepts were made sense of by the Slovak administration, by Jewish witnesses, and by the two organizations representing Jewish survivors in postwar Slovakia, the Association of Victims of Racial Persecution at the Hands of the Fascist Regime in Bratislava and the Central Union of Jewish Communities in Slovakia, both headed by Vojtech Winterstein. The largely anonymous official accounts of the war, with unnamed fascists as the guilty perpetrators and the majority nation as the heroic victim, differed drastically from many of the Jewish narratives written or collected in the postwar period. In many of these early witness accounts, just as in "The Shop on Main Street," the Holocaust was not something that happened to Slovakia but something that took place in Slovakia. Fascists were not anonymous, and neither were they only

---

[58] Stanislav Mičev et al., *Fašistické represálie na Slovensku* (Bratislava: Vydavateľstvo Obzor, 1990), 6.

[59] Jozef Lettrich, "Prvé výročie slovenskej revolúcie," *Čas*, August 1945, 1. Festive issue.

[60] "SNR 1945–1946, Minutes," May 15, 1945, Společná česko-slovenská digitální parlamentní knihovna (The Joint Czech and Slovak Digital Parliamentary Library), http://www.psp.cz/eknih/1945snr/stenprot/003schuz/index.htm. Accessed April 25, 2020.

Germans, but had a name and a face, often one that was well recognizable. I will demonstrate my point through specific examples.

The wartime Slovak state and its institutions were, from early on, crossed out of the vocabulary of the postwar establishment. When Jozef Lettrich, chairman of the legislative Slovak National Council and head of the Democratic Party, opened the festive plenary session of the council on 15 May 1945, for instance, he simply spoke of the "past, a dark past that cannot return."[61] In his speech, Lettrich described the wartime republic as "a fascist regime and a dictatorship," a place where "all civic rights of our people were suppressed." According to this logic, the Slovak nation, which "rather suffered and brought the greatest sacrifices" of life, proved "its unwavering will to defeat fascism at home and abroad."[62] Interestingly but not surprisingly, while the Slovak majority society was portrayed as waiting "for the first opportunity to overthrow the fascist regime with a weapon in hand," little to no mention was given to the participation of Jews and other groups, however defined, in the uprising.[63] Indeed, the nation in the Slovak National Uprising was made into an ethnically exclusive club.

If the participation of Jews in the rebellion was overlooked in the publicly shared representations of World War II, postwar Jewish communities strived hard to include their heroism in the story of the 1944 uprising. Central bodies of postwar Jewish organizations urged local communities to join the yearly festivities surrounding the uprising as "citizens of the Jewish faith who suffered in concentration camps, fought in combat units and joined the Slovak National Uprising."[64] Shortly after the war, at the initiative of the Jewish Agency for Eretz Israel, the Zionist Federation and the Association of Jewish Communities in Bratislava, the Documentation Center for the Central Union of Jewish Communities in Bratislava was founded. Many of the testimonies collected as part of the initiative, some handwritten while most were typed on an official form, testify not only to the communal character of the Holocaust but also give credit to Jewish

---

[61] "SNR 1945–1946, Minutes."

[62] "SNR 1945–1946, Minutes."

[63] "Pred rokom," *Pravda*, September 6, 1945, 2.

[64] Central Archives for the History of the Jewish People (CAHJP), Yeshayahu Jelinek Collection P287 (Jelinek-P287), letter of Jozef Lipa of the Central Union of Jewish Religious Communities addressed to all Jewish communities in Slovakia, not dated, probably from around summer 1954.

involvement in the uprising.[65] Whereas reflecting on their own, personal experiences during World War II, Jewish witnesses presented themselves not solely as victims but heroes as well, being diligent in counting the number of Jewish partisans in their village or town, identifying as many as possible by name and reporting on the circumstances of death of those murdered in the uprising.

It is not that the harm committed against the Jews was forgotten by the postwar administration either, it was deliberately sidetracked, using two main strategies. As elsewhere in Europe, the higher ups, the leaders of the wartime Slovak regime, were removed from the good-hearted nation as a whole.[66] Giving a speech at the annual celebrations in August 1945, Viliam Široký, an influential figure in the Communist Party of Slovakia, representing the ideological antithesis of the Democratic Party, claimed, for instance, that the "Slovak nation has long prepared for the opportunity to undo the shame that the Tiso men have cast on its name, and to do so in front of the whole world and in a timely manner, to atone for the disgraceful alliance with the Germans against the fraternal nations of the Soviet Union, to undo the anti-democratic and anti-Jewish acts of Tiso bandits."[67] As Široký put it, it was Tiso himself and the "*Ludak* leaders who bore full responsibility for everything that happened in Slovakia, including the instigation of Slovakia in the fratricidal war against the Soviet Union; the Slovak bloodshed in German mercenary services; the plundering of Slovak riches by German robbers and the low and inhuman murder of tens of thousands of our citizens of Jewish descent in the infamous death camps."[68] With blame shifted onto "the Tiso men" and "the Ludaks," as members of the Hlinka Party continued to be called, the conscience of the "masses of the nation" remained unchallenged.[69]

Furthermore, crimes of the "past, a dark past," were reduced to a legal matter. The guilt of the Tiso men, including their henchmen who betrayed the nation, was to be settled in the courts. While there might have been guilt as a legal category, notions and emotions of collective guilt or

---

[65] See testimonies donated to the Yad Vashem Archives (YVA), The Documentation Center of the Central Union of Jewish Communities in Bratislava (M.5).

[66] Kubátová and Láníček (2018), 124–38; Hana Kubátová, "On the Image of the Jew in Postwar Slovakia," *The Annual of Language & Politics and Politics of Identity* 9 (2015), 71–85.

[67] Viliam Široký, "Rok od slovenského národného povstania," *Pravda*, August 29, 1945, 2.

[68] "Referát súdr. Vila Širokého o úlohách strany vo výstavbe Slovenska," *Pravda*, August 14, 1945, 1.

[69] Viliam Široký, "Rok od slovenského národného povstania," *Pravda*, August 29, 1945, 2.

responsibility were dodged. This argument can be further illustrated when returning to the May 1945 gathering of the Slovak National Council. What made the session festive was the adoption of "a law on the punishment of all fascist traitors, betrayers, Slovak collaborators and their small helpers."[70] Accordingly, between 1945 and 1948, more than 22,000 individuals were tried in so-called people's courts, either as "fascist occupiers" or "domestic traitors," and almost 9000 received a guilty verdict.[71] In line with shifting the blame onto others, not only the higher ups were blamed, but also the Germans, and, in the Slovak example, the Hungarians as well, since over half of those tried and convicted in the courts were categorized as Magyars.[72] A further 12 percent of those convicted were Germans, meaning only a third of the criminals were either Czech or Slovak. In the postwar rhetoric, the Hungarian occupation of parts of Slovakia was made into "a historically big and unparalleled question," and, as such, the harm committed to the Slovaks could not even be compared "with the injustices committed to the Slovaks by the former regime."[73] Once again, by making the processing of harm a legal matter, and by charging radicals and Hungarians with crimes committed in the past, the moral self-image of the nation went untouched.

Jewish testimonies from the postwar years, whether collected as part of the Documentation Action, established to record the plight of the Jews in the immediate aftermath, or through the competition held by the Yad Vashem, the Holocaust Martyrs' and Heroes Remembrance Authority in Israel in the mid-1950s, were often highly personal, placing former neighbors at the scenes of robbery and betrayal. Again, in contrast to the official discourse, in the Jewish witness testimonies those who took the "piano and other things," those who "betrayed us," those who "stole whatever was possible, clothes, soap from the laundry, wood" had the name of a Gentile neighbor.[74] Indeed, it was the complicity in the theft where the

---

[70] "SNR 1945–1946, Minutes."

[71] Jozef Brandobur, "Čakáme presídlencov," *Národná obroda*, June 15, 1946, 1.

[72] Šindelářová (2015).

[73] Brandobur (1946), 1.

[74] See, e.g., YVA, Testimonies, Diaries and Memoirs Collection (O.33), file number 9387, Memoirs of Peter Eugene Weiss regarding the experience of his family in Liptovska Tepla, the murder of his father and deportation to Theresienstadt; documentation regarding the family and reparation claims, December 3, 1998; YVA, Collection of Memoirs Written for the Yad Vashem Competition (O.39), Memoirs of Stella (Neuman) Maros, born in

official and unofficial narratives clashed, and where the communal aspect of the Holocaust became most visible.[75]

In her comparative account of the reconstruction of Jewish life in Poland and Slovakia, historian Anna Cichopek-Gajraj argues that both postwar administrations lacked something of a moral obligation to correct their wrongs, an obligation resulting from an understanding that they needed to atone for caused injustices.[76] Cichopek-Gajraj mentions the absence of a moral obligation as one of three reasons why postwar governments, in Eastern Europe but also elsewhere, were reluctant to settle restitution claims. Returning stolen Jewish belongings could not only have led to social unrest, officials feared, and rightfully so, but there was also a more general trend towards nationalization that downgraded the whole meaning of private ownership.[77] Whereas Cichopek-Gajraj's arguments support my thesis, her pointing to the question of restitution sheds further light on the nexus between robbery and memory.[78] Indeed, it is here that we see the unwillingness to face the past in its complexity, not only in the sense of allying the country with Nazi Germany but in the very communal exclusion of Jews and, hence, also in the Holocaust.[79]

While it was already the resistance authorities who deemed all property transfers, according to the racial legislation of the wartime state, null and void, and while the central government in Prague attempted to regulate the restitution claims as early as on 19 May 1945, and although the restitution law was introduced on 16 May 1946, the Slovak postwar bodies were reluctant to authorize these laws, making them virtually ineffective on Slovak territory. Repeatedly, every couple of months, institutions representing Jewish victims approached the Slovak but also the central Prague

Ruzomberok, Czechoslovakia, 194, regarding her experiences in Ruzomberok, Zilina, Kalamenová, in hiding in Lubochna and more, December 12, 1955.

[75] Kaja Kaźmierska, "Biographical and Collective Memory: Mutual Influences in Central and Eastern European Context," in *Memory and Change in Europe: Eastern Perspectives*, ed. by Małgorzata Pakier and Joanna Wawrzyniak (New York: Berghahn Books, 2016), 96–112.

[76] Anna Cichopek-Gajraj, *Beyond Violence: Jewish Survivors in Poland and Slovakia, 1944–48* (Cambridge: Cambridge University Press, 2014), 112; Barkan (2006).

[77] Cichopek-Gajraj (2014), 111–13.

[78] See also Dan Diner, "Restitution and Memory—The Holocaust in European Political Cultures," *New German Critique* 90 (2003), 36–44.

[79] Anna Cichopek-Gajraj, "Limits to 'Jewish Power': How Slovak Jewish Leaders Negotiated Restitution of Property after the Second World War," *East European Jewish Affairs* 44:1 (2014), 51–69; Ivica Štelmachovič Bumová, "Židia—spoločnosť—politika (Slovensko 1945–1948)," *Slovenský národopis* 60:2 (2012), 165–74.

administration, sometimes including President Edvard Beneš, being vocal about the guilt and responsibility on the part of both the former regime and the majority society. In the letters, sometimes called protests (*protestný*) or memorable dossiers (*pamätný spis*), Winterstein appealed to those in power, promoting the interests of the postwar Jewish community. While some of the letters were factual, including estimates of those who perished and those who survived, others included drafts of restitution laws, and even others attempted to negotiate specific provisions. What is equally important, I argue, is that these letters also included direct references to "the fascist regime of the so-called Slovak state," and claims that while "the dead cannot be revived," the "perpetrated wrongdoings" of the recent past not only can but need to be corrected. Jewish communities already then, as with many scholars now, saw a link between the wartime complicity of the majority society and the postwar reluctance to return Jewish properties as well as the violence against the Jews that occurred in the aftermath.[80] Winterstein made his point when approaching Lettrich in March 1946, writing that it was an indisputable fact that "in Slovakia, it was the Slovaks and then the Germans who got their hands on Jewish belongings," and that "it is more than morally legitimate and is imperative for the honor of the Slovak nation to atone for the injustice caused by the Slovak government. The Slovak National Council needs to take action."[81]

As the Jewish organizations saw it, judging from minutes of their internal meetings, the tragedy experienced during World War II and the Holocaust did not end with the liberation, and the regime of the wartime state implicated significant portions of the society in the theft, making any atonement difficult. In one of the meetings, dated July 1946, Winterstein took the stand, pointing to the great sacrifices Jews made during World War II and their joining of the resistance in perceptible numbers. Dismissing the popular claims, according to which the Jews, "who were hiding in bunkers" during the war now claim their wealth, Winterstein responded that on the contrary, "the Jews only want their stolen wealth back."[82]

---

[80] CAHJP, Jelinek-P287, protest dossier by Vojtech Winterstein addressed to the Presidium of the Slovak National Council, December 7, 1945.

[81] CAHJP, Jelinek-P287, letter by Vojtech Winterstein addressed to Jozef Lettrich, March 19, 1945.

[82] CAHJP, Jelinek-P287, minutes from the session of the Association of Victims of Racial Persecution at the Hands of the Fascist Regime in Bratislava, July 30, 1946.

Jewish organizations continued to appeal to the authorities through letters, reminding them of the harm committed well up until the Communist takeover in February 1948 that halted any restitution claims for another four decades. Even then, in 1949, a few months after the coup, Documentation Action published its historical survey under the title "The Tragedy of Slovak Jews" (*Tragédia slovenských židov*). While careful in their language and wary of making any generalizations, the communal genocide and trauma was addressed rather directly: "The tragedy of Slovak Jews took place in a state that called itself Christian, thus announcing to the world that it was guided by the principles of love for one's neighbor, that it respected God's commandment and believed in the equality of human beings before the Creator."[83]

CONCLUSION

"The Shop on Main Street" and the debate it triggered, within and outside of Czechoslovakia, point to the implications of the "much-lamented burden of guilt" for postwar societies of Europe, even if those employed persistent avoidance and self-protective strategies to preserve their moral self-image.[84] Whether by exaggerating their role in the anti-fascist resistance, shifting the blame onto others or placing the wartime past in a parenthesis, individuals, groups, and states have inadvertently exposed the lasting effects of a communal genocide.

Whereas much scholarly attention has been aimed at Western Europe, in particular Germany, France and Italy, significantly less work has been done on the effect the Holocaust, especially local complicity and collaboration, had on post-1945 Eastern European societies. The argument often goes that the managing of the past could have started here only following the regime change in 1989. While the 1960s and 1970s are seen as transformative, both for the West and the East, the political "thaw" is often treated in the literature as a diversion and hence largely examined in separation from what preceded and followed. Turning to postwar Slovakia and

---

[83] Jožko Lánik, *Osviecim, hrobka štyroch miliónov ľudí: Krátka história a život v osviecimskom pekle v rokoch 1942–1945* (Bratislava: Povereníctvo SNR pre informácie, 1946); Dezider Tóth, ed., *Tragédia slovenských židov: Materiály z medzinárodného sympózia, Banská Bystrica 25.–27. marca 1992* (Banská Bistrica: DATEI, 1992); Gabriel Hoffmann, *Katolícka cirkev a tragédia slovenských židov v dokumentoch* (Partizánske: Vydavateľstvo G-Print, 1994).

[84] Lars Rensmann, "Collective Guilt, National Identity, and Political Processes in Contemporary Germany," in Branscombe and Doosje (2004), 169.

the ways official and communal actors used and utilized notions of past harm, my chapter shows that the restoring of the moral self-image cannot be separated from efforts on the part of the Jewish witnesses to have past harms recognized and acknowledged.

What made the processing of complicity in the East particularly difficult, apart from the Communist distortion of the past, was the communal character of the Holocaust, and the unprocessed communal trauma it resulted in. This is what "The Shop on Main Street" also highlighted. With its focus on the "little" people like Tono and his wife Evelína, on the then aspiring middle class as well as on the radicals who, however, had both a name and a familiar face, such as Markuš Kolkotský, the movie illustrated the ethnically determined yet entangled experiences of World War II in the many historically multiethnic towns and villages of Slovakia. The responses to the movie then highlighted the broken communal bonds.

This said, at the core of the divided memory of World War II and the Holocaust is the tension between the official explanation of what had happened in the past, and the experiences of the events, as remembered, fostered by Jewish witnesses and institutions representing them. The proximity of collaboration, robbery but also of restitution and memory points to the fact that in order for the healing to begin, the responsibility of the majority society first needs to be made visible, and the communal aspect of the genocide needs to be publicly acknowledged.

CHAPTER 9

"Perpetrator Trauma" in Memoirs of Veterans of the Polish Home Army

Marta Kurkowska-Budzan

INTRODUCTION

Life stories mirror the culture wherein the story is made and told. Stories live in culture. They are born, they grow, they proliferate, and they eventually die according to the norms, rules, and traditions that prevail in a given society, according to a society's implicit understandings of what counts as a tellable story, a tellable life.[1]

The contemporary discourse on politics and culture in Poland is suffused with the ethos of the fight against the German and Soviet

---

[1] Dan P. McAdams, "Identity and the Life Story," in *Autobiographical Memory and the Construction of a Narrative Self: Developmental and Cultural Perspectives*, ed. by Robyn Fivush and Catherine A. Haden (Mahwah, NJ: Lawrence Erlbaum, 2003), 200.

M. Kurkowska-Budzan (✉)
Institute of History, Jagiellonian University, Krakow, Poland
e-mail: marta.kurkowska-budzan@uj.edu.pl

© The Author(s), under exclusive license to Springer Nature Switzerland AG 2022
V. Kivimäki, P. Leese (eds.), *Trauma, Experience and Narrative in Europe after World War II*, Palgrave Studies in the History of Experience, https://doi.org/10.1007/978-3-030-84663-3_9

occupation forces.[2] It has resulted in increased readers' interest in the history of the resistance movement during World War II, with autobiographies, wartime memoirs and interviews with witnesses of history enjoying particular popularity. Such a situation is the consequence of both the politics of memory pursued by the state and of the nature of the contemporary book market. In these publications, readers find not only "drums and trumpets history" but also personal opinions and expression of emotions. An additional factor influencing the high status of autobiographies is the pervasive awareness that the authors of these historical accounts are among the last living representatives of the generation of eyewitnesses of and participants in these events. The generation is referred to as the Generation of Columbuses, for those born after 1918 had to "discover" the reality of the new, independent Poland, while their youth was interrupted by the outbreak of World War II. The name was popularized during the 1960s, having stemmed from the title of a famous novel by Roman Bratny— *Kolumbowie: Rocznik 20* ("Columbuses: Born 1920"). The author created it based on his own experience and that of his coevals involved in the underground movement, in warfare against the Nazi occupation in the Warsaw Uprising of 1944.

The personage of the *Armia Krajowa* (Home Army) soldier of sabotage, and of the Warsaw insurgency of 1944, lies at the core of the Polish memory of the resistance movement during World War II.[3] The Generation of Columbuses remains valid as one of the national myths, a fact that could be attested to by the events of 2013, when it came under symbolic attack. For it is in such a manner that public opinion interpreted the view expressed by Elżbieta Janicka, of the book by Aleksander Kamiński titled *Kamienie na szaniec* ("Stones for the Rampart") about those very experiences of war:

The novel Stones for the Rampart *was published twice during the occupation, for the first time in July 1943. The book was widely read by young people, who received it enthusiastically. It may be regarded as a set of guidelines for patriotic attitudes and its impact has not waned for the seven ensuing decades. Why*

---

[2] I use the term "discourse" as communication including semiotic practice not necessarily restricted to language but to other semiotic modalities. Discourse mirrors society. See Theun A. van Dijk, *Discourse Studies: A Multidisciplinary Introduction*, Vols. 1–2 (London: Sage, 1997).

[3] Barbara Szacka, "Polish Remembrance of World War II," *International Journal of Sociology* 36:4 (2006–07), 8–26.

might that kind of influence seem somewhat worrying? Because it presents as a deeply moral and lifestyle-wise attractive model of military warfare and dying "for the motherland," while disregarding the circumstances, the reality and the burden of violence as well as its moral consequences. In Stones for the Rampart, *death seems a romantic, male adventure.*[4]

In this chapter, I pose a question about the category of trauma found within the relationship between the public discourse encompassing the heroic-romantic model for presenting the wartime experience and the published autobiographical narratives of the veterans of the Polish resistance movement. The memoirs of veterans constitute narrative interpretations of experiences; they comprise "verbalized events."[5] That being so, what position within them is given to the life-threatening, potentially traumatic events, what attitude towards them is assumed by the narrators, and how do these events function within the entire tale?[6] Do they become "tellable stories" nowadays thanks to a trauma theme, or are they the opposite? Lastly, have these narratives been the subject of research by Polish historians in terms of combat stress and the psychological costs of the underground activity? Has trauma been treated as a research category in historical scholarship?

My claim is that a breakthrough moment for the public discourse on the resistance movement in Poland came with the publication of the memoirs of Stefan Dąmbski, a veteran hailing from the south-eastern part of the country. Much like the protagonists of *Stones for the Rampart* and *Columbuses: Born 1920*, he was, as a teenager, a member of the Home Army participating in the armed struggle, and, just like other members, he executed the verdicts of the courts of the Polish Underground State on Nazis and German collaborators. The subsequent editions of Dąmbski's

---

[4] Website https://dzieje.pl/aktualnosci/dr-janicka-z-pan-mit-kamieni-na-szaniec-domaga-sie-analizy (accessed June 2, 2020); Elżbieta Janicka, "'Kamienie na szaniec': Reaktywacja," interview by Paweł Smoleński, *Gazeta Wyborcza*, April 14, 2013, http://wyborcza.pl/magazyn/1,126715,13729897,_apos_apos_Kamienie_na_szaniec_apos_apos__Reaktywacja.html#TRrelSST (accessed June 2, 2020).

[5] Dirven R. Slobin, "Verbalized events: A dynamic approach to linguistic relativity and determinism," *Current Issues in Linguistic Theory* 198 (2000), 107.

[6] Avril Thorne and Kate C. McLean, "Telling Traumatic Events in Adolescence: A Study of Master Narrative Positioning," in Fivush and Haden, eds (2003), 169–85; Jean Talbot, Roger Bibace, Barbara Bokhour and Michael Bamberg, "Affirmation and resistance of dominant discourses: The rhetorical construction of pregnancy," *Journal of Narrative and Life History* 6 (1996), 225–51.

book established the timeline and the dynamic of what I refer to as the contemporary discourse on veterans' memoirs: starting from 2005, when a fragment of Dąmbski's text appeared in the popular historical quarterly journal *Karta*, to the year 2010, when it was issued in print in its entirety by the Karta Centre Publishing Company, and further up to 2018 and 2020 when it was released again by the same publisher. All these editions shared the same title: *Egzekutor* ("The Executioner").[7] In 2011, the Polish Radio broadcast an adaptation of this narrative—a radio play performed by distinguished theater actors, with the telling name *The Stone for the Rampart* that played with the title of Aleksander Kamiński's iconic novel.[8] It was aired again in the autumn of 2018. The scope of the coverage of the debate surrounding *The Executioner* can be attested to by the fact that it caught the attention not only of veterans and historians, but also of authors from almost all major weekly opinion magazines. Trying to answer the research questions posed above, I used the text by Dąmbski as a starting point for a comparative analysis of the memorial narratives by the veterans of the sabotage forces.

Therefore, this chapter has the following structure: in its first section, I present a historical overview of the Polish resistance movement during World War II, concurrently explaining what was involved in the activity of the special courts, whose decisions were executed by members of the sabotage troops, such as the authors of the memoirs. I then go on to sketch an outline of the public discourse regarding the Home Army in the period when the Communists were in power in Poland (1944–89) and of that discourse after 1989, liberated as it was from the institutional censorship and the ideology of the Communist regime. Subsequently, I turn to the presentation of my own research on the memorial narratives. I compare the narrative by Dąmbski with those of other veterans of the Home Army (Polish abbreviation: AK), who also executed the verdicts of the judiciary of the Polish Underground State. I have analyzed the texts which, even if written during the entire postwar period (with fragments being published in the press), were released in book form only after 1989.

The latter date is considered by many to have been the breakthrough for Polish historical discourse; however, in my opinion, of greater

---

[7] Stefan Dąmbski, "Egzekutor," *Karta*, 47 (2005), 67–97; *Egzekutor* (Warszawa: Ośrodek Karta, 2010 / 2013 / 2020).

[8] *Kamień na szaniec*, dir. Katarzyna Michałkiewicz, Polish Radio Theatre, radio premiere: October 26, 2011.

importance was the fact that it marked the moment when the Polish book market started to function in the capitalist system of the economy. This can be seen, for instance, in the fact that some of these autobiographies were issued by newly established, small publishing houses. Their number includes *Prawie życiorys: 1939–1956* ("Almost a Biography: 1939–1956") by Ryszard Bielański and *Ocalone od niepamięci* ("Saved from Oblivion") by Izabella Horodecka.[9] I also analyzed the texts of the memoirs of Stanisław Likiernik, *Diabelne szczęście czy palec boży?* ("Devilish Luck or Divine Intervention?"), and of Jan Kowalkowski, *Likwidacja zdrajców narodu polskiego w Krakowie* ("The Elimination of Traitors of the Polish Nation in Krakow").[10] Of importance for the purpose of comparison with the contemporary discourse are the texts published over the past decade, constituting "remakes" of sorts of the above autobiographies, and entering into a certain dialogue with the originals. These are of hybrid forms: extended interviews featuring elements of the historical essay and of reportage, with ample citations from the earlier editions of the memoirs of their protagonists, Stanisław Likiernik and Lucjan Wiśniewski.[11]

I endeavor to scrutinize how these narratives are bound up with their contemporary discourse. Therefore, I use the notion of a genre which "can be understood as representing some of the cultural resources that are available to individuals as they try to make sense of their lives."[12] Such analysis enables one to understand the "cultural frameworks available to individuals in specific historical and societal contexts."[13] I have also benefitted from the classic model created by Labov and Waletzky referring it to the minor, internal narrative structures which are constituted in the larger memoirs by the descriptions of the sabotage actions.[14] Concurrently, these

---

[9] Ryszard Bielański, *Prawie życiorys* (Zielonka: SI, 1991); Izabella Horodecka, *Ocalone od niepamięci* (Sopot: Aida, 1992).

[10] Stanisław Likiernik, *Diabelne szczęście czy palec boży?* (Warszawa: Czytelnik, 1994); Jan Kowalkowski "Likwidacja zdrajców narodu polskiego w Krakowie," in *Okruchy Wspomnień z Lat Walki i Martyrologii AK,* ed. by Zdzisław Chętkowski (Kraków: Światowy Związek Żołnierzy Armii Krajowej / Oddział Kraków–Wschód, 2002), Vol. 1, 6–59, Vol. 2, 53–107.

[11] Emil Marat and Michał Wójcik, *Made in Poland* (Warszawa: Wielka Litera, 2014); Emil Marat and Michał Wójcik, *Ptaki drapieżne* (Kraków: Znak/literanova, 2016).

[12] More on genres understood as a culturally shared framework of narrative and imagery in Jane Elliot, *Using Narrative in Social Research: Qualitative and Quantitative Approaches* (London: Sage, 2005), 46–8.

[13] Elliot (2005), 58.

[14] William Labov and Joshua Waletzky, "Narrative analysis: oral versions of personal experience," in *Essays on the Verbal and Visual Arts,* ed. by June Helm (Seattle: University of Washington Press, 1967), 3–38.

are passages predominantly narrating life-threatening events, significant due to their potential psychological consequences, and, by definition, essential in the construction of one's "personal myth."[15] In considering the hybrid genres mentioned above, I was interested in the dialogues—the reactions of the protagonists to the questions asked by journalists, as well as the unexpected elements of the structure and content of the memoirs evoked in that manner. Analyzing the content of all texts, I distinguished the main motifs of the narrative, among the most captivating of which there were the issues related to the shaping of one's identity.[16] Similarly, of importance were the reflections developed by the authors regarding the moral dimension of their activity, and in explaining what had led to that period in their lives, and what influence it had on who they are today. In the language used by the narrators, I focused on the metaphors and simi-les which combined their experience with the cultural patterns—valid dur-ing the writing of the memoirs or giving the interview—of "war memories of the veterans of the resistance movement" or those which diverged from it. To demonstrate how the category of trauma fits in the discourse of the historians researching the Polish resistance movement during World War II, I use the example of their opinions expressed in the public debate on the memoirs of Dąmbski.

THE POLISH RESISTANCE MOVEMENT AND ITS UNDERGROUND JUDICIARY

Already in November 1939, the Government of the Republic of Poland (in exile) had made the decision to form an undercover army in the terri-tories of occupied Poland; it was named *Związek Walki Zbrojnej* (ZWZ, Union of Armed Struggle). As a result of the consolidation of early 1942, the ZWZ was transformed into the *Armia Krajowa* (AK). The High Command of the Home Army strived to integrate the efforts made by all the groups fighting against the occupation forces, regardless of political affiliation. At the peak of its development, the Home Army had about 250,000–300,000 soldiers. Such is the standard historical estimate of the

[15] Dan P. McAdams, *The Stories We Live By: Personal Myths and the Making of the Self* (New York: Guilford Press, 1993).

[16] I used computer-assisted qualitative data analysis software (CAQDAS) to code and ana-lyze the content of all the autobiographical narratives.

numbers in the armed resistance movement in Poland, emerging from the archives of official documents. Hence, the Home Army constituted a military organization enjoying constant voluntary enlistment already in wartime conditions. However, the systems of notions imported from military history prove fallible with regard to this historical experience, either as descriptive or as analytical structures. For the undercover military, the experience of hundreds of thousands of—usually young—people meant that instead of fighting in the open, their participation would mean long-term concealment of their military identity and activity in sabotage. The breakthrough came on 1 August 1944 when, resulting from the situation on the Eastern Front of World War II, the High Command of the Home Army decided to launch the Warsaw Uprising. I am going to return to this issue in the subsequent sections of the chapter, as these facts are of key importance for the potential interpretations of the Home Army soldiers' experience informed by the theory of trauma.

The Polish resistance was not only focused on the military effort. Due to the variety and number of initiatives it undertook, and the fact that the main underground institutions had authority delegated to them by state authorities in exile, historians speak of a Polish Underground State rather than a resistance movement.[17] The Underground State had its own judiciary, which also served as a weapon against the occupation. The first courts were established alongside the undercover army. These were the so-called Hooded Courts, whose name was changed in 1941 to Special Military Courts, while in 1942 they came to be accompanied by Special Civil Courts. The objective of the Special Military Courts was "to prosecute and render verdicts in cases of crimes such as treason, espionage, provocation, denunciation, as well as inhumane persecution of and damage to the Polish populace." All these offences could be subject to capital punishment.[18] For obvious reasons under the circumstances of occupation, the prison sentences were impossible to execute. The wider society would learn about those sorts of sanctions for collaboration with the occupation forces from the advertisements issued in the underground press in

---

[17] More on Polish Underground State: Tomasz Strzembosz, *Rzeczpospolita podziemna: Społeczeństwo polskie a państwo podziemne 1939–1945* (Warszawa: Krupski, 2000); David G. Williamson, *The Polish Underground, 1939–1947* (Barnsley: Pen & Sword, 2012); Joshua Zimmerman, *The Polish Underground and the Jews, 1939–1945* (New York: Cambridge University Press, 2015).

[18] Leszek Gondek, *W imieniu Rzeczypospolitej: Wymiar sprawiedliwości w Polsce w czasie II wojny światowej* (Warszawa: PWN, 2011).

a form much like the following: "Every Polish woman and man who for whatever reason is friends with the officers of the Geheime Staatspolizei (Gestapo), or who maintains relationships with them, or spends time in the company thereof will be sentenced under simplified procedure to death by firing squad."[19]

The cases considered by the Special Civil Courts involved broadly understood collaboration with the occupation forces. The following persons were stigmatized and punished:

> *(1) individuals of the subservient type, striving to win the occupant's favor at their every beck and call [...], (2) women flirting with the Germans and frequenting public areas and locales in their company, (3) individuals inviting Germans to home parties or family celebrations, (4) individuals facilitating the organization of German parties and agitating for Polish women participating therein; [...] (8) individuals publicly sneering at or denigrating the Polish Nation, or claiming that our Nation is unable to exist as an independent state, or that the circumstances of today are the result of its own faults.*[20]

The range of punishments imposed by the court in the above cases included: warning (the convict received an official letter), flogging, reprimand, infamy and "damage to property." The latter penalties were given such a form as to ensure that the society was well aware of them. Thus, court sentences were published in the underground press, while women who had socialized with German soldiers had their heads shaven as a sign of their disgrace. The "damage to property" could involve fire being set to a shop or restaurant belonging to a convicted person who had crossed the delicate line separating the "normal" operation of business at the time of occupation from a "subservient" stance.

The cases brought before the courts were dealt with on the basis of the information provided by the scouts of the ZWZ (later the Home Army). Formally, the judiciary of the underground state did not employ an executioner. In the initial phase of the occupation, verdicts were carried out by

[19] The announcement published in *Na Posterunku* ("On Guard"), the press of the Rzeszów Home Army Inspectorate, quoted after Piotr Szopa, "*W imieniu Rzeczypospolitej...*" *Wymiar sprawiedliwości Polskiego Państwa Podziemnego na terenie Podokręgu AK Rzeszów* (Rzeszów: Instytut Pamięci Narodowej, 2014), 51.

[20] From the brochure *Do czynu!* ("Let's Do It!") distributed in southern Poland in 1943, quoted after Waldemar Grabowski, "Cywilne struktury Polskiego Państwa Podziemnego wobec 'akcji czynnej'," in *"Akcja czynna" Polskiego Państwa Podziemnego*, ed. by Waldemar Grabowski (Warszawa: IPN 2007), 65.

various sabotage units of the ZWZ. By the spring of 1941, the German intelligence operation in Poland had been intensified, resulting in an increase in the activity of informers and in the number of denounced members of the covert organizations. Such harsh conditions forced the leaders of the underground to establish a special department to conduct counterintelligence activity in Warsaw and to eliminate the people who could put the conspiratorial network in jeopardy. A two-person detail, known later as the Department 993/W, was formed in Section II of the Home Army Headquarters. The first execution was carried out towards the close of 1941. By 1 August 1944, that is up until the outbreak of the Warsaw Uprising, ca. 150 people had been involved with the unit—among those, the above-mentioned memoirists Wiśniewski, Horodecka and Bielański. The Dept. 993/W performed more than seventy interventions, of which those of a large scale sent shockwaves through occupied Warsaw. Executions of no less than sixty persons sentenced to death were carried out.[21] In the latter half of 1942, the situation in the war theater made the Headquarters of the AK broaden its sabotage activity; hence, appropriate structures came to be established at the district and area commands of the Home Army. These were referred to as the Directorate of Diversion (I use Polish acronym: Kedyw). Kedyw was the organization behind Operation Arsenal in March 1943, during which prisoners were liberated by the soldiers of the Assault Groups of *Szare Szeregi* ("The Grey Ranks"). The event was narrated in the aforesaid novel by Aleksander Kamiński, *Stones for the Rampart*. Kedyw would also carry out executions of German informers and spies, punish collaborators and the so-called *szmalcowniks*.[22] From 1943 on, another author of one of the memoirs in question, Stanisław Likiernik, was a member of "Kolegium A" of Kedyw of the Warsaw District of the Home Army.

In the territories outside of Warsaw and of other large cities, providing the court with a complete three-person line-up, including at least one lawyer, was not an easy feat. With the circumstances of the occupation becoming more restrictive over time, the regulations allowed the troops to deliver and execute verdicts by force of the decision of the leader of an

---

[21] Robert Bielecki and Juliusz Kulesza, *Przeciw konfidentom i czołgom: Oddział 993/W Kontrwywiadu Komendy Głównej AK i batalion AK "Pięść" w konspiracji i Powstaniu Warszawskim 1944 roku* (Warszawa: Radwan-WANO, 1996), 269.

[22] *Szmalcownik* is a pejorative Polish slang expression that was used during World War II for a person who blackmailed Jews who were in hiding, or who blackmailed Poles who protected Jews. More, in Zimmerman (2015).

underground army unit. If "a marked necessity" emerged, a "preventive action with immediate effect" would be resorted to.[23] Depending on the region of the country, special courts terminated their operations between February and May 1945. Scholars have estimated that in occupied Poland these courts dealt with 5000 cases, imposing the death penalty on 3000–3500 occasions, of which ca. 2500 were carried out.[24] The number of such verdicts was growing proportionally to the intensity of terror and the number of members of the Nazi apparatus of repression. Moreover, from 1943 onward, the Home Army wanted the occupation forces to be aware of who was performing the acts of sabotage against them and why; therefore, such information was being disseminated through various avenues. The sentences were also made public in the underground press alongside warnings to the Polish populace about the consequences of collaboration.[25] Within the Rzeszów Subregion of the Home Army, where Stefan Dąmbski served, 500 death sentences were issued, of which 460 were performed.[26] In the same territory, the sum total of floggings carried out was so high that providing even an estimate has proven impossible. Piotr Szopa, a historian of the region has specified that in a report of May 1943, dispatched from the Rzeszów Inspectorate of the Home Army to the Krakow Area Command, there was mention of over thirty instances of punishment by flogging. He admits that "arbitrary application of such punishments was a common occurrence," and it seems likely that the observation could be extended to other regions of the country.[27] Of similar difficulty was the task of estimating the number of head-shaving punishments, which was used predominantly against women socializing and having intimate relationships with the Germans. At the same time, the practice was considered to be efficient as a deterrent to any further activities of the sort.

The special wartime judiciary continues to trigger many discussions. However, these are not centered on the notion of this type of a justice

[23] Bielecki and Kulesza (1996), 12.

[24] Gondek (2011), 114.

[25] It should be mentioned here that the execution of death sentences on officers of the occupation apparatus resulted in the repression by the occupier against the Polish population (mass executions, arrests and incarceration in concentration camps). In most cases, executions of collaborators did not result in retaliation. From 1943 the Home Army wanted to document its actions so that the German occupier was aware of this.

[26] Szopa (2014), 461.

[27] Szopa (2014), 444.

system, but mainly on the mistakes in the execution of sentences it had handed down. Critical opinions are also voiced against the settling of political scores that occurred with the use of the law "on preventive punishment."[28] Only in recent years have such questions been posed, and, in my view, it is an indirect result of the debate stirred up by the publication of the memoirs of Stefan Dąmbski, an executioner of such sentences.

The Postwar Public Discourse on the Resistance Movement

In order to fully comprehend the debate and discussions about the trials and executions, one has to regard them from within the entirety of the discourse on the resistance movement in Poland. After the end of World War II that discourse was influenced by the Communists' struggle to seize power and later to legitimize it. In spite of the fact that their participation in the resistance was marginal to the operation of the Underground State, for forty-five years they resorted to legitimizing their regime precisely on the basis of their military activities, also in the underground, against the Nazis. It constituted "the foundational myth of the victorious war."[29] Between 1944 and 1956, the construction strategy of this myth involved direct, state-sanctioned persecutions of the members of other formations of the resistance movement, particularly of the Home Army and the National Armed Forces. It was accompanied by a brutal propaganda assault, symbolized in a slogan ever present in the bitter memories of the veterans: "the Home Army—a spittle-bespattered dwarf of reactionary forces."[30] After 1956, the ideology of the authorities started to evolve from the revolutionary to national attitudes. The canonic social memory of the war came to include "the experience of the Home Army."[31] Articles and books of memories by the members of the Home Army started to be

---

[28] For example, Bartłomiej Szyprowski, "W imieniu Polski Walczącej," interview by Maciej Rosolak, *Historia: Do Rzeczy*, July 2014, 14.

[29] Joanna Wawrzyniak, *Veterans, Victims, and Memory: The Politics of the Second World War in Communist Poland* (Frankfurt am Main: Peter Lang, 2015), 27.

[30] The slogan comes from a propaganda poster that was distributed as early as in 1945 in Warsaw.

[31] Wawrzyniak (2015), 135–76.

published in the latter part of the 1950s, whereas the 1970s and the 1980s saw a true abundance of such works in print.[32]

Shortly after 1956, in the period of political "thaw" following the Stalinist era, the iconic figure of a young soldier of the Home Army became the central character in popular culture, with the important role now played therein by the cinema.[33] The tragic protagonists of these pictures, the so-called "Home-Army youth," represented the entire generation which, as I have indicated in the introduction, would soon earn the sobriquet of the Generation of Columbuses.

In the ensuing decades of the twentieth century, the soldiers of the Home Army would continue to be present in war films and TV series; however, their image would be that of heroism and triumph. These were young people carrying out actions of sabotage, ready to overcome any challenges they faced in their wartime underground and military activity against the forces of occupation. They did it in the name of freedom and the motherland, but also of their friends and family. Their deeds were motivated by vengeance and hope. If events ever took a tragic turn, it was only for the individuals, never for the community. The nation emerged from the combat victorious.[34] Furthermore, the romantic imagery of the wartime experiences of the youth is set in a specific location: in the capital city. The instances of active sabotage were depicted mainly using the example of Warsaw. These motifs are rich in details of the organization and of everyday life. Due to the fact that war films were classified as historical cinema, the regulations required the producers to employ a historical consultant. Additionally, state censorship was in place, and so were the pre-release screenings of movie productions. Hence, the cinema of the Communist era might be seen as having represented the binding state-defined narrative of World War II.

Besides the institutional censorship, which obviously kept an eye out for inconvenient not to mention "forbidden" topics, the cultural model of the war and Home Army narratives was largely influenced by the veteran movement and its evolution, also directly determined by political circumstances. In 1949, a dozen or so associations were merged into a single,

---

[32] From among the authors referred to at the beginning of this chapter, Izabella Horodecka, aka "Teresa," published fragments of her memoirs already in 1957 and 1958 in the popular magazine *Kobieta Wiejska* ("Countryside Woman").

[33] The canon of Polish culture came to include the films by Andrzej Wajda: *Kanal* (1956), and *Ashes and Diamonds* (1958).

[34] Wawrzyniak (2015), 135–76.

monopolistic Society of Fighters for Freedom and Democracy,[35] which, under the leadership of the so-called partisans, was able, in the latter half of the 1960s, to actually bear influence on the governing of the country. According to Joanna Wawrzyniak, in the 1970s, by virtue of its policy of limited negotiations with various social groups, the Society managed to unify the three myths: that of the triumph over fascism, that of the unity of the resistance movement and that of the innocence of the victims. All three were political in nature, but at the same time they provided the wartime experience with meaning.[36] The transmission of myths occurred through publishing, education and in cooperation with writers and filmmakers. The Society declared its support for all educational and artistic endeavors which would "show the struggle of our soldier against the occupation forces and the combat undertaken by civilians, partisans and the soldiers of the Underground."[37] It also dismissed the existential war films as well as the satirical ones. It resulted in the prohibition of the screening of some films, such as *Agnieszka '46* (dir. S. Chęciński, 1964). This film was based on a novel titled *Agnieszka, córka Kolumba* ("Agnieszka, The Daughter of Columbus"),[38] and showed the inability to return to civilian life of soldiers whose mentality had been altered by the war. Veterans criticized it for "its lack of a heroic message."[39]

The authors of the memoirs I have analyzed worked on them throughout the above-indicated period; however, the complete versions of their works appeared in print only after 1989. The autobiographies were also created in differing circumstances and social milieux. Izabella Horodecka (born 1908), aka "Teresa," created her account as early as 1946, and, as she underscored in the foreword, she had done so at the behest of the commander of Dept. 993/W, where she had served as an officer of intelligence. Ryszard Bielański (born 1922), aka "Rom," who served in the same detail, also wrote down his first memoir on commission—"from a

---

[35] In Polish: Związek Bojowników o Wolność i Demokrację, usually written as acronym: ZBoWiD.

[36] Wawrzyniak (2015), 13, 28.

[37] *Materiały sprawozdawcze z prac Zarządu Głównego i Komisji ZBoWiD za okres grudzień 1964—czerwiec 1965* ("Reporting materials on the activities of the management board of the ZBoWiD"), quoted after Wawrzyniak (2015), 265.

[38] Wilhelm Mach, *Agnieszka, córka Kolumba* (Warszawa: Czytelnik, 1964).

[39] Wawrzyniak (2015), 266. For the important role of films in depicting the troubled war experiences in the postwar era, see also Ville Kivimäki's, Ana Antić's and Hana Kubátová's chapters in this book.

group of friends appointed to explore the history of Dept. 993/W"; he later went on to supplement it in the mid-1980s. Although Lucjan Wiśniewski (born 1925, aka "Sęp" ["Vulture"]) did not decide to release his memoir, he had already had it in typescript form in the 1960s. Since the first postwar months, the members of the 993/W fostered the memory of their common experience. They organized annual meetings, both as official and informal social events, such as joint excursions to a summer house. Knowing the mechanisms that the autobiographical memory abides by, are we to assume that in the case of such close and frequent contacts within the group, what occurred was a certain alignment of the evoked facts and the entirety of the story?

Jan Kowalkowski (born 1921, aka "Halszka" [diminutive of feminine name Halina]) found himself outside the Warsaw community, yet within the scope of influence of the veterans' discourse, as he was a member of the sabotage group of the Home Army in Krakow. His memoir, written down between the 1950s and his death in 1967, was published in 2002 in a journal of a local veterans' association. However, the conditions in which Stefan Dąmbski (born 1925, aka "Żbik I" ["Wildcat I"]) and Stanisław Likiernik (born 1923, aka "Machabeusz" ["Maccabee"]) created their memoirs were different. Both of them had left Poland by 1946 for fear of Communist repression. Dąmbski spent the larger part of his life in the United States, with his first and only visit to Poland coming in the mid-1970s. Likiernik lived in France. We know that Dąmbski did have some contacts with the veterans' community in exile; still, it would be a stretch to speak of a level of closeness similar to that in the Warsaw group. Likiernik, who started to visit Poland already in 1958, kept in touch with his friend, but it was only in the final years of his life that he settled in Warsaw. Both men started to work on their memoirs as mature adults and for personal reasons, both towards the close of the 1970s. According to the family, Dąmbski was prompted by an incurable disease. In the foreword to his journal Likiernik admitted to have been writing persuaded by his son and for him. Having returned to the interrupted narrative several years later, he reflected on another thing—he regretted not having convinced his own father to perform a similar task.[40]

---

[40] "As men and women move into and through midlife, themes of caring for the next generation, of leaving a positive legacy for the future, of giving something back to society become increasingly salient in life stories," McAdams (2003), 194.

THE WAR EXPERIENCE OF "LIQUIDATORS"

"The experience of a Home Army soldier" varies from what could be described as an average "soldier's experience." Even the very "Home Army experience" could hardly be labelled as homogenous, considering the fact that the types of sabotage and the conditions in which they were performed differed greatly depending on the locations and the tasks faced by the resistance movement locally. Members of sabotage and assault units in large cities fought in conditions fundamentally dissimilar to those encountered by the soldiers of regular armies, and they did it on a different basis.[41] Their situation was also unlike that of partisans operating in rural areas. The protagonists of my chapter—executioners of the sentences imposed by the underground courts—could, therefore, be active in quite different circumstances. Nevertheless, they had a lot in common: they enrolled as young volunteers, in time of war, into an army which presented them with tasks completely unlike those they could understand to be the objectives and methods within a "soldier's duty." "We would dream of an open assault – instead of killing people, performing the sentences – of a soldierly assault, face to face," reminisced Ryszard Bielański, a member of the Warsaw diversion unit of the Home Army.[42]

"The performance of executions on provocateurs and traitors is a necessity, a task that should not be avoided," wrote Gen. Stefan Rowecki in "The Guidelines for Sabotage and Diversion Activity."[43] To all military activity the members of the underground referred to as *robota* ("the job"),[44] and the scope of the term included the executions. The wartime euphemism for an execution, encountered also in the documents, was the term "liquidation," whereas "the delinquent" stood for the victim. The procedures for executing a verdict were uniform; still, the practice could differ depending on whether it was to be performed in a large city or in the countryside. In Warsaw, the Underground State had more people at its disposal, hence some units of the sabotage arm could specialize exclusively in carrying out the sentences, as was the case of 993/W and Kolegium A (Likiernik's unit). In Krakow, a much smaller city, and even more so in the

---

[41] Tomasz Strzembosz, *Oddziały szturmowe konspiracyjnej Warszawy 1939–1944* (Warszawa: PWN, 1983), 428–58.

[42] Bielański (1991), 64.

[43] Quoted after Wojciech Lada, "Bo my, proszę pana, po prostu dziurkowaliśmy ludzi," in *Wielka księga Armii Krajowej* (Kraków: Znak Horyzont, 2015), 354.

[44] In his memoirs, Likiernik used a capital letter; Likiernik (1994), 80.

rural areas, the sabotage units of the Home Army performed all the tasks required by the situation, including of course "the liquidation of traitors to the Polish Nation."[45]

The terrorist activity must be escalated – commanded of Gen. Stefan Rowecki midway through 1943 – [...] Intensify the action of eliminating the spies of the Gestapo. [...] To perform the terrorist and liquidation activity mature men of integrity should be selected, ones who do not become depraved. I hereby forbid the commanders to use in such operations young men of less than 20 years of age.[46]

In subsequent months that command was reiterated numerous times.[47] The reservation regarding the minimum age is also telling with regard to the reality of the period. The authors of the memoirs, apart from Horodecka (though she would not pull the trigger), had been born between 1921 and 1925. Wiśniewski and Dąmbski were 16 when they joined the underground forces, Likiernik was 18, Kowalkowski—18, Bielański—20. Dąmbski writes that in his outfit in the region of Rzeszów, "besides officers, I do not remember anyone over 20 years of age."[48]

Even though the sentences were confirmed in writing, the order of execution was given to the executioners orally.[49] A liquidation mission comprised the preparation—that is gathering intelligence about the convict—the identification, the evaluating of the probability of carrying out the execution (so that it would be "rapid and efficient," as Horodecka put it) and the performance of the execution. The memoirs of the members of Dept. 993/W present these features in a strictly professional manner, in line with the written procedures, while the information provided is rich in detail. An execution was attended by a whole team – the scout, the "backup" (i.e., several persons taken to deal with the situation) and the actual executioner—the trigger man. According to the regulations, the eliminator designated by the Command learned about having been selected a day prior to the action. The task itself was announced to the team in advance, and the preparation time for the mission was spent by the members of the outfit in a state of escalated emotions. During that period,

[45] Kowalkowski (2002), 6.
[46] Quoted after Lada (2015), 354.
[47] *Armia Krajowa w dokumentach 1939–1945,* vol. I (London: Studium Polski Podziemnej, 1970–81), 232; Szopa (2014), 351.
[48] Dąmbski (2020), 38.
[49] Lada (2015), 356.

young people would analyze and visualize the "test" they were faced with.[50] A liquidation unit did not possess its own weapon, that was provided directly before the action, by women—the messengers. The course of the execution, as with that of any other underground military action, consisted of three stages: the anticipation (the so-called exposition), the execution and the retreat (the so-called recoil). From the accounts of veterans, we learn that the initial phase could entail extreme mental strain. "The exposition" could take hours on end, while the already armed member of the sabotage unit usually remained in a public place, in the presence of the enemy. The perpetrators had to behave in as natural a manner as possible, while fully aware of the risk of being uncovered at any moment. Consequently, what occurred were instances of instinctive retreat from the location, numb hands losing their grip on the firearm and the sensation of being paralyzed. Kowalkowski, the executioner from Krakow, mentions a situation when his friends at the very last moment proved unable to reach the street where the act was supposed to take place because they had been affected by panic. However, a display of bravery was given by a female messenger who, according to the plan, reached the spot and assisted in the "recoil." Kowalkowski never talks about his own mental fatigue or stress.[51]

Outside of large cities, that is, in the locations where the partisan units of the Home Army were operating, a sentence could be imposed by the commander, while volunteers from his unit came forward to perform the task. As we read in one of the written accounts created for an organization of veterans in 1971, "the job" required people who were "ambitious, selfless, active, morally and physically fit, young, armed, unstintedly devoted to the cause and cohesive as a team."[52] The above passage is representative of all the analyzed narratives, regardless of the time and circumstances of their creation (including also the hybrid narratives). What comes to the foreground in these memoirs is the motif of "professionalism," that is, of the efficiency of the actions, achieved due to the quality of arms, the cooperation within the group, individual aptitude (including the ability to take risks) and the skill in using firearms.[53] However, the same notions pervade

---

[50] Strzembosz (1983), 449.

[51] Kowalkowski (2002), vol. 2, 71–2.

[52] Written testimony of R. Grotowski, 20 February 1971, Archiwum Akt Nowych (AAN), Tomasz Strzembosz Collection (ATS), file 44.

[53] 65 codes common to all autobiographies stood out from the texts during the content analysis. They relate to an average of 300 text pronouns in each autobiography. In each text, the most common codes are: "weapon," "killing technique," and "camaraderie / brother-

the experience and the narratives of all veterans, regardless of the historical period and location, and do not seem particular to the liquidators. A striking feature in the memoirs are the extensive reconstructions of the performed executions, encompassing such reminiscences as the facial expression of the victims, the sounds accompanying the deed and surprising elements of the surroundings of the scene. Even though, in principle, the death penalty was carried out with the use of a firearm—and such imagery of the execution was recorded in films—there were some exceptions to that rule. The reasons were rather mundane—guns would jam because of their poor quality, what mattered in such situations was only the efficiency; hence, actions could end, for instance, with an explosion of a grenade. In Krakow, there are records of executions by hanging and poisoning; such methods were intended to avoid reprisals from the occupation forces.[54]

The cases when the course of the execution differed from the scenarios envisaged in the procedures are discussed in the memoirs; additionally, some reservations might be voiced as to the potential failures in the author's memory. Those authors often happen to be aware of and refer to versions of the events presented by the other persons participating in the action. This demonstrates that the combatant community, whose members maintained direct contacts with one another (as was the case of the people hailing from Warsaw and the members of the local centers of Society of Fighters for Freedom and Democracy, as well as of the veteran communities which emerged therefrom), might have in some way aligned the narratives of their experiences. The authors who wrote their memoirs in Poland do not describe performing sentences other than capital punishment. The sabotage and elimination actions are recorded from the point of view of a participant in or of a witness to the events; however, their evaluation is not personalized. Even the descriptions of the initial execution do not emphasize its unique character, as it constitutes "the first time" only for the author, but not necessarily for the group to which he belongs. Hence, the activity is evaluated from the perspective of the

---

hood." They account for 10 percent of all quotes, or 30 percent of all quotes in each autobiography.

[54] Tomasz Konopka, Paweł Kwasek and Maciej Bochenek, "Okupacja Krakowa 1939–1945 w protokołach sekcyjnych Zakładu Medycyny Sądowej," *Pamięć i Sprawiedliwość* 7/2 (2008), 83–103.

sabotage unit, the resistance movement, or even the entire nation. Jan Kowalkowski, for example, wrote about it in the following manner:

He could no longer betray anyone [...] *He had been the most vile and harmful informant active within the organization* [...] *My duty was over. The following day, I had to send a dispatch to the Command, prepare the act of prosecution for the Special Military Court, attaching the proof of treason with the request to authorize the performed death sentence of the Gestapo agent.*[55]

Kowalkowski carried out at least thirty death sentences. He was considered to be the perfect saboteur—with nerves of steel, courage and organizational skills. Under the surveillance of the Communist secret police, he started a family, found employment. Already at that point, his personal problems had emerged; their nature may only be assumed from the account of the family, who claimed that "he was unable to find his way as a husband and father," and that "his youth which he spent performing executions impacted his entire later life." He stopped working in 1958 and died of cancer in 1967. We know that he would commit his memories to paper in an almost obsessive manner, in every spare moment, on every possible material, even on scraps of pages.[56] At no point on the 200 pages of his account did he reveal his emotions or moments of weakness during the war; he was always able to "save face."

In the breakthrough period of 1989, during the transformation of the political system in Poland, the imperatives of "historical truth" and of filling in the "white spots" came to the fore.[57] The heroes of the resistance movement felt the need to tell the whole truth about the war. They revealed more facts than in their earlier publications, their narrative came to include moral and political reflections.[58] Of course, one must not only

---

[55] Kowalkowski (2002), vol. 2, 55.

[56] Marcin Banasiak, "Jan Kowalkowski 'Halszka' wykonał ok. 30 wyroków śmierci: Demony wojny prześladowały kata zdrajców," *Dziennik Polski*, April 16, 2016, https://dziennikpolski24.pl/jan-kowalkowski-halszka-wykonal-ok-30-wyrokow-smierci-demony-wojny-przesladowaly-kata-zdrajcow/ar/9848750 (accessed January 28, 2020).

[57] Rafał Stobiecki, "Historians Facing Politics of History: The Case of Poland," in *Past in the Making: Historical Revisionism in Central Europe after 1989*, ed. by Michal Kopeček (Budapest: CEU Press, 2008), 179–96.

[58] Horodecka broke taboo and confessed in a television program that she had been ordered to carry out a political assassination attempt on the Polish diplomat; Andrzej M.B.B. Biskupski, *War and Diplomacy in East and West: A Biography of Józef Retinger* (London: Routledge, 2017), 190–220.

consider the political context of that period but also the passage of time, which made the veterans, then approaching their eighth decade, enter the stage of taking stock of their lives. Ryszard Bielański self-published his memoir in 1992. It had been written already during the Communist era, but as he pointed out in the introduction, his account could not have been published "for obvious reasons." His *Almost a Biography* is a tale rich in detail and anecdotes, its genre not dissimilar to that of a picaresque novel. Though in the first part the protagonist is somewhat hidden amidst the group—the narrator speaks on behalf of the nation and the youth undertaking an armed struggle for independence—the story becomes more personal in the second part. The fate of the protagonist is presented as the result of his own industriousness, courage, cunning. Satirical elements can even be noted in the reconstructed scenes of executions, presented with much dynamism, and at times even with a dose of self-irony.[59] It may have been the only way for the author to narrate those events. At the same time, the book features five extensive passages presenting moral reflections on the attitudes of the author's community during the war. For instance:

> *Before leaving for the action, officer cadet "Ali" borrowed my "wis" pistol.[60] When he had returned, he started telling us everything. "Dąbrowa" shot the traitor dead, "Ali" hit his wife in the neck, she was probably dead too now, twice he aimed at their little son, but he had two misfires and decided to let him live. What part the wife had played in her husband's treason I did not know, I had not researched the case. But I certainly did not understand what the boy had to do with any of it. "Ali" claimed that the traitor's den had to be pulled down. I disagreed. Nor did I denounce "Ali." These times were far from normal.[61]*

The narrator analyzes his own and his colleagues' mental breakdown after the death of their commander on the first day of the Uprising,[62] and on two occasions provides a summary of the psychological consequences of the wartime experiences: "the mental constitution of few men, maybe even of no man, could endure such a strain. Despite appearances of outward calmness, I had spent two decades healing myself before I regained

---

[59] Bielański (1992), 128.

[60] WIS (later "Vis", known also as "Radom") was a pistol designed and produced in Poland in the 1930s.

[61] Bielański (1992), 121.

[62] Bielański (1992), 64.

complete mental equilibrium."[63] At the same time, Bielański declares point-blank that it was the war as such that had been the reason behind the poor mental health of an entire generation of youth, including the cruelty of the occupation forces and lives in constant danger; while after the war, it continued with the harassment and persecutions suffered by the members of the Home Army from the Communist authorities. Bielański's colleagues would admit that he had "his own particular way of writing"; however, his book, which was reissued several times, stirred no controversies among veterans.[64]

One can recognize a similarly picaresque convention in the memoirs of Stanisław Likiernik, as suggested by the very title of his book: *Devilish Luck or Divine Intervention?* The author returns to his past "I," using the same narrative strategy as Bielański. He "saves face," and tells a story of victory, but it is devoid of pathos. In it, numerous anecdotes with humorous undertones, recurrent instances of self-irony and satire concerning the reality of the occupation, are intertwined with reportages from the actions (with technical details, such as situation plans of sabotage activity). When the narrator returns to the present, he includes frequent reflections on the nature of meta-memory and moral judgments, of the following kind:

> *In spite of many exhilarating moments, the* [memory of the] *period has become increasingly bitter with the passing years. With many boys and girls killed, with the immense destruction, with so much past and present suffering of millions of people, our actions of sabotage, "our interesting anecdotes" which they have now become could distort the truth of those times.*[65]

Likiernik was one of the two prototypes of the "Columbus" character, from the novel eponymous for the generation, mentioned at the outset of this chapter. From 1946, he lived in France, maintaining contacts with his friends from the war and from his Home Army unit, but in the form of individual and personal relationships. Independent of any veteran communities and organizations, he would express oftentimes bitter opinions—also in many interviews—on the resistance movement and on the experience of his generation. However, his autobiography, even though he did not refrain from talking about executions, did not stir such

---

[63] Bielański (1992), 178.
[64] Marat and Wójcik (2016), 155.
[65] Likiernik (1994), 81.

controversies nor did it give rise to such emotional reactions among readers, historians and veterans as the memoirs of Stefan Dąmbski, a Home Army liquidator from a remote province.

CONFESSION WITHOUT ABSOLUTION

Stefan Dąmbski came from a wealthy, aristocratic family from southern Poland. His mother died when he was still a child. His father left the country not long before the outbreak of the war. Stefan and his brother had been brought up by an unmarried aunt. They were being educated at a boarding school in Lviv. Stefan joined the resistance movement at 16, like many boys of his age, as indicated in the accounts of other memoirists. He did so, influenced by the ideals instilled in the youth by their prewar education. Dąmbski writes about the matter in a different vein than the other authors. Admittedly, Likiernik was the first to critically claim: "From the perspective of today, our upbringing was extremely romantic and filled with patriotic slogans."[66] Still, the ethos of the prewar upbringing and the symbols that accompanied it were diligently preserved in the veterans' community:

> *They shaped our personalities, and hence also such an attitude. Here is the Holy Mass in our school and a standard-bearer enters. Everything glimmers: sabres, eagles, helmets and belts. We were watching it as if it were God himself. It stayed with us, followed us to the underground, to the partisan warfare.*[67]

On the other hand, Dąmbski recognizes it as the source of his personal drama and that of his entire generation and he voices an accusation:

> *When you shot a man speaking the same language as you, a person you had often known for years, it was rather difficult to explain yourself before your conscience. In the name of what – what was it that made us perpetrate the deeds that would amount to almost a murder in a civilized world? Were we doing it "in the name of the Motherland," or maybe it fell within the range of the so-called military activity? We were to be blindly obedient, as required by our inbred patriotism. It was our duty to show the world that the Poles would never give up and that "for our freedom and yours" they would die with a smile on their faces. However, in reality, they often murdered anybody, who was not on*

---

[66] Likiernik (1994), 12.
[67] Józef Mioduszewski quoted by Bielański in the introduction, Bielański (1992), 8.

their side or who disagreed with their ideals − with the full approval of the Command.[68]

[...] I reached this animal state mainly because of the upbringing I had received in my youth − in the atmosphere of patriotic exaggeration.[69]

The content of his autobiography includes elements which also constitute all the other accounts left by the Home Army soldiers and liquidators: the story of joining the resistance movement, the initiation action, the first execution, the detailed reconstructions of subsequent military actions, the description of the risks and of the elements indicating the professionalism of the sabotage force, the facts evoking a strong "brotherhood-in-arms," such as the profile of the Commander and of colleagues and the attitude towards the enemy.

What makes Dąmbski's narrative stand out from among the other memoirs is its extremely expiatory nature. The author admits to having spent much time after the war analyzing his life. Through writing his memoirs, he wants to settle accounts with his past self, a task he attempts to achieve in a twofold manner: through the structure of his tale and through direct assessment of his deeds and stance. Like the authors mentioned above, Dąmbski recalls the past by making use of anecdotes. His style is that of a crime novel about mobsters. He reaches deep into his memory to evoke the smallest, drastic details of the executions. On the other hand, he never mentions the activity that he could be proud of, in which he had participated as attested to by historical research, such as railway sabotage, airdrops, partisan battles. He systematically records his emotions during each of the executions (joy, excitement, satisfaction of a job well done, cold blood) and confronts them with the image of the victim. He describes the looks, clothes and facial expressions of even anonymous casualties (such as the Soviet soldier asleep at the side of the road, whom he murdered by hammering a nail into his skull). The scenes of murders are intertwined with equally detailed scenes from the everyday life of the partisans, of which the author selects almost exclusively the images of getting drunk and partying together.[70] Such series of events

[68] Dąmbski (2020), 130.

[69] Dąmbski (2020), 131.

[70] He writes about his initial execution differently from all other actions. He uses the present tense in the same way, but here the evaluation and the narrative coda are at the beginning: "It didn't occur to me that in a few hours I should shoot a man, that I have to deprive

narrated in the present tense reminds one of an action film on a loop, with too rapid a pace, too realistic and brutal to remain bearable.[71] Narrating some memories, Dąmbski pauses for a moment. He endeavors to understand who he was at that period: "At that time, I did not care about my life, just like I did not care for the life of others. Not having graduated from any school, I was a nobody in my civilian life, while here in the Home Army I had a large gun on my belt and I could play the big shot."[72] Occasionally, he looks for a justification:

> *I treated my duties seriously and – being a specialist in eliminating people – I performed the sentences entrusted to me without emotions, with a stoic composure, enjoying the fact that my services were needed. I was well aware that without people like me the sabotage forces could not exist.[73] [...] Yet, even the likes of me came across jobs that gave rise to great remorse, the memory of which would torture me for years on end.[74]*

Scrutinizing his past self, Dąmbski does not give himself absolution: "My dreams had come true; I had become remorseless ... I was worse than the most vile animal. I found myself at the very bottom of the quagmire of humanity."[75] His memories end with the words: "It is too late today to ask for anybody's forgiveness, there is no way to bring people back to life."[76]

The readers' reactions to the fragments of Dąmbski's diary, first published in 2005, clearly indicated that his story crossed the line of the accepted framework for memorial narratives about the resistance movement. As mentioned by the publisher: "The text [...] came as a shock to many readers unable to believe that it was an account of the facts and not a piece of original fiction by the author."[77] The brutality of the scenes presented by Dąmbski does not serve any of the accepted models that the

---

of life a human being [...] I apparently considered this to be a perfectly normal thing, something that had to be done, a mere patriotic duty." Dąmbski (2020), 17.

[71] I would like to thank prof. Rafał Wnuk for his remark on the fact that Dąmbski was writing his memories immersed in American pop culture, which must have influenced the way he constructed his narrative.

[72] Dąmbski (2020), 63.

[73] Dąmbski (2020), 27.

[74] Dąmbski (2020), 121.

[75] Dąmbski (2020), 29.

[76] Dąmbski (2020), 131.

[77] Zbigniew Gluza, "Od wydawcy," in Dąmbski (2020), 10.

reader might have been prepared for. The descriptions of the acts of murder do not function as a justification for the collective vengeance for the cruelty of the enemy. Dąmbski does not hide behind such argumentation. There is no trace of romanticism to his narrative; what remains is the point of view of a teenager demoralized by the war. This is who the protagonist of Dąmbski's autobiographical tale is, this is the role he consistently assumes when reaching into his memory.[78] In the memoirs by Likiernik and Bielański, it is the enemy that bears the responsibility for the wartime demoralization of young people; first the Germans, later the Soviets. Bielański writes:

> War is cruel. This one, however, exceeded the norm of cruelty many times. The rules of the game were imposed by the Germans. Our life was worth as much as the bullet was worth [...]. Traitors of various sorts caused huge human losses, a sea of suffering and destruction. They had to be exterminated without mercy. A man in the war gets wild. [...] Today, more than forty years after the described accidents, we have a different judgment, a different view. But then hatred blinded us. Especially hatred of traitors.[79]

Gustaw Budzyński, another executioner from Warsaw who carried out sixty death sentences, says: "The occupational forces, the Germans, the aggressors, made us gradually assume collective responsibility as an acceptable means of inter-human activity. It was something we would not have been able to even imagine before 1939."[80] Even though Dąmbski recognizes as the cause of his personal tragedy not only the war, but also the prewar upbringing and the system of values transmitted in the interwar school; ultimately, he takes all the blame onto himself. All who lost their lives by his hand are personally his victims; he feels the pangs of his individual conscience. He does not seek comfort in the common experience of the Generation of Columbuses. Nor does Dąmbski present himself as the victim of wartime stress or trauma, in spite of the fact that his "anecdotes"

---

[78] See the concept of "an imago"—an idealized personification of the self that functions as a protagonist in the narratives; Dan P. McAdams, "Love, power, and images of the self," in *Emotion in Adult Development*, ed. by Carol Zander Malatesta and Carroll E. Izard (Beverly Hills, CA: Sage, 1984), 193.

[79] Bielański (1992), 122.

[80] Gustaw Budzyński in a television documentary *Karą będzie śmierć*, dir. Marcin Szumowski, Telewizja Polsat, 2014, https://www.youtube.com/watch?v=KkFuoXqMkuw (accessed January 28, 2021).

tend to present situations that could easily be labelled as heavily stress-inducing, if not downright traumatic. Besides the descriptions of "killing techniques," his narrative predominantly features passages presenting situations of direct danger to the life of the author or that of the partisan unit in which he served.[81] Several years of living in the circumstances of constant peril, either on the move or in hiding, in the forest, notoriously malnourished, dirty, lousy—that was the everyday life of the soldiers of the Polish underground during World War II. All of the above Dąmbski had experienced by his 20th birthday, for he turned 20 in July 1945.

As a non-psychologist, I am not inclined to present my interpretations and suspicions regarding the consequences of having experienced that sort of events at such a young age. I limit myself to signaling the things that I can observe in the text of his autobiography. In it, the author alternates between two language registers and, so to speak, between his different selves: that of the teenager and that of the man towards the close of his life (it is worth remembering that at the time of writing, he was suffering from a terminal illness). Reconstructing the situations, he narrates them "with his feet planted in the past." He is a confrontational teenager, devoid of terror, of the fear of death; instead, there is the joy of killing, as unfathomable for the reader as that might be. Much like Likiernik, Bielański and Kowalkowski before him, the author appears to be "saving face." However, it is not a "face" that the reader is willing to take notice of or accept. Voices after the first publication of fragments of his memoir accused Dąmbski of assuming a "pose," of "playing an actor's role," of "embellishing the story" and "exaggerating." A letter to the publisher included the following sentence: "Instead of making himself into a hero of the Home Army, the author made himself into a cruel sadist."[82]

The debate that has surrounded the book—with opinions being voiced by veterans and historians, as well as by authors writing for opinion magazines—centered around the motifs of "historical truth" and the problem of "wartime demoralization." The experts invited to write various articles and visit TV shows referred to facts, archival documents and accounts by other veterans; and by way of comparison with the state of knowledge and

---

[81] The content analysis of Dąmbski's text showed that the codes that I associated with combat stress, such as: reconstructing a sense of threat, situations of high risk of one's own death occurred in 16 narrative units. 42 times the author expresses self-analysis and moral reflection, 8 times remorse is expressed directly.

[82] Irena Filipowicz, "Letter to the publisher," in Dąmbski (2020), 143.

with the image of the resistance movement, they "corrected" the content of Dąmbski's memoirs.[83]

Historians, for that matter, doubted that Dąmbski could have been recruited by a partisan outfit at such a young age, not to mention that he might have been ordered to perform death sentences, for it is a well-known fact in light of the afore-cited documents—the commands—that it would have been against all regulations. Furthermore, the book caused an outrage among the Home Army veterans. They claimed that Dąmbski had fabricated the whole story, that he intended to take credit for performing many "heroic deeds" related in the book. One of the journalists referred to the veterans' reaction as "the measure of the tragedy and of the moral havoc wreaked and instilled in people by the war."[84] The questions recurred as to whether it could have happened at all, and whether Dąmbski was a pathological case of a soldier of the Home Army. Another question to have been directly formulated was whether the book could undermine the image of the Home Army.[85] Every opinion given by the various authors commenced with an expression of shock at the naturalist depictions of the killings. It can be observed that depending on the political and ideological leaning of a given magazine, some journalists would emphasize the negative view of patriotism formulated by Dąmbski, while others would attribute sadistic tendencies individually to the author. Historians treated the text of *The Executioner* as historical material, taking a stance on the matter of wartime demoralization, addressing it at the level of evaluating the entire World War II, those responsible for its outbreak and for its course.

At this juncture, it is worth remembering that in Polish research into experience and memory—both individual and collective—trauma is a category that emerged as early as 1946 within psychiatry and psychology, and subsequently in the form of a "cultural trauma" in sociology and culture

[83] For example: Dariusz Stola, "Przemoc chwalebna," interview by Piotr Lipiński, *Duży Format*, October 28, 2010, http://wyborcza.pl/duzyformat/1,127290,8570820,Prze moc_chwalebna.html (accessed January 28, 2021); Andrzej K. Kunert interviewed by Michał Wójcik, Cafe Historia, https://vod.tvp.pl/video/cafe-historia,egzekutor,685494 (accessed January 28, 2021).

[84] Sz. Hołownia, "Egzekutor z AK," *Newsweek* 43/2010, https://www.newsweek.pl/ egzekutor-z-ak/szkdbmz (accessed January 28, 2021).

[85] Piotr Lipiński in an interview with Dariusz Stola, "Przemoc chwalebna," *Duży Format*, October 28, 2010, http://wyborcza.pl/duzyformat/1,127290,8570820,Przemoc_ chwalebna.html (accessed January 28, 2021).

studies.[86] In Polish historical literature, however, the interpretive category has only appeared in recent years, and even then in only very few books.[87] Of course the debaters did not overlook the facts mentioned by the publisher in the foreword to the book, namely that after his emigration to the United States Stefan Dąmbski found it difficult to adapt to the requirements of family life, eventually, suffered from a terminal illness, committed suicide, and that his journal abruptly ends mid-sentence.[88] Nevertheless, only the cultural anthropologist, Joanna Tokarska-Bakir, was able to recognize, not only in the facts but also in Dąmbski's narrative, the suffering, the "deterioration before the reader's eyes of the authorial subject."[89] She noticed it behind the overtly rhetorical mask, and wrote that such cynical confessions "might just as well have been divulged by a child soldier from the Congo."[90]

Dąmbski had no contact with veterans' organizations in Poland, although he did maintain a relationship with Polish veterans in exile in the United States. He was not influenced by the Polish culture of romantic and tragic heroism, and the state canon of remembrance of World War II was distant to him. Dąmbski spent his entire mature life in the United

---

[86] Stefan Baley, Stanisław Batawia, Maria Kaczyńska and Maria Żebrowska used the term "war complex" for the symptoms identified later by American psychologists as post-traumatic stress disorder (PTSD): Stefan Baley, "O pewnej metodzie badań wpływów na psychikę młodzieży," *Rocznik Psychiatryczny* 37 (1949); Stefan Baley, "Psychiczne wpływy drugiej wojny światowej," *Psychologia wychowawcza* 1–2 (1948); Maria Kaczyńska, "Psychiczne skutki wojny wśród dzieci i młodzieży," *Zdrowie Psychiczne* 1 (1946).

[87] The most cited example is Marcin Zaremba, *Wielki strach—Polska 1944–1947: Ludowa reakcja na kryzys* (Kraków: Znak, 2008). The mental condition of soldiers in various periods of antiquity, representations of trauma in historical literature and reflections on the potential of oral history for interdisciplinary research on the trauma of soldiers of World War II—these are the topics discussed in the publication *Psychologia boju na przestrzeni dziejów: Człowiek w doświadczeniu granicznym*, ed. by Michał Stachura (Kraków: Towarzystwo Wydawnicze "Historia Iagellonica," 2017).

[88] Jerzy Klechta was the only journalist, who used the "trauma" term in his commentary on Dąmbski's autobiography; Jerzy Klechta, *Dramat bohatera*, https://studioopinii.pl/archiwa/2065 (accessed January 28, 2021).

[89] Joanna Tokarska-Bakir, "Historia i antropologia: Trudne sąsiedztwo," in *Historia dziś: Teoretyczne problemy wiedzy o przeszłości*, ed. by Ewa Domańska, Rafał Stobiecki and Tomasz Wiślicz (Kraków: Universitas, 2014), 281; see also Joanna Tokarska-Barki, "Egzekutor z Grossem w tle," *Dwutygodnik*, March 10, 2011, https://www.dwutygodnik.com/artykul/1922-egzekutor-z-grossem-w-tle.html (accessed January 28, 2021).

[90] Tokarska-Bakir (2011), https://www.dwutygodnik.com/artykul/1922-egzekutor-z-grossem-w-tle.html (accessed January 28, 2021).

States, where especially in the 1990s PTSD was gaining attention in the public discourse. It can be said that, unlike his peers who lived in the People's Republic of Poland and had few means to express and share their traumatic experiences, he had the chance to express his trauma in words. He did it in his own way, sometimes using the language of American popular culture. It is not known whether he was under the care of therapists, but it seems likely that he wrote his memoirs while treating that as self-therapy.[91]

A TELLABLE VETERAN'S LIFE

Four years after the publication of *The Executioner*, a book was released to commemorate the 70th anniversary of the outbreak of the Warsaw Uprising. It featured an extended interview with Stanisław Likiernik. The protagonist narrates to a pair of journalists, Emil Marat and Michał Wójcik, what we could already have learned from his published autobiography (the third, supplemented edition was issued in 2010); additionally, he answers their oftentimes provocative questions. The authors of the interview emphasize the fact that Likiernik served as one of the prototypes for the titular character of the novel *Columbuses: Born 1920*. In the afterword to their book, they refer to the social phenomenon of Bratny's novel and specify who in their view deserves to be called a member of the Generation of Columbuses. In this context, Marat and Wójcik from the outset attempt to induce Likiernik to reveal his emotions—both those from years ago and those of today. They follow the motifs featured in the memoirs of Dąmbski. Likiernik answers bluntly and with much bitterness: "It is true that killing people is not good for your health when you are twenty. Still, it is also true that killing can be very easy. This is the tragic aspect of it all: being able to kill with no remorse."[92] He goes on to talk about the exalted patriotism taught in the prewar schooling, which had certainly shaped his—very naive at the beginning of the war—understanding of how a Polish person should behave. At times, Likiernik speaks in a manner reminiscent of Dąmbski: for instance, "In such circumstances, killing a man is not as shocking as you might imagine. I did kill him, but it was like snapping my

---

[91] For more on the therapeutic effects of writing in the literature, see, for example, James W. Pennebaker, "Theories, therapies, and taxpayers: On the complexities of the expressive writing paradigm," *Clinical Psychology: Science and Practice* 11 (2004), 138–42.

[92] Marat and Wójcik (2014), 44.

fingers. A trifle. It is very unfortunate what I am saying here, but that is how it is. It didn't cost me absolutely anything."[93] And later, "You cannot realize what a feeling it was – to finally stop being the hunted animal, to turn into the hunter. 'The job' was like going to the cinema to watch a good film. Not a burdensome duty, but sheer joy."[94]

Some outraged readers of Dąmbski's book considered the fact that he had described war actions in the style of film scenes to be a proof of his demoralization and cynicism.[95] Marat and Wójcik opened their interview with the topic of the "film-like quality" surrounding the war, the resistance movement, the Warsaw Uprising. In the dialogue with Likiernik, references to film discourse recur again and again. Even the interviewee comments on things like the manner of holding the weapon "just like in a Western," or describes an act of sabotage using a film convention. There are also allusions to Polish films, both those mentioned here in the opening and the most recent ones, including the TV series which influenced the modern-day perception of war and the sabotage forces under the German occupation.[96] The film scene never appears as something that has ever triggered traumatic or unpleasant memories in the interlocutor (cf. Ville Kivimäki's chapter in this volume). Despite these similarities, the book did not cause as much of a stir as the memoirs of Dąmbski. The readers ultimately came to accept not only the facts, that is the very existence of the Home Army executioners, and their being very young, but also even the form of the narrative—the naturalism of the descriptions of murders, a specifically cynical point of view of the narrator and it being presented in the convention of a film.

Marat and Wójcik decided to pursue this avenue and released already in 2016, in one of the largest publishing houses in Poland, their book *Ptaki drapieżne: Historia Lucjana Wiśniewskiego, likwidatora z kontrwywiadu AK* ("Birds of Prey: The Story of Lucjan Wiśniewski, Eliminator of the Home Army's Counter-Intelligence"). This time, the front cover did not feature an archival photograph of the main character (which was virtually

---

[93] Marat and Wójcik (2014), 46.

[94] Marat and Wójcik (2014), 54.

[95] "A wonderful black Opel is coming. This time the road is empty. The car arrives majestically in front of our basement. I see four people in German uniforms. 'Now!'—I scream—and the avalanche of fire blows towards the car! We shoot at the height of the windows. The Opel, in slow motion, makes a slight left turn and falls into a ditch. I noticed that a few seconds earlier the rear door of the car opened, from which a wounded Nazi jumped out onto the road. He even tried to get up, but at that moment a short series from our machine gun calmed him down forever." Dąmbski (2020), 52.

[96] Dąmbski (2020), 42, 51, 63.

a rule up until then), but a black-and-white still frame from the 1958 movie *Zamach* ("Assault," dir. J. Passendorfer). The dynamic picture presents three young saboteurs in action, armed. The book focuses on the activity of the Dept. 993/W (the same one that Bielański and Horodecka served in), while at its core there are the memories of Wiśniewski, who participated in circa 60 acts of elimination. The extended interview was complemented by extensive passages cited from the written accounts by Wiśniewski and his colleagues,[97] and the authors also added much material themselves. The book is a historical reportage, in which besides the mentioned witness relations, use was made of archival documents. Blurbs on the back cover scream at the reader slogans such as: "A Hero. An Avenger. An Executioner"; "In an honest conversation, 'Sęp' discusses how he and his teenage peers from 'the Bird patrol' [...] transformed, from nestlings into birds of prey, defenceless boys, the merciless soldiers." In the interview, Wiśniewski among other things tells the story of how he sent out on a "job" a 15-year-old or 16-year-old boy, because the latter "was raring to shoot some."[98] Wiśniewski joined the resistance while not yet 17. He recalls his first execution: he shot a woman in the back of her head.[99] He addresses the issue of ("silly" and "youthful") competition among the saboteurs for military decorations—the Crosses of Valor.[100] He provides information on acts blatantly contrary to the regulations, for instance, the prohibition on carrying firearms on a daily basis.[101] The authors of the book devoted an entire chapter to the issue of material remuneration for the work in diversion. They avail themselves of accounts drawn from archives, while Wiśniewski furnishes the details, discussing not only the payments for executions, but also shop robberies that members of his troop happened to commit.

The facts narrated by the protagonist of *Birds of Prey* belong to the same category and are a testament to the same phenomena as those described by Dąmbski, which had become the subject of heated debates among historians. Marat and Wójcik make attempts to document the facts with materials drawn from many sources. This is therefore much more than merely the memory of a single veteran, crushed by trauma and the

---

[97] Manuscripts in the University Library Archive in Warsaw.
[98] Marat and Wójcik (2016), 23.
[99] Marat and Wójcik (2016), 33.
[100] Marat and Wójcik (2016), 104.
[101] Marat and Wójcik (2016), 120.

subsequent years of loneliness in exile. Nor would it be easy to accuse Wiśniewski of confabulating or displaying pathological character traits. He is a witness validated by his continuous postwar activity in the Warsaw community of the Dept. 993/W veterans. No representative of the media, no one from among historians and authors was "shocked," "terrified" or "appalled" by the content of the book, or by the manner in which the tale has been constructed, even though it is a story firmly embedded in contemporary discourse, and in the popular culture of today. The autobiographical narrative of Wiśniewski constitutes a component of the work, and the interviewee yields himself to the convention. Much as they did in the interview with Likiernik, the journalists ask questions or comment on the protagonist's opinions by referring to films and other pop-cultural artefacts. Owing to that, Wiśniewski is able to tell the story of his life in relation to them.

Consequently, what the reader receives is a "life like a film" or, to top that, "life better than a film." Marat and Wójcik present the veterans of the Dept. 993/W as a group united during and after the war, all the way up to the present, drawn together by something more than mere brotherhood-in-arms. From the book we can learn that they continued to meet each other throughout the entire postwar period, starting in 1946—at every Christmas. While promoting their book, the publishing house and the authors willingly resort to using a photograph taken in the 1980s in Wiśniewski's summer garden plot, which shows a group of eight smiling, relaxed men and women in sunbathing suits, wearing sun hats. The caption under the photograph reads: "Gentle old people—executioners of wartime court sentences." What keeps the group together are their extraordinary secrets, still undiscovered, their unique experiences, their distinguished professionalism.[102] After all, they are the counter-intelligence, "the gentlemen performing the dirty jobs," a secret "executioners' club."[103] The interlocutor accepts such a style of conversation, when he says, for instance: "in this line of work one does not talk much."[104] Both sides jocularly continue on this Bondian path. In the interview, Wiśniewski had an opportunity to adjust his autobiographical narrative to the modern discourse, even though he did not achieve it entirely single-handedly.

---

[102] For example, when Wiśniewski says that the Security Office wanted to recruit him to work in 1946, journalists react: "Well, as an instructor? Because none of them knew as much about the job as you and colleagues from 993/W did." Marat and Wójcik (2016), 265.

[103] Marat and Wójcik (2016), 160 (caption to photo 5), 182, 183.

[104] Marat and Wójcik (2016), 184.

However, one may venture to say with much certainty that it was he who decided not to beat the patriotic drum. His longer utterances convey very few reflections on morality, when not provoked by direct journalists' questions. He was able to rationalize whatever he had done during and after the war. "I do not feel guilty about anything," he says.

CONCLUSION

Every autobiography is an assemblage of theories of the self and self-representation; of personal identity and one's relation to a family, a region, a nation; and of citizenship and a politics of representativeness (and exclusion).[105] Contemporary literary and culture studies present the genre of autobiography as a hybrid: equally applicable to the past, present, to what is your own, and what is someone else's; it is at once documentary and fictitious.[106] My claim is that during the recent decade in Poland, we have witnessed, as mentioned at the outset of this chapter, a growth of public interest in wartime memories of veterans, and that, as a result, these have undergone alterations, which may be traced by researching the content of the memoirs published during the past decades, particularly the last thirty years. I consider the issue to be an important one because, as indicated by Dan McAdams, who follows Anthony Giddens and Charles Taylor, "the unique problems that cultural modernity poses for human selfhood require modern men and women to become especially adept at assimilating their lives to culturally intelligible stories."[107] The memories of the oldest generation alive are the lesson for the generation of today in what a narrative of wartime experiences ought to look like, but at the same time they are subject to adaptations to contemporary genres. Such a system of genres as described by Tzvetan Todorov functions as the "horizon of expectation" for readers and as models of writing for authors.[108]

---

[105] Charlotte Linde, *Life Stories: The Creation of Coherence* (New York: Oxford University Press, 1993), 3–20, 98–127.

[106] Philippe Lejeune, "The Autobiographical Pact," in *On Autobiography*, ed. by Paul John Eakin, trans. Katherine Leary (Minneapolis: University of Minnesota Press, 1989), 3–30.

[107] Dan P. McAdams, "Personality, modernity, and the storied self: A contemporary framework for studying persons," *Psychological Inquiry* 7:4 (1996), 295–321; McAdams (2003), 202; Anthony Giddens, *Modernity and Self-identity: Self and Society in the Late Modern Age* (Stanford, CA: Stanford University Press, 1991); Charles Taylor, *Sources of the Self: The Making of the Modern Identity* (Cambridge, MA: Harvard University Press, 1989).

[108] Tzvetan Todorov, *Genres in Discourse* (Cambridge: Cambridge University Press: 1990), 10.

Roger Luckhurst identifies trauma as a "conceptual knot" in the contemporary discourse: "It has been turned into a repertoire of compelling stories about the enigmas of identity, memory and selfhood that have saturated Western cultural life." With his tale of a tragic life and a lacerated conscience, Stefan Dąmbski wanted to leave a moral message. However, in contemporary Poland, where popular culture rapidly devours historical themes and transforms them into spectacles—of historical re-enactments, "patriotic hip-hop music" and computer games—the brutalism of Dąmbski's narrative and his type of a protagonist had proved nothing more than just another bit of fodder. The publishing of Dąmbski's memoirs gave rise to an updated model of narrating the experience of World War II, but, paradoxically, against the author's intentions. In contemporary Poland, a "tellable life" of a veteran continues to be a manly adventure. Contrary to the heroic romanticism, sacrifice and drama present in the narratives created in previous political and cultural epochs, present-day veterans' stories are filled with "fast and effective" characters feeling no pangs of conscience when all is said and done. This genre offers no room for expiation and healing traumas.

Acknowledgment The chapter is based upon research supported by National Science Center, project no. 2015/19/B/HS3/01761.

CHAPTER 10

Environmental Trauma in the Narratives of Postwar Reconstruction: The Loss of Place and Identity in Northern Finland After World War II

Outi Autti

INTRODUCTION

The final stages of World War II meant a dramatic change in the lives of people living in Northern Finland. From the summer of 1941 until the autumn of 1944, a large number of German troops were deployed in the area, fighting together with the Finnish army against the Soviet Union. Then, in September 1944, the Finnish government signed an armistice with the Soviet Union. For Northern Finland, this meant that areas in Salla, Kuusamo and Petsamo were lost. The treaty also ordered Finland to expel their former German "brothers in arms," an army of 200,000 men,

O. Autti (✉)
School of Architecture, University of Oulu, Oulu, Finland
e-mail: Outi.Autti@oulu.fi

267

V. Kivimäki, P. Leese (eds.), *Trauma, Experience and Narrative in Europe after World War II*, Palgrave Studies in the History of Experience, https://doi.org/10.1007/978-3-030-84663-3_10

from all Finnish territory within two weeks' time.[1] To empty the area ahead of forthcoming military operations, the civilian population of Northern Finland got an evacuation order from the Finnish army headquarters. For some, this was not the first evacuation order: during the Winter War of 1939–40, the inhabitants of eastern parts of Lapland were evacuated westwards.[2] At first, the Germans helped civilian refugees by offering transportation southwards.[3] Hostilities between Finns and Germans began in earnest at the beginning of October 1944, as the tight timeline made a peaceful retreat impossible. In addition, there was a serious threat of Soviet occupation in Northern Finland and of a new war against the Soviet Union.[4]

For the refugees, the departure was quick and sudden. The evacuation was successfully completed in Lapland in two weeks. In 1944, the population of Lapland was around 143,500. About 56,500 persons were evacuated to Sweden and 47,500 elsewhere within Finland, mainly Ostrobothnia in the west.[5] In the receiving communities, the evacuees were placed partly in farmhouses and yard buildings, partly in public buildings and refugee camps.[6] Some of the evacuees used their personal contacts and sought their way to relatives or friends independently, while

---

[1] Oula Seitsonen and Eerika Koskinen-Koivisto, "'Where the F… is Vuotso?': Heritage of Second World War Forced Movement and Destruction in a Sámi Reindeer-Herding Community in Finnish Lapland," *International Journal of Heritage Studies* 24:4 (2018), 421–441; Marianne Junila, "Wars on the Home Front: Mobilization, Economy and Everyday Experiences," in *Finland in World War II: History, Memory, Interpretations*, ed. by Tiina Kinnunen and Ville Kivimäki (Leiden: Brill, 2012), 191–232.

[2] Interview data Lapland War (LW), 2013–18, in possession of Outi Autti; Onerva Hintikka, *Pako Lapin sodasta* (Helsinki: Maahenki, 2015).

[3] Veli-Pekka Lehtola, "Second World War as a Trigger for Transcultural Changes among Sami People in Finland," *Acta Borealia* 32:2 (2015), 125–47; Veli-Pekka Lehtola, *Surviving the Upheaval of Arctic War: Evacuation and Return of the Sámi People in Sápmi and Finland During and After the Second World War* (Inari: Kustannus-Puntsi, 2019); Veli-Pekka Lehtola, *Saamelainen evakko* (Inari: Kustannus-Puntsi, 2004).

[4] Erkki Rautio, Tuomo Korteniemi and Mirja Vuopio, *Pohjoiset pakolaiset: Tietoa ja tarinoita Lapin sodasta ja lappilaisten evakkotaipaleelta* (Oulu: Pohjan väylä, 2004); Hintikka (2015); Marja Tuominen, "Lapin ajanlasku: Menneisyys, tulevaisuus ja jälleenrakennus historian reunalla," in *Rauhaton rauha: Suomalaiset ja sodan päätyminen 1944–1950*, ed. by Ville Kivimäki and Kirsi-Maria Hytönen (Tampere: Vastapaino, 2015), 39–70.

[5] Martti Ursin, *Pohjois-Suomen tuhot ja jälleenrakennus saksalaissodan 1944–1945 jälkeen* (Oulu: Pohjoinen, 1980), 29–32.

[6] Interview data LW.

others defied the evacuation order and stayed behind, hiding in the forests and the wilds.

When withdrawing towards Northern Norway, the German troops systematically destroyed not only all their own military installations but also civilian infrastructure and practically everything within their reach. Railways, roads, telephone lines and bridges were destroyed. Province capital Rovaniemi was burned to the ground and almost 15,000 buildings were destroyed elsewhere in sparsely populated Northern Finland. Over 24,000 domestic animals and 20,000 reindeer were lost.[7]

As soon as it was possible, Lapland War refugees started to return to their homes—with the exception of the inhabitants of Salla, Kuusamo and Petsamo, areas that were ceded to the Soviet Union. Refugees from these areas lost their home environment and had to be settled elsewhere. The last Germans crossed the border between Finland and Norway on 27 April 1945. Even with the withdrawal of the Germans, some of the refugees could return to their homeland as the frontline advanced northward. Nevertheless, the return was often delayed because of the destroyed infrastructure and burned out homes, but also because of land mines and other explosives that were being planted by the withdrawing Germans. The return home was eagerly awaited, but the homecoming, with the sight of so much destruction, came as a shock. Oula Seitsonen and Eerika Koskinen-Koivisto write about a twofold feeling of "shock and joy" when the refugees returned home: the material and cultural environment was destroyed, but the important physical features of the environment, such as fjells, rivers, and familiar landscapes were left.[8] People had to start their lives again from scratch. The housing situation was poor, dozens of people had to live in tiny saunas or barns. Most of the refugees returned by July 1945, at the latest. The last returns continued until the end of 1947, however, and, due to various reasons, such as illnesses, some people came back even later.[9]

Nevertheless, it was not just wartime destruction that shook the foundations of the human-environment relationship in the area—the huge postwar modernization project in Northern Finland was a direct consequence of the war years and changed the physical and cultural environment of the area profoundly. Marja Tuominen writes that the war in

---

[7] Ursin (1980), 383–5.
[8] Seitsonen and Koskinen-Koivisto (2018), 430.
[9] Tuominen (2015), 58; Interview data LW 2013–18.

Lapland harmed not only material but also mental conditions and complicated efforts at developing the province for decades. The effects of the war were to be seen in the landscape and the economy of the area, but the impacts were also mental and social.[10] More traumatizing environmental changes were caused by postwar reconstruction work that included damming the rivers Kemijoki and Iijoki for electricity production (Fig. 10.1). The Kemijoki is the largest watercourse in Finland, extending through almost all of Lapland. It was one of the most significant salmon rivers in Europe and the Iijoki was one of the most important ones in Finland.[11] After the war, the production of electricity was generally seen as a common, nationwide goal since the country was suffering from a severe shortage of energy. Finland had lost a substantial part of its hydropower to the Soviet Union, and energy was needed in industrialization and postwar reconstruction.

Reconstruction work made Northern Finland a laboratory of modernization, and the hydro-power production intensified the work in that laboratory. The damming caused a massive environmental change in the area, changing not only the landscapes but also the socioecological and cultural dynamics of local communities. As operational fish passages were neither planned nor built, substantial salmon fishing cultures were rapidly eliminated along both rivers.[12] The focus was on engineering and economic growth; environmental and cultural values were overlooked, and the experiences of local people neglected.[13] Postwar reconstruction also changed the traditional cultural landscapes of Lapland. The building stock from the traditional timber constructions—now mostly destroyed—was replaced with modern, type-planned houses, which responded to the practical

[10] Marja Tuominen, "Lapin sodan tuhot ja jälleenrakennus," in *Lappi: Maa, kansat, kulttuurit*, ed. by Ilmo Massa and Hanna Snellman (Helsinki: SKS, 2003), 102–4.

[11] River Kemijoki is 550 km long and its basin covers an area of 51,000 km². River Iijoki has a length of 370 km and a basin area of 14,191 km².

[12] Outi Autti, "Aina vaan tuli iso lasti herroja: Elämäntavan muutos Kemijoella," in *Lappi palaa sodasta: Mielen hiljainen jälleenrakennus*, ed. by Marja Tuominen and Mervi Löfgren (Tampere: Vastapaino, 2018), 308–33; Outi Autti, *Valtavirta muutoksessa—vesivoima ja paikalliset asukkaat Kemijoella*, Acta Universitatis Ouluensis E136 (Oulu: University of Oulu, 2013b); Kai Hoffman, *Pohjolan Voima 1943–1993* (Oulu: Kaleva, 1993); Leena Suopajärvi, *Vuotos- ja Ounasjokikamppailujen kentät ja merkitykset Lapissa* (Rovaniemi: Lapin yliopisto, 2001); Kustaa Vilkuna, *Lohi: Kemijoen ja sen lähialueen lohenkalastuksen historia* (Keuruu: Otava, 1975).

[13] Outi Autti and Timo P. Karjalainen, "The Point of No Return: Losing Salmon in Two Northern Rivers," *Nordia Geographical Publications* 41:5 (2013a), 45–57.

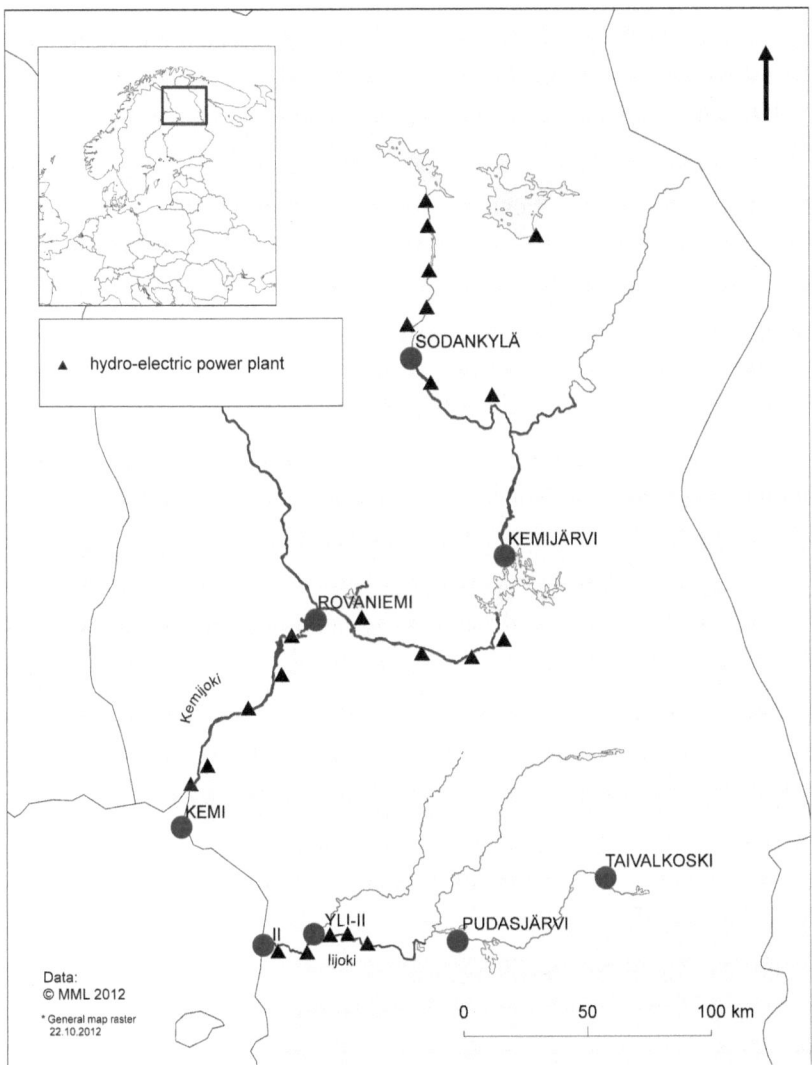

Fig. 10.1 The research area: the biggest municipality centers and hydro-electric power plants in Northern Finland. (Map by Juhani Päivärinta, Outi Autti and Anu Soikkeli)

needs that prevailed immediately after the war. New building stock brought equality into living but at the same time changed the traditional landscapes.[14]

Histories of places, communities and families are connected and they live in the material objects of the environment. Places, landscapes and material objects that relate to human existence in the place are packed with narratives, memories and emotional experiences.[15] The loss of significant town and village landscapes, home yards, buildings and personal property can be traumatizing and weaken people's place attachment. In a rapidly changed and newly built environment, people's place relation becomes contradicted, as the landscape no longer mirrors the histories of local people, families and communities, nor their activities.

In this chapter, I study *environmental trauma* and its various aspects that lean on theories on human-environment relationship and place attachment. My empirical data consist of qualitative interviews conducted among people living in Northern Finland. I examine the traumatic nature of postwar environmental change in a northern community whose residents have a strong bond to the natural world and have experienced several changes in their home environment.

The origin of war-related traumas can often be traced to different war experiences, such as actual warfare and battles, loss of loved ones, witnessing the horrors of war, forced moves and the threat of all these events. Even though the causes and phenomena behind an environmental change and war-related destruction are different, the traumatizing effects can be very similar. My argument is that much of what is nowadays considered to be war-related trauma can also be found as active processes elsewhere. For example, various development projects that alter the environment can activate trauma processes that are very similar to war-related trauma. And, as with Northern Finland, the environmental damage can also be indirectly war-related and initiated by the economic demands of national reconstruction in the postwar period.

---

[14] Anu Soikkeli, "Tyyppitalojen aika: lappilaisen asumisen muutos," in Tuominen and Löfgren, eds (2018), 143–63.
[15] Tuominen (2015), 54.

ENVIRONMENTAL TRAUMA CONNECTS
TO THE ENVIRONMENTAL PAST

In this chapter, trauma refers to psychological trauma caused by a shocking event that creates severe stress. Loss, grief and suffering are closely related to trauma. Changes that cause losses sometimes result in long-lasting grief and suffering. In the case of a prolonged or delayed symptom, one can speak of post-traumatic stress disorder. Environmental trauma can be caused by natural disasters or man-made ecocides, such as wars, or the exploitation of natural resources. To define an event as an origin of environmental trauma, it must include aspects that have changed or threaten the physical environment and negatively affect the lives of people. The adhesion to the physical environment differs environmental trauma from directly war-related and cultural trauma.[16] Environmental trauma can, however, become a cultural trauma when the consequences touch upon the human sphere of life more broadly or affects larger communities. Changes in the physical environment, including the natural and cultural environment, affect people in various ways. We hope for stability and sustainability in our environment, we form emotional attachments to various features of our environment, we carry the places we grew up in and live in with us, and our home environments are closely linked to our identity.[17] Rapid and large-scale changes may shake the cornerstones of our identity and cause emotional imbalance as well as varying degrees of crisis and trauma.

In addition to physical nature, the environment also has social, economic, cultural, ethical and aesthetic dimensions. Moreover, environment can be understood not only as a physical environment, or specific place or area, but also in an abstract sense. Ann Kaplan writes about climate change where she talks about the abstract element of climate trauma and

[16] Jeffrey C. Alexander, "Toward a Theory of Cultural Trauma," in Jeffrey C. Alexander, Ron Eyerman, Bernard Giesen, Neil J. Smelser and Piotr Sztompka, *Cultural Trauma and Collective Identity* (Berkeley: University of California Press, 2004), 1–30; Ron Eyerman, "Social Theory and Trauma," *Acta Sociologica* 56:1 (2013), 41–53.

[17] Steven Feld and Keith H. Basso, "Introduction," in *Senses of Place*, ed. by Steven Feld and Keith H. Basso (Santa Fe, NM: School of American Research Advanced Seminar Series, 1996), 3–12; Gillian Rose, "Place and Identity: A Sense of Place," in *A Place in the World*, ed. by Doreen Massey and Pat Jess (Milton Keynes: Open University Press, 1995), 87–132; Edward Relph, *Place and Placelessness* (London: Pion, 1976); Yi-Fu Tuan, *Topophilia: A Study of Environmental Perception, Attitudes, and Values* (Upper Saddle River, NJ: Prentice-Hall, 1974).

pretrauma, since climate change consequences are not yet fully known.[18] Environmental trauma can also be activated by the threat of an environmental disaster or ecocide. Sometimes the threats can be long-lasting. In climate change adaptation research, the values of individuals and communities, narratives and place relations, have recently become increasingly important.[19]

Jeffrey C. Alexander writes that cultural trauma can occur "when members of a collectivity feel they have been subjected to a horrendous event that leaves indelible marks upon their group consciousness, marking their memories forever and changing their future identity in fundamental and irrevocable ways."[20] The horrendous event that Alexander refers to can obviously be an environmental catastrophe. Environmental trauma can take collective and individual forms, and the experience can differ between individuals and groups, depending, for example, on their personal histories and future intentions, or the scale of the change.[21] Doreen Massey sees residents of a certain area as heterogeneous in many respects, and different groups' ideas of place and its identity can differ significantly.[22] There are different ways of participating and contributing to a place, and the ways places are used is under constant negotiation on different levels. Cultural trauma is strongly connected to collective memories and social processes, as the causing event threatens the existence and the identity of a group. In order to become a cultural trauma, the event must be culturally narrated as such. However, environmental trauma is contextualized: at its minimum, it can remain an individual experience that sometimes is left without expression. An event or change has shaken the individuals' connection to their home environment or to some significant feature of it. The magnitude is varied, dynamic and wide: the cause of trauma can be shocking for someone even if someone else does not notice any change. It can be a loss

---

[18] Ann E. Kaplan, *Climate Trauma: Foreseeing the Future in Dystopian Film and Fiction* (New Brunswick, NJ: Rutgers University Press, 2016).

[19] See, for example, W. Neil Adger, Jon Barnett, Katrina Brown, Nadine Marshall and Karen O'Brien, "Cultural Dimensions of Climate Change Impacts and Adaptation," *Nature Climate Change* 3 (2013), 112–17; Helene Amundsen, "Place Attachment as a Driver of Adaptation in Coastal Communities in Northern Norway," *Local Environment: The International Journal of Justice and Sustainability* 20:3 (2015), 257–76. DOI: https://doi.org/10.1080/13549839.2013.838751

[20] Alexander (2004), 1.

[21] See Anna Wylegała's discussion on individual and collective trauma in this book.

[22] Doreen Massey, "The Conceptualization of Place," in *A Place in the World*, ed. by Doreen Massey and Pat Jess (Milton Keynes: Open University Press, 1995), 45–86.

of an important feature in the environment, or a large-scale environmental disaster. In this sense, environmental trauma differs from the definition of cultural trauma: in some cases, no historical evidence remains of the causing event and there are no grand narratives about it. The existence of it, at its minimum, can be a single, personal, negative, environment-related experience.

Environmental change can affect people directly and indirectly. Direct trauma impacts concern people who have personally experienced the changes and suffer from the consequences, such as a loss of the home environment. Indirect impacts can be economic, political, cultural or social consequences that affect people who have, or have not, directly experienced the change. For example, when an environmental change negatively impacts the sources of livelihood, the consequences can be wide and long-lasting, also affecting future generations who have not personally experienced the original cause of the trauma. Long-term impacts and social processes also make environmental trauma transgenerational. Natalie Clark et al. write about direct and indirect (cultural) pathways from biodiversity to human health. Biodiversity change can directly affect health, for example, through transmission of diseases. Indirect impacts happen through cultural pathways: loss of biodiversity affects the provision of cultural goods, after which there are fewer opportunities to realize and place cultural values upon those goods.[23] This reduces our wellbeing and negatively impacts our health.

The nature of change and its starting points play a role in coping with the trauma: whether the causing event is natural, economic or political makes a difference. Environmental conflicts concerning, for example, large-scale mining projects or other disagreements regarding land use incorporate questions about power and injustice. Such projects, evidently harming the environment, bring benefit to many but harm others, often locals. Coping with a natural disaster, for example, an earthquake, is more likely to evoke a sense of communality, making coping and fixing the consequences more of a collective responsibility. However, current environmental changes are often complicated mixtures of natural and man-made origins.

---

[23] Natalie Clark, Rebecca Lovell, Benedict W. Wheeler, Sahran Higgins, Michael Depledge and Ken Norris, "Biodiversity, Cultural Pathways, and Human Health: A Framework," *Trends in Ecology and Evolution* 29:4 (2014), 198–204. DOI: https://doi.org/10.1016/j.tree.2014.01.009

The experience of environmental trauma can become central in recognizing a community's moral responsibility. It can play a key role in empowering people, in recognizing their voices and rights and in identifying power relations. Environmental trauma has the potential to provide links between cultures: our own trauma experiences may find words from similar experiences elsewhere, and understanding the pasts of others will add to our ability to more broadly understand the fragility of human-environment relationship. Through that concept, we can identify the disconnections between man and environment and how they affect human wellbeing.

Environmental trauma as a concept is a framework within which it is possible to understand environment-related human pain and feelings of injustice. At its worst, environmental trauma attaches to important place-based aspects of life; it threatens the sources of livelihood, emotional bonding with the environment, a sense of collectivity, personal and family history, community history and memories. Environmental trauma can open up new perspectives and understandings of environmental change both past and present. It is connected to the concept of eco-anxiety, the sense of global dread and lack of control, usually referring to current and predicted climate change.[24] The materials to be used in research may include oral and written histories, data produced by ethnographic inquiries, archive material, literature, films, music and other cultural representations. The artistic expressions of environmental trauma may prove especially fruitful when looking for deeper explanations, as traumatic experiences are often surrounded by silence. Sometimes language alone falls short: people do not find words, justification or common support for their traumatizing experiences.

Possible research areas may include human-environment relationship studies, environmental conflicts and power relations, environmental activism or morbidity/health studies. When studying environmental conflicts, the power relations easily blur the view: it is important to notice the competing narratives, their connections and justifications. Those who have experienced environmental trauma, especially that related to land-use conflicts, often find no space in dominant discourses. It is important to pay attention to the contextual factors, starting from how the relationship

---

[24] Susan Clayton, Christie Manning, Kirra Krygsman and Meighen Speiser, *Mental Health and Our Changing Climate: Impacts, Implications, and Guidance* (Washington, D.C.: American Psychological Association / ecoAmerica, 2017).

between human beings and nature is perceived in the society—can one use nature indefinitely and believe the new technology will repair the damages, do we search for balance with nature, or do we see nature as stronger than man?

THE CONNECTION BETWEEN PEOPLE AND PLACES

The human-environment relationship is complex but at the same time so obvious that the relationship is often not considered.[25] The environment is taken for granted and people do not always recognize their place attachment or the importance of the environment to their wellbeing. The bond between the human and the environment gets attention when something changes in the environment, or the danger of change threatens the existence of a person or a group. A person's identity and idea of self are constructed in relation to places and to acting within those places, whether we acknowledge it or not. We are connected to our environment by many invisible ties. Our experiential, meaningful relationship with the surrounding world is built on the basis of place.[26] The environment dictates our actions in a visible way through, for example, the quality of climate and soil; however, many subtle, multidimensional levels exist in our relationship with the environment. Places influence our actions; we give places meanings and we build emotional bonds. The environment does not reflect only people's practical and technological abilities but also our cultural and societal needs, hopes and points of interest.[27]

By place, I mean to refer to the human living and operating environment, which, in addition to the physical characteristics of the place, includes social, cultural, economic and historical features at different levels. John Agnew has presented three aspects of place: physical location,

[25] Jeff E. Malpas, *Place and Experience: A Philosophical Topography* (New York: Cambridge University Press, 1999); Barbara B. Brown and Douglas D. Perkins, "Disruptions in Place Attachment," in *Place Attachment*, ed. by Irwin Altman and Sentha M. Low (New York: Plenum, 1992), 279–304.

[26] Malpas (1999); John Agnew, "Space: Place," in *Spaces of Geographical Thought: Deconstructing Human Geography's Binaries* ed. by Paul Cloke and Ron Johnston (London: Sage, 2005), 81–96; Edvard Relph, "Place," in *Companion Encyclopedia of Geography: The Environmental and Humankind*, ed. by Ian Douglas, Richard John Hugget and Mike Robinson (London: Routledge, 1996), 906–24.

[27] Malpas (1999).

activities at the place and sense of place.[28] Places have their unique meanings. According to Tim Ingold, the experiences of people who spend time in a certain place influence the nature of the place. The sense of place is shaped by the views, sounds and scents, which in turn relate to the local activities. Our environment reflects not only the practical and technological capabilities of the community but also our culture and society, our needs, our aspirations, our preconceptions and our dreams.[29]

The connection between a place and a person becomes apparent in identity: through identity, we define ourselves, and a strong meaning given to a place may become a central part of a person's identity. The strongest place-related experiences are associated with places where a person has grown up and spent his childhood.[30] We build a relationship with our environment bodily, through sensory experiences, while moving around and through various activities.[31] Identity is built on lived experiences and on subjective feelings related to everyday knowledge, but at the same time, those experiences and feelings are anchored to wider networks of social relationship. Accompanying this are the past and the social, economic and cultural present.[32] *The environmental past* of a person consists of "places, spaces, and their properties which have served instrumentally in the satisfaction of the person's biological, psychological, social and cultural needs."[33]

The concept of *place attachment* captures aspects of place and emotional connection. Leila Scannell and Robert Gifford see place attachment as a multidimensional tripartite model with a person, psychological process and place dimensions. Personal memories and important experiences form the basis for the attachment. At the group level, it comprises the collectively shared symbolic meanings of a place among different cultures, genders and religions. Culture links its members to places through shared

[28] Agnew (2005).

[29] Tim Ingold, *The Perception of the Environment: Essays on Livelihood, Dwelling and Skill* (London: Routledge, 2000), 192.

[30] Malpas (1999), 9.

[31] Anne-Mari Forss, *Paikan estetiikka: Eletyn ja koetun ympäristön fenomenologiaa* (Helsinki: Yliopistopaino, 2007).

[32] Rose (1995); see also Maria Vittoria Giuliani and Roberta M. Feldman, "Place Attachment in a Developmental and Cultural Context," *Journal of Environmental Psychology* 13 (1993), 267–74; Shmuel Shamai, "Sense of Place: An Empirical Measurement," *Geoforum* 22 (1991), 347–58.

[33] Harold M. Proshansky, Abbe K. Fabian and Robert Kaminoff, "Place-identity: Physical World Socialization of the Self," *Journal of Environmental Psychology* 3 (1983), 59.

historical events, experiences, values and symbols, the meanings of which are transmitted to subsequent generations. Place dimension is the place itself with two levels: social and physical place attachment. People are attached to places that facilitate social relationships and group identity, but also to physical features of places that provide amenities or resources to support personal goals.[34] Places are part of personal histories: Barbara B. Brown and Douglas D. Perkins find place attachment promoting and reflecting stability, signifying long-term bonds between people and their homes and communities.[35]

Environmental trauma closely connects to environmental past and place attachment, which contribute not only to personal and collective identities, but also to human health and wellbeing. A body of research has shown how biodiversity has significant positive effects on wellbeing.[36] Biodiversity is threatened by modernization and the maintenance of a modern ethos that requires an increasing use of nature.[37] Changing conditions often cause wider environmental, cultural and social consequences and threaten our connection to our environment, affect emotional place attachment, environment-related activities and cultural identity. These disconnects, breaks and disassociations from nature cause anxiety and may affect mental health, which may also lead to impacts on physical health. If a person has a strong connection to the environment, any changes or uncertainty can lead to anxiety, distress, grief and depression.[38]

[34] Leila Scannell and Robert Gifford, "Defining Place Attachment: A Tripartite Organizing Framework," *Journal of Environmental Psychology* 30 (2010), 1–10.

[35] Brown and Perkins (1992).

[36] Marjo Tourula and Arja Rautio, *Terveyttä luonnosta* (Oulu: Thule-instituutti / Oulun yliopisto, Metsähallitus & Oulun seutu, 2014), http://www.oulu.fi/sites/default/files/content/Terveytt%C3%A4_luonnosta.pdf, retrieved on 10 March 2020; Clark et al. (2014).

[37] Klaus Eder, "The Cultural Code of Modernity and the Problem of Nature: A Critique of the Naturalistic Notion of Progress," in *Rethinking Progress*, ed. by Jeffrey Alexander and Piotr Sztompka (Boston: Unwin Hyman, 1990).

[38] Amy Kipp, Ashlee Cunsolo, Kelly Vodden, Nia King, Sean Manners and Sherilee L. Harper, "At-a-Glance: Climate Change Impacts on Health and Wellbeing in Rural and Remote Regions across Canada – A Synthesis of the Literature," *Health Promotion and Chronic Disease Prevention in Canada Research, Policy and Practice* 39:4 (2019), 122–6; Brown and Perkins (1992).

Materials and Methods

The following analysis is based on ethnographic fieldwork conducted during three different research projects in 2009–10 and 2013–18.[39] The data consist of 2 written memoirs and 82 interviews carried out with persons living along or near the Rivers Kemijoki and Iijoki in Northern Finland. The rivers run across and through sparsely populated areas, where the settlements are concentrated on riversides: the rivers formed transportation routes, provided salmon and favourable areas for small-scale farming. Local cultures in the research area have traditionally obtained their living from many different sources, as the cold climate has made the area marginal, for example, in terms of agriculture. People have relied on small-scale farming, fishing for migratory fish, reindeer herding, forestry, hunting and berry-picking for their sustenance. Through these activities, local people developed specific local knowledge about the area and created a strong relationship with their home environment.[40]

The interviewees had experienced dramatic changes to that physical, cultural and social environment. In their narratives, the informants recounted how they connect to and yet are disconnected from their environment. They distinguished the eras of war, evacuation and reconstruction. Two key experiences defined their narratives: the Lapland War (1944–45) and the postwar reconstruction work, including the damming of the northern rivers that still continues. The interviewees belonged to 2 generations: 49 of them were elderly persons (born in the 1920s, 1930s and early 1940s) and 33 belonged to a younger generation (born in the late 1940s, 1950s and 1960s). The older generation talked about their experiences during World War II and the Lapland evacuation, the era of reconstruction, and the damming of the rivers. The younger generation had no personal experiences of the war. Thirty-one of the informants were female, 51 were male. The names of the interviewees in this chapter are pseudonyms.

The interviews were recorded on audiotape and transcribed verbatim. The analysis, based on qualitative content analysis, included studying three sets of interviews and looking for descriptions of human-environment

[39] For example, Giampietro Gobo and Andrea Molle, *Doing Ethnography*, rev. ed. (London: Sage, 2017 [2008]).
[40] Outi Autti, "The Wise Salmon that Returned Home," in *Shared Lives of Humans and Animals: Animal Agency in the Global North*, ed. by Taina Syrjämaa and Tuomas Räisänen (London: Routledge, 2017), 179–91.

relationship and changes experienced in the environment.[41] In terms of this chapter, one important difference between the two river areas must be considered: when it comes to the Lapland War, the Kemijoki area, especially the surroundings of the province capital Rovaniemi, was destroyed by German troops, while Iijoki area did not suffer such war damage. I have analyzed the sources, features and experiences of environmental trauma and their connections to human-environment relationship. My aim has been to study not only the immediate, individual experiences of environmental trauma, but also the long-term effects of coping with trauma and the collective memory culture in the communities that have faced traumatic experiences.

THE RETURN TO DESTROYED HOMELANDS

As the frontline of the war moved towards the border between Finland and Norway, the refugees slowly began to return to their homes. Those who could return felt happy to be able to do so, especially after the rumours about a possible Soviet occupation of Northern Finland. "It was a common perception, and the Germans also suggested, that there would be Soviet occupation. There was a rumor that we would not return, that when you leave, you leave for good."[42]

Those who returned from Sweden noticed the difference in the standard of living. After five years of war, there was a lack of everything in Finland; after spending many months in prosperous Sweden, the change in the circumstances was prominent. "It was quite a change in the circumstances, immediately when we came to the Finnish side of the border. The food was also different from that in Sweden. We went for a meal in Tornio, and the bread was as black as bogey's shit. The rest of the food was not worth much either."[43]

The returning refugees were aware that the Germans had destroyed their home province, as they had seen photos in the newspapers and received letters from people who had returned earlier. Still, the views of

[41] Hsiu-Fang Hsieh and Sarah E. Shannon, "Three Approaches to Qualitative Content Analysis," *Qualitative Health Research* 15:9 (2005), 1277–88.

[42] Interview data LW/M/O (Lapland War, 2013–18; M=male; F=female; O=older generation; Y=younger generation).

[43] Veikko Kerätär, *Evakkoreissu*, Yläkemijoen historia, https://ylakemijoenhistoria.wordpress.com/keratar-veikko-evakkoreissu/, retrieved on 10 March 2020.

devastation were shocking: buildings burned to ashes, bridges and roads blown up.

The whole town was just a sea of pipes [...] Some stone buildings were upright, but one could see from their windows and sooty walls that they had been burned. The railway station yard was full of charred and warped carriages and other scrap. We saw people living in the cellars of burned houses [...] The bridge that had been built the previous summer had been blown up: only the stakes of the bridge poles came out of the water. The entire ferry area was full of blasted materials, exploded concrete and bridge remains. On the roof of a burnedout stone house there was a cigarette-advertising sign left, saying "Klubi will cheer you up."[44]

In his written reminiscences, Toivo Saunavaara described his return vividly, but many of the informants had difficulties finding words to communicate their experiences. Many told about the destruction of buildings and the depressing views of destroyed homes in a declarative way, not articulating their feelings. The informants at the time were children or young persons, unable to always understand all the contextual factors of events. Some informants, on the other hand, were very emotional even though the memories were hard to verbalize. Tauno, born in 1925 and who had participated in the Lapland War, started to explain how he returned home while his family was still in evacuation, but the memory of an empty, destroyed village was too much for him. He started to cry heartbreakingly and could not go on with his story.

The war had so destroyed the area that it was difficult for the returnees to identify familiar places. While Toivo Saunavaara travelled to his home village, he saw how everything had changed:

The houses [in the village] had been burned, only a few houses failed to burn. Even though we knew about the destruction, I could not even imagine the scale of the change. It seemed the scenery was not the same, nor was it, as the trees on the hill had been cut and other large trees had been felled to create a firing line. Only our food cellar had not burned down, attempts had been made to light it, but only the shelf had burned a bit. The door of the drying barn was in one piece, as it had been carried into a ditch to serve as a base for a machine gun. In the

---

[44] Toivo Saunavaara, *Muisteluksia evakkomatkasta Ruotsiin vuosina 1944–1945*, Yläkemijoen historia, https://ylakemijoenhistoria.wordpress.com/evakkomatka-ruotsiin-ts/, retrieved on 10 March 2020.

middle of the yard were the remains of a campfire with burnt iron from the spinning wheel.[45]

Service infrastructure, such as hospitals and schools, were also damaged. Liisa was 15 years old when she returned from her evacuation journey from Southern Finland. She remembered the first winter after the war, when the children went to school in cold, temporary barracks, wearing outdoor clothes during classes. The war had destroyed not only homes but also personal properties and household effects. There was also a shortage of clothes: some informants recalled wearing shoes made of paper. Reorganizing life was difficult: people cabined in small saunas or temporary bunkers where dozens of people would share small rooms. The reconstruction of new houses required inventiveness because in practice no building supplies or tools were available. Some residents had managed to hide tools and other goods before the evacuation, but many had thought it was pointless as it was not known whether they would return. Some belongings were packed and shipped to safety according to an evacuation order, but that property was seldom returned. Marja Tuominen writes that losing homes and personal belongings broke people's bond to their past. This bond, important for one's identity, is tangled with material objects and recreated in them through memories and emotions.[46]

The war had turned familiar places into an environment of danger. German troops had heavily mined the area, and despite de-mining, many accidents happened that injured or killed people. The de-mining continued until 1948, but accidents still happened up into the 1960s.[47] Wartime explosives continue to be found in the area even today. The informants remembered how they had to avoid places that had not been cleared of mines yet. Kerttu returned to her hometown of Rovaniemi when she was eight years old, but because of the mine danger the family had to live elsewhere with relatives for months. She recalled how painful it felt to look at her home area and not be able to go there.[48]

Explosives were easily found before the mine clearers had finished their work. Young boys especially played dangerous games with explosives:

[45] Saunavaara (2020).
[46] Tuominen (2015), 54.
[47] Tuominen (2015), 52.
[48] LW/F/O.

The Germans had a big warehouse in the neighborhood, so there were terribly many mines. We played with them; it was only good luck no bigger accidents occurred. We had a big shotgun shooter; it was this size [shows with his hands]. *There was a firing pin in the front, so we thought it would explode whatever it hit. But I suppose it was wet when we threw it against a pine tree* [laughs], *oh good heavens. And then there were pretty many flares from a cannon, and we shot them in the air after crafting a hole in the cartridge case and making the gunpowder look like macaroni. We set them on fire, and they exploded. Yes, we boys were in danger, and it was a wonder that we weren't hurt. I know many who were.*[49]

Focusing on work and positive things was an important way to overcome the difficult situation. There was no time for moaning and groaning: one had to get a shelter, food and income. "Everything looked so horrible, like where have we come to? and what will come of this? but the answer was just to start working."[50] By concentrating strongly on the activities instead of feelings of loss, the landscape became a taskscape.[51] Starting from a scratch was perceived as a better option than contemplating having lost everything—the returnees compared their situation to the ones who were not able to return to their homelands. When Toivo Saunavaara's family discussed their situation on the ruins of their home, the family members comforted each other by highlighting the good points, looking to the future confidently: they were able to return home, peacetime was there and with hard work their home would soon be in better shape than ever. Toivo's little brother comforted his crying mother: "We still have heaven and earth."[52]

In the middle of a demanding situation the social environment strengthened. People turned to each other and helped one another, and a sense of community and attachment became stronger between community members. Living in want also caused frictions, but all in all the common challenge united people. The home environment was still badly damaged, but the social environment recovered sooner. "It was wonderful to meet my former schoolmates and get to go to the same class with them again. That

---

[49] LW/M/O.
[50] LW/M/O.
[51] Ingold (2000), 195.
[52] Saunavaara (2020).

was a good thing, but it was shocking to see the city in such a condition, and the ruins of my own home."[53]

Social relations affected people's moods positively, and twinkles of light started to appear. Before the war, young people especially used hills, beaches and other natural sites for social gatherings, and these places were still there. Asko talked about the significance of Ounasvaara hill in Rovaniemi—a traditional place for young people's social events and get-togethers:

> Ounasvaara hill affected our spirits and moods, the traditional midsummer bonfire for example. It was a meeting place, we used to ski there in the spring, and it was a common place of memories. When we returned home, people were searching for each other, and Ounasvaara was one of the places to meet.[54]

Wartime and reconstruction affected the interviewees strongly. They felt they had lost their youth as they were not able to live the normal life of a child and a young person. "The carefree childhood of an 11-year-old boy was over, and reconstruction began. I no longer imagined that when this or that job was done, I could go play on my own as I had previously thought."[55] Young people still tried to look for opportunities to socialize with their peers or do things young people used to do. Eino was 16 when he was evacuated; he had walked the cows from his home village to Sweden with other young shepherds. Along the way, the group stayed overnight in farmhouses, and local girls had come and asked the shepherds to follow them to a nearby place where they could dance. "We did not go; we were so tired. But every now and then people tried to live a normal life."[56] Also Anna tried to do normal things. She had returned from the evacuation at the age of 16 and was anxious to get her hair done with a permanent wave. As soon as the road to the town was more or less cleared of mines, she got a lift from a local policeman, travelled to town and searched for a barrack she had heard of. She got herself her first permanent home in February 1945.[57]

---

[53] LW/F/O.
[54] LW/M/O.
[55] Saunavaara (2020).
[56] LW/M/O.
[57] LW/F/O.

RE-DESTRUCTION OF LAPLAND

During the Lapland War, the Germans had destroyed a bridge at the mouth of Kemijoki River. The rebuilding of the bridge in 1948 had a long-lasting and wide-ranging impact on the landscape and culture of Lapland because the construction included a dam and a power plant named Isohaara. Since the completion of Isohaara, a total of 17 large hydroelectric plants and 2 large water reservoirs have been constructed.[58] Damming the Kemijoki was one of the largest hydropower construction projects in Europe.[59] Harnessing the Iijoki started with the construction of the Pahkakoski power plant in 1959. In 1971, the last of the five power plants was completed.[60]

The damming caused severe damage. It radically changed the water environment and the species it had contained as well as the landscape and the usage of the river. Damming represented a deathblow to salmon migration. Many people had to give up their traditional livelihoods, such as agriculture, fishing or reindeer herding. Homes, farms and grazing grounds were left under water, power plant structures or new roads. In the worst cases, people lost both their homes and their livelihoods. However, the locals also gained many advantages: the construction work offered employment, the infrastructure and standard of living developed and new bridges and roads shortened distances.[61]

Although locals were aware of the construction plans, they could not believe that environmental change could be so dramatic. As the dammed water rose, shores, homes and villages were covered by water. Many places significant to locals were also left beneath the power plant structures and new roads. Below the dam, the river became dry, and using the river became impossible. Due to landscape changes, it was sometimes difficult to understand that the location was still the same one. The informants

[58] Suopajärvi (2001); Kemijoki: Power plants and production, https://www.kemijoki.fi/en/power-plants-and-production-2.html, retrieved on 10 March 2020.

[59] Vilkuna (1975); Hoffman (1993).

[60] Jarmo Rusanen, *Role of the Local People in the Utilization of Water Resources: A Case Study of the River Iijoki in Northern Finland* (Oulu: Pohjois-Suomen maantieteellinen seura, 1989).

[61] Autti (2013b); Timo Järvikoski, *Vesien säännöstely ja paikallisyhteisö* (Turku: Turun yliopisto, 1979); Matti Luostarinen, *A Social Geography of Hydro-Electric Power Projects in Northern Finland: Personal Spatial Identity in the Face of Environmental Changes* (Oulu: University of Oulu, 1982).

remembered lost places in detail. The places were gone, but the emotional bond with them remained strong:

There were seven houses that were left under water, my home was one of them. There were meadows, and the village road... many saunas on the riverbank. The water rose and reached the forest, and the whole landscape was lost. In terms of the scenery, it was really terrible.[62]

I was away from here almost 18 years. When I returned, I started to cry. Everything looked so horrible, you see the riverbanks were just bushes [...] Dying, something dying. It is a dying land.[63]

Over here was a fishing spot, and the log floaters' house was kind of a cultural sight. Apparently, no one has even a photo of it, it was a remarkable building. And the whole milieu, the smell of tar in it [...] it was a good place to fish for grayling. My father used to know the names of all the reefs, bigger rocks and the river neckline. Today, such places can be found nowhere.[64]

Experiencing environment is multisensory.[65] In addition to visual landscape changes, the informants also described the changes in sounds and scents. The clean, fresh scent of a free river was gone, replaced by fusty smells from a still backwater. The rivers became quiet as the rapids were no longer roaring. The changed soundscape was traumatizing, especially for people who lived near rapids; they were used to the constant roar, or singing, of the rapids, as they described it. Many interviewees reacted strongly to unexpected changes in the soundscape. When the rapids became silent, people had difficulty getting to sleep. Hannele described the sound of the rapids as her "birth music" and the river itself as the stream of life. Sudden silence struck her ears.[66] One informant compared the sudden silence to a situation where one had to learn to walk again; another compared the

---

[62] Interview data Kemijoki 2009–10, in possession of Outi Autti. KEMI/F/O.

[63] Interview data Iijoki 2009–10, in possession of Outi Autti. II/M/O.

[64] KEMI/M/Y.

[65] Vivienne Walkerdine, Aina Olsvold and Monica Rudberg, "Researching Embodiment and Intergenerational Trauma Using the Work of Davoine and Gaudilliere: History Walked in the Door," *Subjectivity* 6 (2013), 272–97, https://doi.org/10.1057/sub.2013.8; Marja Sirkkola, *Multisensory Environments in Social Care: Participation and Empowerment in Sociocultural Multisensory Work* (Hämeenlinna: HAMK, 2010).

[66] KEMI/F/O.

change to an apocalypse or a solar eclipse. For Lauri the situation was shocking:

> *The water was raised in the fall of 1971, and back then, on weekdays, I was in upper secondary school in Rovaniemi [nearby town]. It was quite shocking for me to go home when the water had risen during the week and the rapids had become silent. I was used to hearing the constant, buzzing sound of the rapids. And sometimes one could hear it inside the house too, but now it was just quiet. It was a very shocking experience for me. And it had happened while I was away. It was like learning how to exist without hearing the sound of the rapids.*[67]

The environmental change affected activities: swimming, boating and fishing became impossible or difficult. The changed riverbanks, beaches and stream conditions were described as strange, even scary. The hydropower constructor was in no hurry to fix up the environment back to being safe and accessible, so hazards arose. One's home environment had become different and odd, shores, routes and paths had disappeared. People had to get used to the changed qualities of their environment and to learn how to act in its new frames; the other option was just to concentrate on other things.

In addition to changes in the physical environment, the damming dramatically altered the environment on other levels as well. In the informants' narratives, the memories, activities, and aesthetics of the river landscape were woven into the environmental history of the area. The river was of both material and spiritual importance. A free river is a very different natural and cultural environment compared to a built one. It is aesthetic and adventurous; it is often metaphorically spoken of and it plays an important role in the wellbeing of local people. As a mental landscape, a free river is independent, powerful, dynamic and in constant motion. The informants declared sadness for the river breathing its last. They also expressed sorrow for the fate of salmon, as it reminded them of their own powerless situation.[68] The visible signs of the salmon-fishing culture and the social system around it vanished quickly from the landscape. The experiences, knowledge and skills related to fishing and other uses of the river which had earlier been shared between generations, suddenly became

---

[67] KEMI/M/Y.
[68] Autti (2017), 189.

irrelevant. This separated the worlds of the older and the younger generations and created a gap between them.

Hydropower construction and the changes to the landscape shifted agency out of the hands of the locals, and the objectives of the activities were no longer determined by them. Along with the end of many river-related activities, local peoples' participation became marginal or disappeared altogether. Strong involvement in the environment was gone and people became bystanders in their own environment. A dammed river only existed for one purpose, energy production. The role of the locals was a tiny part in the great machinery, and the new role was not as satisfactory as the previous one. Consequently, citizens' interest in the changed environment weakened as they felt they had no say nor any share in matters concerning the river. Place attachment and the feeling of belonging weakened, which had a negative impact on both personal and collective identities.[69] People turned their backs on the river that was now owned and controlled by the hydropower producer.

IMPACTS ON HEALTH AND WELLBEING

Negative, rapid environmental change can directly affect human health through diseases or contamination but also indirectly through cultural change.[70] My data revealed connections between environment and mental, social and physical health. The violation of people's home environment and sense of place was a traumatic, war-like experience. Environmental change weakened the sense of belonging significantly, and this affected the wellbeing of people.

Our environment, places and landscapes provide countless, visible and invisible links to local history, family histories, our own personal history and social networks, but also to places that no longer exist. The informants associated the feelings of longing and sadness with the memory of lost places and activities. They also associated other people's depression, melancholy, sudden heart attacks and even suicides with the change in the environment. Veli-Pekka Lehtola has studied the forced migration of

[69] Tuuli Lähdesmäki, Tuija Saresma, Kaisa Hiltunen, Saara Jäntti, Nina Sääskilahti, Antti Vallius and Kaisa Ahvenjärvi, "Fluidity and Flexibility of 'Belonging': Uses of the Concept in Contemporary Research," *Acta Sociologica* 59:3 (2016), 233–47.

[70] Clark et al. (2014).

indigenous Sami people during the Lapland War.[71] He writes that after the evacuation to the southern parts of Finland, the Sami started to "die of homesickness." Sometimes it was difficult to distinguish stomachache from homesickness. The Sami were used to the shelter of forests and fells in their homeland, and the desolation and the flat expanses of the lowlands felt oppressive.

Many informants likened the river change with war. Damming the rivers continued the traumatization that had started earlier, as the following dialogue between the interviewer and an informant shows:

Outi: *Did you miss the old environment after all these changes that the damming caused?*

Informant: *Well, we experienced lots of changes after the war, we returned from evacuation and everything was just ashes, we tried to start from scratch, so the damming was just …*

Outi: *Yes, another brick on the wall.*[72]

Those who witnessed the excavator's work and the diverting of the water from the old riverbed described these events as shocking. In general, the interviewees used strong expressions when describing the change. The words "catastrophe," "shock," "destruction" and "nightmare" were much used when describing the first feelings. Environmental change was portrayed as a deep insult that easily made those who endured the losses bitter.

Some interviewees expressed the feelings of sadness and shock, but, for many, verbalizing was difficult. Silence and denial in the data collected were the first clues to the existence of trauma. The difficult things might not have been addressed, they did not want to be remembered or it was just difficult to find words. Peter Leese writes in the introduction to this volume that mental wounds may be difficult to admit because they expose one to stigmatization. The inability to cope with the change created a silent, hidden crisis. Some informants denied that the change had any effect at all; some were in the process of adjusting through internal negotiations and justifying the change on its merits, while others depicted a deep emotional wound and bitterness that has continued to this day. In some of the interviews, heavy silence was present as a painful, primitive

---

[71] Lehtola (2015); Lehtola (2018).
[72] KEMI/F/O.

and devious means of adjustment.[73] This painstakingly overpowering effort to adapt was manifested in those who denied the loss and turned their backs on the river. They had no means, or even words, to cope with the difficult issue. Those who tried to adjust were in a better position health-wise: they had actively tried to adapt to the situation and articulate their feelings of sorrow, longing and loss.

Environmental trauma has long trails, especially when your home environment constantly reminds you of the change. In her chapter, Anna Wylegała writes about *living with the dead*, the necessity of continuing to live in places contaminated by violence. Many of my informants described how difficult it is to get rid of bitterness, when the changes are still visible in the everyday environment. Rauli said his soul is crying silently for the lost river nature: "It really broke my heart so terribly [points at his heart], and it is still broken. Many decades have passed since the river has been lost, but still it wrenches my heart so badly."[74]

After the interview, Rauli called and wanted to share more of his feelings. I have written in my research diary, "Rauli told me on the phone that environmental change has caused him heart ailments and sorrows. He said he will be sorrowful for as long as he lives."[75] Other interviewees also spoke of how the change of the river still continues to cause anger: "It was such a treasure, that river, so it is no wonder you get depressed when you go there."[76] The grief was linked not only to its starting point, the damming, but also to the long period of traumatization, the sense of injustice and the powerlessness to deal with the matter.

TRANSGENERATIONAL ASPECTS OF ENVIRONMENTAL TRAUMA

Marja Tuominen writes that wars tend to continue to exist as a psychic reality in people and cultures, even after the actual wartime. As a psychic reality, such memories can live on for generations.[77] The informants that had personally witnessed the dramatic changes often tried to protect their children; by not talking about their losses, the parents tried to ensure that

[73] Jay Winter, "Thinking about silence," in *Shadows of War: A Social History of Silence in the Twentieth Century*, ed. by Efrat Ben-Ze'ev, Ruth Ginio and Jay Winter (Cambridge: Cambridge University Press, 2010), 3–31.

[74] KEMI/M/O.

[75] Outi Autti, research diary, April 2013.

[76] KEMI/F/O.

[77] Tuominen (2003), 104–5; Tuominen (2015), 69.

the next generation would not need to mourn the same things. Similarly, in the introduction Peter Leese writes about the reluctance to articulate damaging pasts in favour of a better future. However, the younger generation was still affected, because they saw the powerlessness and sadness of their parents. The younger generation understood what the river and the fishing culture had meant to their parents. When the rich culture suddenly disappeared, they saw their parents' grief and the struggle to adapt. Environmental trauma became transgenerational in a socially mediated process.

The long trails of environmental trauma also became evident in the interviews of the members of the younger generation. Many of them reflected upon the experiences of their parents:

> *They had two focal experiences, this older generation, first the war and then the damming of the Kemijoki. The war was already a significant experience on an emotional level. And after that, a centuries-old, or even a thousands-of-years-old culture suddenly dies. It is put into the service of an effective economy, for the good of society. These people were not able to specify their experiences. It was such an insult, a violation they could never deal with.*[78]

The older generation also talked about how their parents tried to hide the severity of the wartime situations and their personal suffering from their children. During the evacuation, the informants were very young, and often perceived the challenges as adventurous. However, they nevertheless paid attention to the melancholy of their parents. Kerttu was eight years old when she returned from the evacuation journey with her family. The home site was burned down, and later their land was expropriated because of the hydropower construction. Kerttu sees that these events on their behalf caused her father's short life: "It was too hard for him, too much to take, just to see everything falling apart around him."[79]

Many interviewees linked their parents' physical illnesses to environmental change. The interviewees were very strongly influenced by such experiences at the emotional level. Juhani told of his father, who fought to get compensation money for the loss of salmon for the riverside residents. He had traveled to meet MPs and ministry officials in Helsinki, where he had suffered a heart attack. A week later, back home, he suffered another

[78] KEMI/M/Y.
[79] LW/F/O.

attack and died. Juhani considered that death a result of the loss of the salmon culture and the powerlessness it caused.[80] Tapani described how his father had ached about the environmental effects of damming the river and losing land through expropriation. He had tried to repair the environmental damage himself by digging new wells. "Yes, my old father was in a tight spot. One could see how he suffered. He was so headstrong; he said he will either dig a new well or cry and dig it. That is what he said, but he died before he saw any new wells."[81]

Martta understands environmental change caused her mother's premature death:

> *My mother suffered from it terribly* [starts crying]. *It is difficult to talk about it. Mentally, it has been an awful situation. And they had no intention to fix the damage. So, the river was dry enough for me to take the baby buggy to the other side of the river and back. That caused the death of my mother, in my opinion. She was 60 years old* [cries]. *I have understood that in some areas there were suicides. The life was so [...] shocking.*[82]

Pekka told about his father, who confronted an enormous excavator. He could see no other option but to walk in the river:

> *I remember my father, my father [...] he was [...] He was in the river, he walked in the river to stop the excavator's work. That you will not start the construction. I remember as he walked in the rapids his trousers were all wet. And he managed to stop it; in 1968 the builders had no planning permission yet, and after that my father went to the police to seek help.*[83]

In the 1950s, an unparalleled structural change began in Finland. Young people left their traditional livelihoods and moved to cities in Southern Finland or Sweden. In Northern Finland, the change was hastened by the electrification of the river, leaving the inhabitants less time to adapt.[84] The salmon fishing culture had died and modernization and mechanization reduced the need for labour. These changes created a gap

---

[80] KEMI/M/O. See also Anna Wylegała's data examples where sudden heart attacks and deaths are linked with unbearable war experiences.
[81] II/M/Y.
[82] II/F/O.
[83] II/M/Y.
[84] Järvikoski (1979); Autti (2013b).

between the generations. The older generation had grown up within the traditional system: fishing, hunting, working at logging sites and crofting. These livelihoods were taught by the parents, and they felt they were important links in the chain of generations. The older generation was prepared to teach their skills and knowledge to their children. Suddenly, the situation in the physical and cultural environment became very different and continuing with the traditional lifestyle became impossible. The life-worlds of the generations separated: "We have a fishing culture here, hundreds of years we have done dam fishing and trapping. But the world of the younger generation is different. I belong to the generation that still can fish with traps and dams, but my son does not know how to do it."[85]

The change in the society left the older generation with a feeling of uselessness: their skills and knowledge were no longer needed.[86] The younger generation was also at a crossroads. They had to find new life paths that the older generation had not taken. Their home environment was destroyed and subordinated to serving the good of the whole society. They witnessed their parents' frustration and sense of uselessness and felt rootless and ashamed of their rural background themselves. The sense of belonging was shattered for both generations. A phrase *"En ole mistään kotoisin"* was often used in the interviews. The sentence has a dual meaning: "I come from nowhere / I have no home," and "I am no good."

CONCLUSIONS

The lives of the people in the research area have traditionally been tightly entwined with nature. Their home environment has offered various meanings. The natural environment has formed a foundation for place relation: it has determined the possible livelihoods and ways of living, for example, the ways of transportation and mobility. The cultural environment—visible activities of individuals and communities that shape the environment—includes, for instance, the built environment, the cultivation and other use of land, but also the family and community histories. The value of the cultural environment is based on its temporal and spatial stratification, reflecting the cultural stages and the changes in the interaction between man and nature. In the interview data, the social environment was based particularly strongly on the chains of generations, local histories and

---

[85] II/M/Y.
[86] See Danuté Gailiené's "Case study A" of farmer V.B. in this book.

continuity, as many families had lived in the area for generations. Social relationships and cultural practices were described in a way where past and future generations were conjoined, and this strongly impacted the interviewees' perceptions of themselves, their identities and their senses of belonging.

The aesthetic environment consists largely of the visual landscape but is also multisensory. In the interviews, the soundscape and the fresh scents of the rapids were highlighted. The cognitive understanding of the diversity of the natural environment also played an important role. Some of the more intangible issues that the surrounding sites offered included the symbolic and emotional meanings, memories, importance of silence, purity of nature and open spaces. Such an environment provided stress relief and spiritual experiences. Brian W. Eisenhauer et al. refer to the category of emotional bonds as personal fulfilment, which can also be considered as part of identity formation.[87] Places can become essential in terms of emotional attachment and can be viewed as much more than a simple physical resource.

Environmental trauma in this study is connected to the importance of the home environment at many different levels. Before modernization presented the ideology of man ruling nature, the subject positions of the human-environment relationship in the study area were different. Even though the locals used natural resources for living, they considered themselves more as an extension of nature. Nature was considered to be a provider for life, and it was also given spiritual meanings.[88] This dependence and viewpoint increased the intensity of environmental trauma.

The discussed environmental changes in Northern Finland took place at the same time as the structural change in the society. A remote, sparsely populated area became a laboratory of modernity. On one hand, the developments accelerated the rise in living standards, but, on the other hand, features of the local cultural environment were lost. Moreover, those losses affected personal and social activities and hastened a cultural change, which in other more stable circumstances is usually slower and includes more friction. The rapid change in Northern Finland did not

---

[87] Brian W. Eisenhauer, Richard Krannich and Dale Blahna, "Attachments to Special Places on Public Lands: An Analysis of Activities, Reason for Attachments, and Community Connections," *Society & Natural Resources* 13 (2000), 421–41.

[88] Autti (2017).

provide enough time for adjustment, and this accelerated the process of trauma.

The findings show that place attachment is a powerful motivator for adaptation to a changing environmental and social context. Wartime destruction and environmental change caused by river damming have one significant difference that impacts the experiences and the coping with trauma. After the war, most people in Lapland were able to return to their homelands and start over in a familiar environment. Local people were strongly involved in the reconstruction work, but when it came to river damming, their position was no longer active. Environmental changes caused by hydropower production were permanent and excluded local people from their home environment, breaking or weakening their place attachment and sense of belonging. However, the experiences were not homogenous among the locals. Ville Kivimäki writes that the process of cultural trauma includes breaks and silences.[89] Peter Leese adds, "the presence and persistence of traumatic memories depends on the subsequent life-story of the teller, on the material and political conditions within which the troubled recollection returns."[90] There is rarely a shared view of experiences of trauma: in my data, some people adapted to the changed situation quickly, but for some the change and finding the words to express their experiences was still very difficult. The long trails of trauma became evident as some of the interviewees contacted me afterwards, revealing that talking about their traumatic experiences with me had activated a process of analyzing their own experiences and memories.

This chapter shows that the traumatic effects of war were not only limited to wartime and to the actual physical violence. It introduces environmental trauma as a complementary concept that is connected not only to environmental change but also to the complex, multidimensional human-environment relationship, often regarded as self-evident. The concept enables clarifications of matters that remain too loose when operating with the concept of cultural trauma. An environment-based perspective provides a different insight into the process and dynamics of trauma, while it considers individuals' diverse backgrounds, intentions and commitments to their environment. The concept constructs new meaningful sets of influences on events, structures, feelings and actions that have previously

---

[89] Ville Kivimäki, "Sodanjälkeisiä hiljaisuuksia: Kokemusten, tunteiden ja trauman historiaa," in Tuominen and Löfgren, eds (2018), 34–57.

[90] See Peter Leese's introduction in this book.

seemed disconnected. The destruction caused by the Lapland War is a shared environmental trauma which the rapid reconstruction work that changed the landscape could not compensate for. Instead, the damming of the rivers was an epilogue of destruction. The transgenerational aspect of environmental trauma adds to our understanding of how trauma is socially mediated, how it affects collective memory cultures, and how long-lasting it can be. The interviewees mourned the environmental trauma on behalf of the previous generations, and the trauma was thus passed on.[91] Experience of trauma also spreads horizontally, reaching new audiences. Along both northern rivers, most current activists demanding river restoration and the reintroduction of migratory fish, for example, have not personally ever seen the rivers free.

The change in the environment awakened the locals to seeing the value and significance of their environment, both materially and mentally. At the time however, the concern for environmental and social changes was minor. Culture and identity are difficult to include in economic and public policy issues and their loss, as well as the loss of the sense of place or community, are not easily compensated for.[92] Modernization increased material wellbeing, but technological and economic development do not compensate for all welfare. The depression, bitterness and morbidity resulting from environmental trauma reflect the value of the human environment as well as its importance as a building block of personal and collective identities. Locals gradually started to voice their views and environmental concerns as well as demands for restoration projects. Environment-related activism has improved the involvement of the locals and reinforced their place relation, sense of belonging and place attachment.

Acknowledgement I wish to thank Dr. Marjo Tourula for her contribution to this work. Our discussions are much appreciated. This work has been supported by the Academy of Finland (grant number 310855).

---

[91] On *postmemory*, see, for example, Marianne Hirsch, "The Generation of Postmemory," *Poetics Today* 29:1 (2008), 103–128.

[92] Adger et al. (2012).

CHAPTER 11

Suicide Rates as a "Social Thermometer": Reading the Traumatized History of Lithuania

Danutė Gailienė

INTRODUCTION

As Peter Leese and Mark Micale note in their introductory chapters to this volume, little has been written about the psychological aftermath of World War II, especially in Central and Eastern Europe and the Baltic States. Researchers register the strong presence of traumatic experiences, but there is inadequacy of language and other means to express and share it due to social, cultural and historical reasons.

It seems even less possible to talk about any objective indicators that might reflect the impact of historical traumas on the mental health of the society. However, after years of working in the field of suicidological research, it has become increasingly clear to me that the suicide rate of a

D. Gailienė (✉)
Institute of Psychology, Vilnius University, Vilnius, Lithuania
e-mail: danute.gailiene@fsf.vu.lt

© The Author(s), under exclusive license to Springer Nature
Switzerland AG 2022
V. Kivimäki, P. Leese (eds.), *Trauma, Experience and Narrative in Europe after World War II*, Palgrave Studies in the History of Experience, https://doi.org/10.1007/978-3-030-84663-3_11

country is precisely the indicator of the psychological state of that society. High suicide rates indicate widespread psychosocial stress and psychological pain in a country as well as few coping and assistance resources. Empirical epidemiological studies have confirmed that the dynamic of suicide prevalence in the Baltic States is well explained using Émile Durkheim's sociological theory of suicide.[1]

What does closer examination of the Lithuanian situation look like? In the twentieth century, Lithuania experienced dramatic historical and cultural shifts. An independent European state with very low suicide rates during the interwar period, Lithuania became one of the leading countries of the world in suicides in the 1990s, overtaking Hungary, the country that had long been in the lead. How is it possible to understand such a radical shift in the mental health of a society?

Upon close examination of epidemiological data, the dynamics of the Lithuanian suicide rates throughout the twentieth century read like a history textbook—all the historical breaks and traumas are reflected in the suicide rate curves (see Fig. 11.1).

Ever since the interwar period, Lithuania has undergone major historical upheavals—it lost its independence, was occupied thrice, experienced long-lasting Soviet domination and restored its independence by peaceful resistance in 1990.

As two criminal regimes of the twentieth century—the Soviet Union and Nazi Germany—divided Europe, Lithuania was passed over to the Soviet sphere of influence in September 1939. Accordingly, it was occupied by the Soviets in 1940; repression and Sovietization of the country arrived more or less immediately. In 1941, Germany and the Soviet Union went to war with each other, and the Red Army was pushed out of Lithuania by the Nazis. German occupation, including persecution of disloyal citizens and genocide of the Jews, lasted until 1944, and in the summer of that year, Lithuania was again occupied by the Soviet army. The second Soviet occupation lasted until 1990, when Lithuania declared the restoration of its independence. After that, a period of radical social transformations followed, which also proved a great challenge to individuals and society. The suicide rates perceivably dropped after 2004, when Lithuania joined the Western alliances, the EU and NATO (Fig. 11.1). Thus, Lithuania was a disrupted society—socially, politically, mentally and

---

[1] Airi Värnik, Liina-Mai Tooding, Ene Palo and Danuta Wasserman, "Suicide and Homicide: Durkheim's and Henry & Short's Theories Tested on Data from the Baltic States," *Archives of Suicide Research* 7 (2003), 51–9.

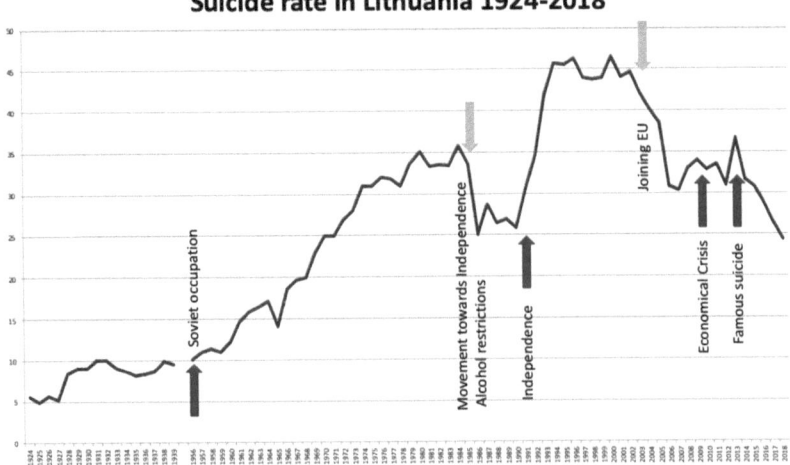

Fig. 11.1 Suicide rates in Lithuania 1924–39 and 1962–2018. (Source: Paulius Skruibis, Paper presented at the International Association for Suicide Prevention conference in Derry, 2019)

emotionally—from World War II until the early 2000s. The fluctuations in the suicide rates indicate the extent of despair and social disintegration caused by the historical trauma. However, the Lithuanian experience also demonstrates the ability of a society to overcome the effects of historical traumas.[2] Once the traumatization and the historical perturbations are over, the conditions emerge for a healing of the society; psychosocial stress decreases, and that has also been reflected in the significant decrease in suicide rates over the past 15 years.

SOCIOLOGICAL VIEW OF SUICIDE AND SUICIDE RATE AS *SOCIAL THERMOMETER*

The sociological theories of suicide provide a theoretical explanation of the association between the shifts in the society and suicide rates. For a long time, they have promoted the idea that suicide is mostly determined

[2] Danutė Gailienė, "When Culture Fails: Coping with Cultural Trauma," *Journal of Analytical Psychology* 64:4 (2019), 530–47, DOI: https://doi.org/10.1111/1468-5922.12519

by social circumstances—social, economic and cultural factors. It has been established that suicides significantly increase during times of social shifts and economic recession. Therefore, suicide rates may be considered a quantitative index, a barometer of a society's moral health.

Émile Durkheim (1858–1917), who created the classic sociological theory of suicide,[3] consistently developed the idea that the prevalence of suicide in a society is primarily determined by the social circumstances, the general moral and psychological climate in a society. In this way, the suicide rate may be considered to be a *social thermometer* that indicates the "social temperature," the mental health of the society or its groups. More specifically, according to his student, the French social philosopher Maurice Halbwachs, "the number of suicides [in a region] can be considered a sort of thermometric indicator which informs us of the condition of the mores and moral temperature of a group."[4]

Durkheim's theory indicates two forces that maintain the social order and protect society from chaos: *social integration* and *social regulation.* Social *integration* connects an individual to the society through social norms and values. Social *regulation* defines the extent to which people's aspirations and behaviors are regulated by the social norms and rules. If the balance of these social forces is optimal, suicide rates remain low. Meanwhile, if they are unbalanced, that leads to one of the following threatening conditions—either extreme individualism or anomie. The state of extreme individualism emerges due to weakened social integration and creates the conditions for *egoistic* suicide. The individual feels like he or she does not belong in a community or in social groups. This can lead to becoming depressed due to excessive individuation. Weakened social regulation, on the other hand, causes a state of anomie, or normlessness, and creates the conditions for *anomic* suicide. When a society or social group undergoes a crisis and disorganization, the rules that regulated human behavior are no longer valid, the established hierarchy of norms falls apart, and, since new traditions have not yet emerged, culture fails in its protective function; it no longer sustains the feeling of community and safety.

Besides egoistic and anomic suicide, Durkheim described two more types of suicides: altruistic and fatalistic suicides. *Altruistic* suicides are

---

[3] Émile Durkheim, *Suicide: A Study in Sociology* (New York: Free Press, 1979 [1897]).

[4] Maurice Halbwachs, *The Causes of Suicide* (London: Routledge & Kegan Paul, 1971 [1930]), 6.

caused by too much social integration, when individuation is hardly present. An individual must obey the customs, norms, traditions of the community. In earlier times, such customs were the cause of wives' suicides after the death of their husbands, or servants' of their lord. But heroic suicides (e.g., Christian martyrs, kamikaze pilots, suicides in political protest), "[…] with the spirit of renunciation and abnegation as their immediate and visible cause,"[5] and military suicides may also be attributed to this category. The last in the classification list, the *fatalistic suicide*, is not a clearly described category. It also happens under conditions of excessive social regulation, when an individual's life is too narrowly defined by norms, repressions, so much so that the person has no freedom of choice (e.g., obligatory suicides of slaves). Sometimes these two categories of suicides are not easily distinguishable.

Durkheim observes that economic crises and societal shifts, both positive and negative, increase people's suicidal tendencies, because they reduce social integration and social regulation. Durkheim's theory is often applied to explain how the processes on the social level are associated with suicide.[6]

Mortality data on Lithuanian residents have been registered according to international standards since the early 1920s.[7] Figure 11.2 shows significant fluctuations in suicide rates which coincide with periods of historical trauma: the fall of the independent state of the interwar era, the Soviet occupation and liberation from it, the radical sociopolitical transformations after the restoration of independence.

THE INTERWAR PERIOD AND THE HISTORICAL TRAUMAS DUE TO WORLD WAR II

After the fall of the empires post–World War I, independent states were emerging in Europe, and Lithuania also declared its independence on 16 February 1918. It was decided that Lithuania should be a democratic

[5] Durkheim (1979), 239.

[6] Lise Thibodeau and James Lachaud, "Impact of Economic Fluctuations on Suicide Mortality in Canada (1926–2008): Testing the Durkheim, Ginsberg, and Henry and Short Theories," *Death Studies* 40 (2016) 305–15, doi:https://doi.org/10.1080/0748118 7.2015.1133727

[7] Domantas Jasilionis, "Sociodemographic determinants of urban-rural differences in mortality in Lithuania," summary of Ph.D. thesis (Kaunas: University of Technology, Institute for Social Research, 2003).

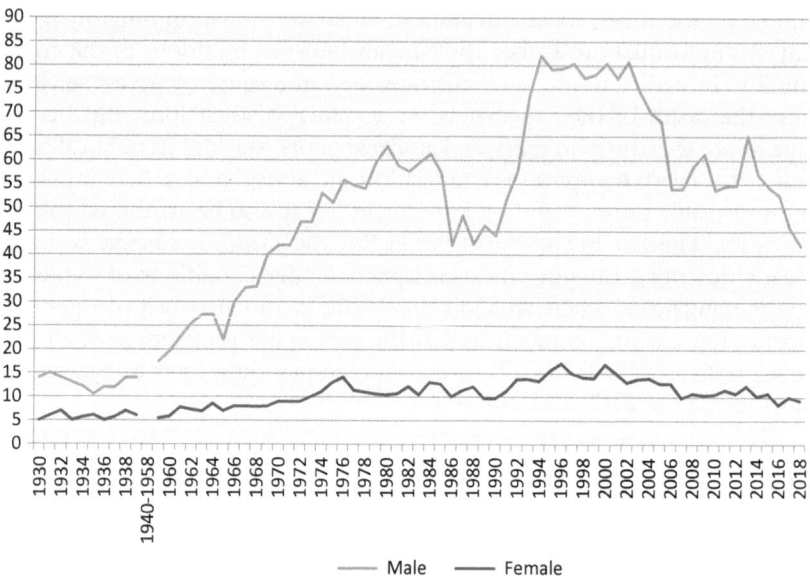

Fig. 11.2 Lithuanian male and female suicide rates over two periods—pre-war (1930–39) and postwar (1962–2018)

parliamentary republic. Over the couple of decades of independence, the country became stronger politically, economically and culturally. The "social thermometer" thus indicates the mental health of the society to have been quite strong. Suicide rates were low (Fig. 11.2), the average suicide rate for 1924–39 was 8.1 per 100,000 population. Lithuanian suicide rates were similar to those of its Catholic neighbor Poland and much lower than in Protestant Latvia and Estonia on the same Baltic coast.[8] This is typical of European countries of the period: suicide rates of Catholic countries were lower than those of Protestant ones. As he observed this tendency, Durkheim formulated his statement about the protective function of religion. He said that belonging to a religious congregation is a protective factor against suicide. According to Durkheim, Catholics are better protected than Protestants and Jews. Durkheim related it to the

---

[8] Danutė Gailienė, "Suicide in Lithuania During the Years of 1990 to 2002," *Archives of Suicide Research* 8 (2004), 389–95.

stronger social cohesion and social integration among Catholics. Like in most European countries, in Lithuania at the time, male suicide rates were twice as high as those for females (Fig. 11.2), and urban suicides were twice as prevalent as rural ones.

As World War II began in 1939, Lithuania was occupied by the Soviet Union in 1940. A year later, the Red Army was driven out by the Nazis, and in 1944, the Soviet occupation was again installed. There are no reliable data about the suicide rates during the first Soviet occupation (1940–41) and the Nazi occupation (1941–44). However, during the second Soviet occupation (1944–90), the mortality rates were registered, and it was done quite well.[9] Reliable data regarding the prevalence of suicide have been collected since 1962, but they were long classified. Researchers could only access some of the publications of demographic statistics stamped "for agency use." But they, too, did not contain detailed information and presented mortality data only in very broad strokes.[10] The reason was the Soviet propaganda that maintained that all social evils are overcome in a country of mature socialism. Therefore, the data regarding suicides, murders, work-related accidents, cases of cholera and plague were strictly forbidden and classified. This data only became accessible to researchers and to the public at the very end of the regime.

However, historical documents reveal that at the beginning of the second Soviet occupation, a lot of *resistance suicides* took place. These were suicides of guerilla fighters, and Durkheim's theory classifies such suicides as altruistic: "[…] some may doubtless be said to have yielded to altruistic motives, such as soldiers who preferred death to the humiliation of defeat […] or unhappy persons who killed themselves to prevent disgrace befalling their family."[11] As the second Soviet occupation was approaching in 1944, a rather well-organized armed resistance began in Lithuania and lasted for more than a decade. The Lithuanian population at the time had already experienced the brutal first Soviet occupation; therefore, this time they actively resisted Sovietization. Members of the resistance movement therefore avoided mobilization in the Red Army and joined instead the guerilla war against the Soviet Union. This war destroyed the Soviet propaganda myth that Lithuania joined the Soviet Union voluntarily. The

---

[9] Danuta Wasserman and Airi Värnik, "Reliability of Statistics on Violent Death and Suicide in the Former USSR, 1970–1990," *Acta Psychiatrica Scandinavica* Suppl. 394 (1998), 26–33.

[10] Jasilionis (2003).

[11] Durkheim (1979), 228

majority of the people arrested and deported to Siberia and other eastern parts of the USSR in 1945–47 were guerilla fighters, their supporters and those who evaded service in the Red Army. Family members of the guerilla fighters were also arrested and deported.

More than 20,000 guerilla fighters died. The guerilla war lasted until 1953 when the Soviet security troops captured and killed Jonas Žemaitis, the commander-in-chief of the Lithuanian guerilla fighters; but isolated resistance activities flared up for ten more years. The last member of the guerilla resistance was surrounded by the KGB and the army forces in 1965; he refused to be taken alive and shot himself. The Lithuanian guerilla fighters had sworn an official oath not to surrender alive in order not to betray their comrades. Besides, in order to protect their loved ones, they often chose suicide by explosion: "He tried to escape under the cover of his own fire, but he was wounded. He didn't want to be captured alive, so he pulled the ring of a grenade and raised it to his face. Later, thousands of Lithuanian guerilla fighters would kill themselves in this way – they would try to destroy themselves beyond recognition so that the MGB could not further persecute their loved ones."[12] The guerilla war is a very important part of Lithuanian history and historical consciousness. The example of the heroic suicides of the guerilla fighters is just as firmly rooted in the collective memory. To the guerilla fighters, the choice of suicide was a serious moral problem caused by the negative Christian attitude towards suicide on the one hand and the fact that suicide was unavoidable on the other.[13] Interestingly, in order to justify suicide, a Medieval episode of the resistance against the Teutonic Knights was employed: the fall of the legendary Pilėnai Castle.[14] This is the most prominent instance of suicide carried out by losing warriors in the history of Lithuania. It was recorded in 1393–94 in the chronicle of Wigand von Marburg (1394/1996).[15] Ever since the Romantic period, this suicide has been established in the collective imagination as a symbol of self-sacrifice in the struggle for the freedom of the country and the nation.[16] The altruistic suicides of the

---

[12] Nijolė Gaškaitė, *Pasipriešinimo istorija: 1944–1953 metai* (Vilnius: Aidai, 1997), 47.

[13] Danutė Gailienė, "Why are Suicides so Widespread in Catholic Lithuania?" *Religions* 9:3 (2018), 71, doi: https://doi.org/10.3390/rel9030071

[14] Justinas Lelešius-Grafas, *Partizanų kapeliono dienoraštis* (Kaunas: Į laisvę fondas, 2006).

[15] Vygandas Marburgietis, "Naujoji Prūsijos kronika. 1394," in *Baltų religijos ir mitologijos šaltiniai* (Vilnius: Mokslo ir enciklopedijų leidykla, 1996), 1, 458–70.

[16] Darius Baronas and Dangiras Mačiulis, *Pilėnai ir Margiris: istorija ir legenda* (Vilnius: Vilniaus Dailės akademijos leidykla, 2010).

guerilla fighters, associated with the heroic myth of Pilėnai, affected the societal consciousness and reduced the taboo towards suicide, thus weakening the prevalent Christian attitudes in a way, and legitimizing suicide. During this modern critical period in the history of Lithuania, the idea of heroic suicides re-emerges as real actions: in 1972, for instance, a self-immolation in political protest took place, as resistance against the Soviet occupation was undertaken. In 1986–90, during the period of liberation from the Soviet Union, again political actions of self-immolation or threats of self-immolation spread. At the time, suicides in the Lithuanian press were much more romanticized than in the Western European countries.[17] It later developed into a certain attitude of acceptance, especially among politicians,[18] and for a long time it became an impediment to creating a national suicide-prevention strategy.

An international study of the cultural traits of the process of suicide indicates that the psychological structure of Lithuanian suicide notes is similar to that of the participants in a political protest who self-immolated in South Korea, including traits of extreme psychological pain and helplessness and the blaming of an outside subject.[19] Even today in Lithuania, the topic of the guerilla fighters' suicides often arises in discussions about whether or not suicide is excusable.[20] Thus, the narrative of resistance suicides, including the idea that suicide may be compatible with Christianity, creates a certain attitude of heroizing and acceptance. In turn, the attitudes regarding suicide are one of the significant factors of self-destructive behavior. Another important factor that reduced the protective power of religion was the Soviet atheization politics, which reduced religious practices and the activities of religious communities.

[17] Sandor Fekete, Armin Schmidtke, Elmar Etzersdorfer and Danutė Gailienė, "Media Reports on Suicide in Hungary, Austria, Germany and Lithuania in 1981 and 1991," in *Suicide Prevention,* ed. by D. De Leo, A. Schmidtke and R. F. W. Diekstra (Dordrecht: Kluwer Academic Publishers, 1998), 145–56.

[18] Birthe Knizek, Heidi Hjelmeland, Paulius Skruibis, Reinhold Fartacek, Sandor Fekete, Danutė Gailienė, Peter Osvath, Ellinor Salander Renberg and Rudolf Rohrer, "County Council Politicians' Attitudes Toward Suicide and Suicide Prevention: A Qualitative Cross-Cultural Study," *Crisis* 29:3 (2008), 123–30.

[19] Antoon Leenaars, Danutė Gailienė, Susanne Wenckstern, Lindsey Leenaars, Jelena Trofimova, Ieva Petravičiūtė and Ben Park, "Extreme Traumatisation and Suicide Notes from Lithuania: A Thematic Analysis," *Suicidology Online* 5 (2014), 33–46.

[20] Jonas Eimontas and Danutė Gailienė, "Apie savižudybes rašančių žurnalistų požiūris į specialistų rekomendacijas ir jų laikytis palankūs ir nepalankūs veiksniai," *Psichologija: Mokslo darbai* 49 (2014), 34–43.

Later, the spread of self-destruction in the society was affected by yet another social factor associated with historical trauma: the use of alcohol as a means of overcoming psychosocial stress.

THE SOVIET OCCUPATION AND LIBERATION

The second Soviet occupation of Lithuania lasted for several decades. The totalitarian regime controlled all areas of life. Censorship, isolation from other countries, destruction of community and religious groups, a forced single ideology, the restriction of all the democratic liberties weakened and weighed upon people. The "social thermometer"—the suicide rates— indicate increasing social disintegration. These steadily grew throughout the second Soviet occupation; and they more than doubled from 16 suicides per 100,000 population in 1962 to 36 suicides in 1984. Compared to the interwar period, suicide rates in Lithuania increased nine or ten times. As we can see (Fig. 11.2), historical traumas affected men more; their suicide rates "responded" with greater sensitivity to radical psychosocial changes. The female rates varied less. During this period, the ratio of male/female suicide rates increased from two to six; thus, men were six times more likely to die of suicide in Lithuania than women.

The urban/rural rate ratio also shifted radically. Suicides became more prevalent in rural areas. Unlike in interwar Lithuania, where urban suicide rates were twice as high as rural ones, in the Soviet era suicide rates became twice as high in the country as in the city. This trend was observed in all the Eastern European countries: during the communist era, suicide ceased to be exclusively a phenomenon of the large cities and spread ever more into the countryside.[21]

Upon closer examination of historical reality, it becomes apparent that the countryside, and country men in particular, suffered from the Soviet occupation regime more than others. During the interwar period, Lithuania was an agrarian country with a traditional structure of society and family. The man was the head of his household and his family. The Soviet regime destroyed these essential foundations of male existence in no time. The most powerful men—the large farmers and their grown-up sons, teachers, priests and other educated people—were deported or went "to the woods" to become guerilla fighters; the majority of them died, and

---

[21] Ilkka Henrik Mäkinen, "Suicide mortality of Eastern European regions before and after the Communist period," *Social Science & Medicine* 63 (2006), 307–19.

the survivors remained scared and passive. In accordance with the Soviet politics of "collectivization," private property was taken away, people were forced to join "collective farms" (*kolkhoz*). There was no room for either economic or cultural initiative, to say nothing of political engagement: everything was regulated and controlled by the regime. There were no informal communities—parishes, free organizations had all been forbidden and destroyed. Ideological education of children was taken over by the state: the ideologized system of education, rather than the family, dictated the concept of history and values that the rising generation would inherit. It appears that consumption of alcohol was the only escape. This was especially true since state policy was also encouraging that. A drunk husband and his wife, who bears all the burdens of home and family by herself, became the typical image of lives lived in the Soviet villages.

After the war, alcohol became an important stress management tool. Diaries and documents of the time contain impressive testimonies regarding the spiritual state of the society and the prevalence of drinking. Sometimes historians assign the study of diaries and personal records to the sphere of the theory of history referred to as microhistory. A microhistorical view of particular historical episodes may reveal the reflections of the great social and cultural processes taking place around them.[22] From the perspective of psychological research, contemporary testimonies are much more valuable than retrospective stories or autobiographies, as they are less affected by selective memory / forgetting, self-censorship and other similar factors.

For example, here is an inscription from the diary of Lionginas Baliukevičius-Dzūkas, Dainava County guerilla leader, dated 24 March 1949,[23]

poverty all over! No sliver of hope for a nicer life. The only entertainment is samagonas [home-made liquor], *often followed by fistfights. Samagonas simply rules the village. Everyone is making and drinking it, even children. The nation is drowning in blood, tears, darkest despair, and apparently samagonas alone brings comfort and temporary peace. The idiots, criminalists* [i.e., criminals], *freaks, embezzlers, prostitutes and retards these goddamned years are going to bring Lithuania! Some say the years of the bolshevik occupation and the*

---

[22] Eligijus Raila, *Lietuvystės Mozė: Jono Basanavičiaus gyvenimo ir ligos istorija* (Vilnius: Naujasis Židinys-Aidai, 2019), 10.

[23] Lionginas Baliukevičius, *Partizano Dzūko dienoraštis. 1948 m. birželio 23 d.–1949 m. birželio 6 d* (Vilnius: LGGRTC, 2014), 112.

struggle will harden the nation. The steel will remain, they say. Maybe there will remain some like steel, the ones who melt and become hardened in this fight. But they will be few. A lot of steel will be used up in the fight. What will remain will be pieces upon pieces of rusted and bent iron, and even more than that, there will be clay. Here's the evidence. The best part of the nation is fighting and dying or ending their days in exile and prisons. The fighters are all the idealists, the most precious blossom of the nation, who fear not to lay their head down for their homeland. They fight and they die, as there is no struggle without sacrifice, just as there is no freedom without struggle and devotion. What remain are cowards, sycophants, drunkards, mindless minions of the bolshevik machine, schemers, hypocrites.

Vaišvilkas, an officer at the guerilla headquarters, also observes in his report to higher guerilla authorities regarding the moods of the residents in early 1950:[24]

As for vices of the city folk, one must emphasize that they are plentiful and mostly caused by the moods and morals of the people … One of them is drinking, which is widespread both among the intellectuals and other residents. Uncertain life in the future, loss of clear meaning of life and work, pessimist moods regarding the fate of our nation – all of that has led to the so-called life for today. People search for something to help them forget the bitter reality and drown in oblivion. They find alcohol.

Ksavera Veriankaitė, who was an underground Catholic nun,[25] also wrote in her diary on 3 March 1951,[26] "I'm all out of ideas on how to treat the Lithuanian for his intoxication. It is widespread and shoved at us at every step. If it goes on for long, whoever is not killed by the bullet or Siberia, will be finished off by drinking."

Thus, forced collectivization and almost complete destruction of private property undermined the very foundations of the villagers' existence: it severed the traditional connections of community and family, encouraged alcoholism, drove people to despair. The story of the farmer V. B. represents a rather typical tragedy of the time:

[24] Baliukevičius (2014), 197.
[25] All convents and religious institutes, monasteries and friaries were closed and forbidden under Soviet rule, only a few continued their activities in secret.
[26] Ksavera Veriankaitė, *Viskas praėjo* (Kaunas: Naujasis amžius, 2009), 134.

Case Study A

V. B.'s father was a poor villager who owned little land, and his own greatest desire in life was to have his own farm. He married a woman who was older than him and came from a rich farmers' family from whom they acquired a large farm, which they managed successfully. V. B. had a special passion for horses and loved his own very much. As the Soviet collectivization began, his farm and all of his land were confiscated, the family was allowed to stay in one part of the house while the rest was turned over to the kolkhoz. All adult family members had to "sign up" for the kolkhoz. One of his daughters tells in her memoir:

> *After the war, the Russians came over again and started taking away farm animals. They took our beautiful horses, the cows, they left just the sheep. After some time, they come into our yard with our horses. They were skinny, starving, all bones, sores on their sides. My dad came over, held the horse's head, he's crying, and the horse's tears are flowing too ... And our beautiful yard is full of cows, there's dung everywhere. Strangers in charge, cursing, walking around wherever they want. My dad is all knocked sideways. He is no longer the lord of his dream, his homestead that he worked so hard to make beautiful. If he needs to go somewhere, he must ask the brigadier for permission and for the horse. They even took his bicycle away. With all the stress, my dad's health quickly turned poor.[27]*

He started drinking a lot, developed an addiction. When drunk, he became very aggressive and violent towards his wife and children. During one of his binges, he hanged himself in the basement of his house.

The countryside was once again psychologically deprived due to the large yearly outflows of the younger population (aged 18–39) to urban areas;[28] and the people who lived in the *kolkhozes* tried to send their kids to the cities, hoping for better prospects for them, so that they wouldn't have to suffer the life of a slave in the *kolkhoz*.

In general, ideological control in every area was characteristic of life under the Soviets. There were no democratic freedoms. Studies carried out in Lithuania after regaining independence have shown that even when people felt they had some freedom of choice during the Soviet times, in some cultural areas, for example, the regime was very carefully monitoring

---

[27] Unpublished memoirs.

[28] Statistics Lithuania, Official statistics portal, retrieved from: https://osp.stat.gov.lt/ (15 February 2020).

and controlling all activities and developments.[29] The stuffy, confined atmosphere in society tended to generate a great deal of psychological stress, and the destructive results of coping with that stress—alcohol abuse, self-mutilation—grew more prevalent.

Artists generally perceive the "moral temperature" of their surrounding reality with a high degree of sensitivity. The suicides of artists are also a sign of an epoch. Understandably, creative personalities are often more sensitive people than others, but the role of social circumstances in suicide stories of the prominent Soviet Lithuanian artists appears critical—it included censorship, limited creative freedom, sensitivity to politicized judgments and alcohol as a way to reach oblivion. Laimonas Tapinas, writer and journalist, wrote a retrospective documentary book about his student times and the life paths of his fellow students, the Vilnius University Lithuanian Language and Literature class of 1962. It reveals both the atmosphere of the time and the tragic fates of prominent literary talents:

Case Study B

> *We hated the system – it's true. But it's impossible to live even in the most hateful system if all you carry is the feeling of hatred. We had to find some way to exist. [...] I've come close to the limit so many times, both physically and morally, when one breath is all out, and the next one isn't coming in. So many of us, choked by phone calls from "there," [the KGB] shocked, directly touched by the sophisticated violence, the mechanism of oppressing human beings, used all kinds of ways of evasion, afraid not for ourselves, but for the sake of others – families, friends or colleagues.[30]*

Of the small group of students of literature, maybe 20 in total, as many as 5 later took their own lives—by jumping from the balcony of their home, drowning, succumbing to fatal alcohol poisoning. Characteristic of the biographies of each are displays of their greater literary talents and creative ambition, traits of character—sensitivity, melancholy, extreme ambition, vulnerability to criticism—and evidence that they were wounded by censorship and rejection. The medical documents of artistic suicides also contain evidence of the shockingly poor state of the mental health support system.

---

[29] Arūnas Streikus, *Minties kolektyvizacija: Cenzūra sovietų Lietuvoje* (Vilnius: Naujasis židinys-aidai, 2018); Nerija Putinaitė, *Nugenėta pušis: Ateizmas kaip asmeninis apsisprendimas tarybų Lietuvoje* (Vilnius: Naujasis židinys-aidai, 2015).

[30] Laimonas Tapinas, *Prarasto laiko nebūna* (Vilnius: Alma littera, 2004), 82.

Case Study C

L. K., already well known and a very talented writer, experienced very difficult episodes of melancholy. His loved ones managed to convince him to ask for help. At the city psychiatric hospital, he was counseled by a psychiatrist. He was prescribed outpatient treatment, with medication and a follow-up appointment a month later, when he again received a new prescription of medication. There was no psychological support or psychotherapy, because, at the time, such specialists were non-existent in the healthcare system. His condition did not improve and, after some stress, it grew especially bad. The day before his suicide, his family sees his state, his great exhaustion, his depressed and suicidal thoughts, so they call an ambulance and convince him to go to the hospital. The check-up is superficial, the doctor on duty simply gives him a sedative and sends him home. That same night he kills himself.[31]

The claustrophobic atmosphere of Lithuanian society in these years was further exacerbated by a suicide of political protest in 1972: high school student Romas Kalanta immolated himself in the city of Kaunas, in protest against the occupation of Lithuania. Suicidological research has established that self-immolations are extremely rare in Western culture.[32] Self-immolations come from the Buddhist and Hindu tradition. The wave of political protest by public self-immolation first arose in Vietnam in 1963, when the Buddhist monk Thich Quang Doc immolated himself in protest against religious persecution, and at least seven other monks followed suit.

But from the 1960s on, suicides in political protest against the system also became much more frequent in the communist bloc. Even though quite a number of them have taken place, they have not attracted significant interest among researchers. One of the few historical analyses reveals that they indeed were suicides of protest—considered, meticulously prepared—and carried out after carefully choosing a symbolic location for the act and ensuring the spread of information regarding motives. In the majority of cases, the actions of the protesters consistently followed their dissident activities.[33] In 1969, the Czech student Jan Palach immolated

---

[31] Tapinas (2004).

[32] John T. Maltsberger, "Laur's Final Display: Suicide by Fire," *Suicide and Life-Threatening Behavior* 33:4 (2003), 448–51.

[33] Łukasz Kamiński, "Siwiecas, Palachas, Kalanta—suvokti nesuvokiamą," *Naujasis Židinys-Aidai* 3 (2019), 19–24.

himself in Prague in protest against the Soviet military intervention in the Prague Spring uprising; a year earlier, the Polish philosopher Ryszard Sywiec immolated himself in Warsaw in protest against the Soviet aggression in Prague and the occupation of Poland. The same year, 1968, the Ukrainian Vasyl Makuch immolated himself in the center of Kyiv. The Hungarian high school student Sándor Bauer followed the example of Jan Palach and immolated himself in 1969; in Riga, the student Ilja Rips attempted self-immolation the same year. In 1976, Oskar Brüsewitz, a pastor from the communist German Democratic Republic, immolated himself, and a couple of years later he was followed by the pastor Rolf Günter. In 1987, the Ukrainian dissident Oleksa Hirnyk and the Crimean Tatar Musa Mamut immolated themselves. In almost every case, their followers also chose the same method of suicide.[34]

After the self-immolation of Romas Kalanta, political protests in society grew much stronger, but so did the response of the regime. Suicide rates kept growing. In 1986, the Lithuanian suicide rate suddenly dropped from 36 suicides per 100,000 population to 25, that is, they decreased by nearly a third, or 31 percent. This is a special case in the history of suicidology. Such a prominent and sudden drop in the rate across the Baltic and Slavic republics of the Soviet Union has almost no match. Between 1984 and 1989, the suicide rate in the whole of the Soviet Union dropped by 34.5 percent—from 5.3 percent in Armenia to 37.9 percent in Belarus.[35] In Lithuania, the shift affected male suicides much more than female ones: the rate of male suicides dropped by 14 percent, whereas the female ones by only 1.4 percent. These years marked the beginning of *perestroika* in the Soviet Union. The processes of democratization were growing stronger. Transparency became greater, historical truths were gradually being acknowledged and anti-alcohol campaigns began. The hope of freedom grew very strong. Lithuania, followed by the other Baltic nations, replaced initial aspirations for democratization with more radical ones: for complete independence from the Soviet Union. After a few years of mighty political effort, Lithuania declared the restoration of the independent Republic in 1990, whereupon it experienced and survived the armed

---

[34] Danutė Gailienė, "Suicides in Lithuania: Sociocultural Context," in *Lithuanian Faces after Transition: Psychological Consequencies of Cultural Trauma*, ed. by Danutė Gailienė (Vilnius: Eugrimas, 2015), 198–216; Kamiński (2019), 22–4.

[35] Airi Värnik, *Suicide in the Baltic Countries and in the Former Republics of the USSR* (Stockholm: Gotab, 1997).

aggression of the Soviets on 11–13 January 1991. Finally, in the summer of 1991, Lithuanian independence was acknowledged by the international community.

THE PERIOD OF RADICAL REFORMS

The restoration of independence brought about radical social, political and economic reforms in the country. It was a great challenge. Even though the restoration of independence was a positive change, and the majority of the population enthusiastically supported it, the shifts were also associated with traumatic experiences known as *pains of transition*[36]— unemployment, inflation, loss of social status, corruption, crime and so on. The resources were lacking, not just material ones, but also the knowledge and know-how necessary for suicide prevention.

The suicide rates rose dramatically. From 1990 to 1996, suicide mortality in Lithuania grew by 82.4 percent. The suicide rate in 1996 reached nearly 47 per 100,000 population. Suicide rates for 1998–2002 remained very high (the average rate for the period is 44.6 suicides per 100,000 population), the male rates were 5–6 times higher than the female rates (Fig. 11.2).[37] Average life expectancy for men decreased to 62.5 during those years. Male suicide rates grew more than female ones (3.9 percent and 2.8 percent per year, respectively).[38]

These conditions lasted for more than ten years. In the early 1990s, Lithuanian suicide rates overtook the Hungarian ones, which had been the highest in the world for three decades. For a brief time between the "Hungarian" and the "Lithuanian" periods, Sri Lanka took the top position with 47 suicides per 100,000 population.[39]

Only in 2005 does the suicide rate begin to slowly drop. A prominent social event marking the beginning of this period is 2004, when Lithuania joined the Western alliances of the EU and NATO. For the first time in

[36] Piotr Sztompka, "Cultural Trauma: The Other Face of Social Change," *European Journal of Social Theory* 3:4 (2000), 449–66.

[37] Danutė Gailienė, "Suicide in Lithuania during the Years of 1990 to 2002," *Archives of Suicide Research* 8 (2004), 389–95.

[38] Jadvyga Petrauskienė and Ramunė Kalėdienė, "Mirtingumas dėl savižudybių Lietuvoje ir jo demografiniai, socialiniai bei teritoriniai netolygumai," *Nacionalinės sveikatos tarybos metinis pranešimas 2001* (Vilnius, 2002), 37–9.

[39] Peter Värnik, "Suicide in the World," *International Journal of Environmental Research and Public Health* 9 (2012), 760–71, doi: https://doi.org/10.3390/ijerph9030760

years, 2005 saw a suicide rate below 40 per 100,000 population. Since 2002, the average suicide rate in Lithuania has dropped by 47 percent (to 24.3 per 100,000 in 2018). Thus, the social thermometer seems to indicate that the moral health of the society is improving. The society is becoming more mature, its attitudes are shifting and adequate forms of help for people with psychological difficulties have become more available.

A quarter of a century after the restoration of the country's independence, we carried out a complex study in order to evaluate the present psychological condition of the people: how they survived the restoration of their independence and the radical transformations that followed, how their present psychological state correlates with historical experiences and subjective judgments of them.[40] The study covered a representative sample of three generations of Lithuanian citizens with varying historical experience. The oldest generation (average age 67) spent the greater part of their lives under the Soviet occupation; the middle generation (average age 47) lived both during the occupation and in independent Lithuania; and the youngest generation (average age 23) grew up in independent Lithuania. What all three groups had in common was their generally positive attitude towards the restoration of independence and the social transformations that followed. The evaluations of the youngest generation are the highest. Also, in all three generations there is a correlation between the positive attitude towards the social transformations and identification with family history. Interestingly, the historical experience of repressions as experienced within the family has had the greatest influence on the evaluation of the changes brought about by independence in the youngest generation rather than in either the middle or the oldest one. Present differences in the psychological state of the people are mostly related to personal resources, like education and subjective evaluation of one's financial situation (as opposed to objective income).[41] So, once again we see how particular epidemiological indicators sometimes record not just the extent of particular problems but allow some insights into the general moral condition of the society.

---

[40] Gailienė, ed. (2015).

[41] Rasa Bieliauskaitė, Dovilė Grigienė, Jonas Eimontas and Nerija Grigutytė, "Evaluation of Changes Brought About by Independence on Three Generations in Lithuania," in Gailienė, ed. (2015), 48–85.

CONCLUSION

Thus, the fluctuations in Lithuanian suicide rates correspond to significant historical breaking points and confirm the hypothesis of the importance of suicide rates as a social thermometer, as postulated in classic works of sociology. One might say that the fluctuations in the Lithuanian suicide rates indicate yet another "cost" of historical traumas. By destroying the stable cultural fabric of the society, such traumas create the conditions for extreme self-destruction—suicides. The destroyed social integration means the destruction of community and a loss of sociocultural support. People feel lonely and hopeless. Furthermore, some of the people feel so desperate, and even like a burden to others, that they come to see suicide as their only solution.

But the effect of the opposite processes is just as strong: the sudden radical drop in Lithuanian suicide rates in the mid-1980s, when suicides decreased by a third in a single year, coincided with the beginning of the processes of democratization and the liberation movement. Hope emerged that a better life would be possible, and once again people experienced community and togetherness.

In the Lithuanian case, the traumatization was burdensome and long-lasting: the occupations lasted for five decades. The studies of long-term effects of such traumatization are beginning to indicate that adapting to the regime was in fact more harmful psychologically than even the direct experience of repressions.[42] The increase in suicide rates indicates that the mental state of the society over those decades was constantly deteriorating, and the despair growing. The cultural attitudes about the acceptability of suicide as a possible escape emerged. The use of alcohol was also spreading as an escape method, a way of overcoming psychosocial stress. It significantly contributed to that physical self-destruction, suicide.

The Lithuanian case also indicates that the cultural attitudes and patterns stemming from historical traumas shift rather slowly and remain inert. Even today, the attitudes towards, and the stigmatization and psychiatrization of suicide are quite strong, although they are relics of the Soviet era. There also still exists a quite powerful stereotype with respect to self-sufficiency: about overcoming difficulties on one's own and feeling

[42] Danutė Gailienė, "The 'Captive Mind' Is Worse Than Repressions: Psychotraumatological Study of Historical Trauma in Lithuania," *Rocznik Antropologii Historii* 9:12 (2019), 159–76, DOI https://doi.org/10.25945/rah.2019.12.011

shame and weakness in asking for help.[43] Even today, the extent of male suicide in Lithuania can in large part be explained by the psychological patterns that emerged in the period of Soviet rural life.[44]

The Lithuanian case is also the case of overcoming historical traumas. On the one hand, we can see that the effects of such traumas are long-lasting and inert: the Lithuanian suicide rates only began decreasing more than a decade after the liberation from Soviet occupation. But we can also see that after the traumatization was over, and the democratic regime was restored, the conditions required in order to overcome the deepest psychological effects of the historical trauma emerged as well.

[43] Said Dadašev, Paulius Skruibis, Danutė Gailienė, Jolanta Latakienė and Antanas Grižas, "Too Strong? Barriers from Getting Support Before a Suicide Attempt," *Death Studies* 6 (2016), DOI: https://doi.org/10.1080/07481187.2016.1184725

[44] Domantas Jasilionis, Pavel Grigoriev, Daumantas Stumbrys and Vlada Stankūnienė, "Individual and Contextual Determinants of Male Suicide in the Post-Communist Region: The Case of Lithuania," *Population, Space and Place* 26:8 (2020), https://doi.org/10.1002/psp.2372

PART III

Coda

CHAPTER 12

Towards a History of Trauma in Central and Eastern Europe After World War II: A Coda

Mark Edele

INTRODUCTION

Central and Eastern Europe are still haunted by World War II. From Russia in the east to Germany in the west, from Finland in the north to Bulgaria in the south: everywhere the memory of this war, its violence and destruction are embedded in collective memory and, more often than not, in demography and the landscape as well. In many places in this region, history wars are raging over how to properly remember this war. More and more often, states legislate what can and cannot be said about this past.

M. Edele (✉)
School of Historical and Philosophical Studies, University of Melbourne,
Parkville, VIC, Australia
e-mail: mark.edele@unimelb.edu.au

V. Kivimäki, P. Leese (eds.), *Trauma, Experience and Narrative in
Europe after World War II*, Palgrave Studies in the History of
Experience, https://doi.org/10.1007/978-3-030-84663-3_12

World War II, then, is not just of academic interest. It is the "war that nobody can forget."[1]

That, of course, is one of the definitions of "trauma": an event that cannot be forgotten; an experience which haunts years or decades after it was lived through; a happening that cannot be laid to rest; a past that cannot become history. As Peter Leese points out in the introduction to this volume, the concept of trauma has moved from a preoccupation of specialists into everyday speech. This popularization came with a growing lack of precision. Increasingly, the term means anything that makes us uncomfortable, agitated or uneasy. As Leese writes, in the twenty-first century, trauma "is a failing concept because it has become so widely embraced, because it increasingly seems present at all time and in all places." We're all traumatized now, which devalues the concept as an analytical tool for war experience and its aftermath.

And yet, as historians of the twentieth century, we cannot do without "trauma." The wars of that terrible century left people hurt, landscapes scarred and societies wounded. The harm was physical, but it was also psychological. Survivors went prematurely grey, had nightmares, drowned their memories in drink or conspicuous consumption, spoke incessantly about this past or said nothing about it. The ubiquity of psychological harm has sparked a scholarly literature in particular about World War I and Vietnam, less so about other wars. Strikingly little is written about the psychological aftermath of the greatest conflagration of the century: World War II.

This volume is an important step towards closing this gap in the literature. It performs four moves beyond the extant body of scholarship: it transfers the study of trauma from the West to the East; it shifts it from World War I to World War II; it broadens the subject of study to include civilians; and it tries to come to grips methodologically with how

---

[1] Julie Fedor, Markku Kangaspuro, Jussi Lassila and Tatiana Zhurzhenko, eds, *War and Memory in Russia, Ukraine and Belarus* (Cham: Palgrave Macmillan, 2017). I owe the phrase that World War II was the war nobody can forget in Eastern Europe to a conversation with Shaun Walker. See also his *The Long Hangover: Putin's New Russia and the Ghosts of the Past* (Oxford: Oxford University Press, 2018). For an introduction to the wider East-European context see Ivan Torbakov, "Divisive Historical Memories: Russia and Eastern Europe," in *Confronting Memories of World War II: European and Asian Legacies*, ed. by Daniel Chirot, Gi-Wook Shin and Daniel Sneider (Seattle: University of Washington Press, 2014), 234–57.

historians can approach trauma in contexts where the discourses surrounding it are muted.

As a commentator on this volume, I come to the task somewhat from the sidelines. I am not a scholar of trauma or of Central and Eastern Europe more generally, but a historian of the Soviet World War II and of its consequences. As such, my comments are both slanted somewhat towards Soviet history and come from the sidelines of this discussion, in which I'm an observer rather than a participant.[2] My comments focus on four areas: methodological pitfalls this volume successfully avoids; the problem of unearthing trauma before the discourse of "trauma" was securely established; problematic attempts of post-war societies to deal with mass trauma (what I call "toxic therapy"); and where research could go from here.

METHODOLOGICAL PITFALLS

To begin with methodological problems, any history of psychological harm caused by war has to avoid two pitfalls. More widely appreciated is anachronism: the imposition of the investigators' own sensibilities onto past times and places. Contributors frequently comment on the problematic practice of imposing a diagnosis of Post-Traumatic Stress Disorder (PTSD) on contexts which did not know this conceptual tool. Another analytical trap, however, is equally counterproductive: the move to the other extreme, to what could be called radical historical constructivism. If people do not have a language expressing a certain experience, as the argument goes, they don't have the experience.

It is one of the theses of this volume that both anachronistic diagnoses and radical historical constructivism are untenable in the history of trauma. War caused psychological harm to people in times and places which were not equipped with the language we have today. At the same time, however, all contributors resist the temptation to simply, and rather mechanically, "apply" the concept of "PTSD." Instead, they read sources carefully, closely, and creatively to move somewhat closer to understanding the

---

[2] Mark Edele, *Soviet Veterans of the Second World War: A Popular Movement in an Authoritarian Society, 1941–1991* (Oxford: Oxford University Press, 2008); idem, *Stalin's Defectors: How Red Army Soldiers Became Hitler's Collaborators, 1941–1945* (Oxford: Oxford University Press, 2017); idem, *Stalinism at War: The Soviet Union in World War II* (London: Bloomsbury, 2021).

emotional harm World War II caused in Central and Eastern Europe. The result is both an affirmation of the experience of trauma and a demonstration of the contingent and varied ways in which the psychological distress of wartime is worked through in the aftermath. The most striking example for this contextualization is probably the phenomenon of "partisan hysteria" explored by Ana Antić, but other contributors make similar points: trauma there was, but it expressed itself in specific ways in specific post-war societies.

Trauma Before "Trauma"

The chapters assembled in this volume thus conclusively prove that there was trauma in Central and Eastern Europe after World War II despite the absence of full-blown discourses about it. "Late Stalinist society managed the aftermath of wartime violence and destruction remarkably successfully," writes Robert Dale in his contribution. "But this should not blind us to the enormous material damage, emotional dislocation, and the psychological fallout of war." Building on the path-breaking work of Benjamin Zajicek and taking issue with the radical constructivism of Catherine Merridale, Dale explains the extent to which frontline trauma could be articulated in post-war society.[3] He shows that the notion that war trauma either did not exist or was enveloped in silence is based on ignorance of the sources: both veterans and those entrusted with their care spoke about the experience, sometimes more, sometimes less, explicitly. Future research will need to come to terms with the role civilians—especially women—played in this process,[4] but also if and how non-combatants articulated their own suffering (in the Soviet Union, like elsewhere in Eastern Europe with the exception of Finland, civilian casualties far outran the military body count). What historians thus need to explore, in Antić's words, is "how narratives of psychological loss and pain were articulated indirectly – in broader cultural and public spheres."

---

[3] Catherine Merridale, "The Collective Mind: Trauma and Shell shock in Twentieth-Century Russia," *Journal of Contemporary History* 35:1 (2000), 39–55; Benjamin Zajicek, "Scientific Psychiatry in Stalin's Soviet Union: The Politics of Modern Medicine and the Struggle to Define 'Pavlovian' Psychiatry, 1939–1953," Ph.D. thesis (University of Chicago, 2009).

[4] For a starting point: Anna Krylova, "'Healers of Wounded Souls:' The Crisis of Private Life in Soviet Literature, 1944–46," *Journal of Modern History* 73:2 (2001), 307–31.

Ville Kivimäki makes a similar point. He shows how careful and creative reading of the evidence can unveil the reality of traumatic aftermaths. In what amounts to a carefully constructed "critique of the criticism of PTSD," he develops a list of "central tenets of traumatic memory" in the Finnish case, which dovetails well with Dale's observations for the Soviet equivalent: the intrusion of unwanted memories; dreams and flashbacks; various physical symptoms. Stressing experience over language, he argues, "the phenomenon of posttraumatic memory can be empirically found and studied in sources from earlier times, too."

Kivimäki's dictum that "traumatic symptoms are not simply born out of changing psychiatric paradigms and conceptualizations" could well serve as a motto for this book: other contributors make similar observations. Anna Wylegała's reconstruction of the "collective or communal trauma" suffered by communities in Eastern Galicia is particularly impressive in this respect. The multi-level assaults on groups and individuals swept up even bystanders in perpetration—"a blow to the basic tissues of social life." The violence damaged not just individuals but "the bonds attaching people to each other." Social ties were pulverized by the relentless onslaught. Instead of communities, she finds groups "of entangled individual bystanders" unable to predict who will attack whom next. All-encompassing fear and existential loneliness were central parts of this war experience—with long-lasting effects.

That few Central and Eastern European societies developed a sustained discourse about trauma in the aftermath of World War II was surely in part a result of this very ubiquity of the phenomenon. In a world where the borders between front and home front were blurred, where civilians suffered as much, often more than soldiers, where genocide was so pervasive that even those who tried to ignore it could not block it out—in such a world the boundaries of the group of trauma sufferers were so indistinct that singling out "patients" from "the population" would have been virtually impossible. Any "therapy" would have to envelop entire societies and the relations between them—an all-encompassing task.

Toxic Therapy

We learn from this book, however, that this task was in fact attempted. Sometimes implicitly, sometimes more explicitly, the contributors to this volume point to the existence of society-wide "therapies" for the psychological wounds of war. In most societies, a discourse of the war emerged which tried to unite society behind a monolithic story of heroic suffering and victory. The most famous example is the Soviet war cult, a state-sponsored complex of symbols, rituals, commemoration dates and grandiose memorial complexes, which can be read as a way to acknowledge the enormity of the suffering while channelling it into regime-stabilizing directions.[5] In Russia, this Soviet discourse has survived, purged of some of its Soviet content and ethnicized as "Russian." In Ukraine, it has been replaced, at least in part, by a new cult of the Organization of Ukrainian Nationalists (or OUN) and its military wing, the UPA—a resistance movement with a dual history of fighting against foreign occupation and violence against those not deemed of the nation (Poles, Jews, and Ukrainian "traitors" and "collaborators").[6]

Antić develops a similar diagnosis for Yugoslavia, where "narratives of collective endurance and resilience" drowned out acknowledgments of "traumatization, weakness, and suffering." Yugoslav "Black Wave" cinema of the 1960s and 1970s, as well as Serbian war novels of the 1980s were symptoms of the return of the repressed traumas of war. Finland, too, developed a post-war culture which was "post-traumatic" in nature, as Kivimäki argues.

These collective attempts at therapy, however, were toxic. Like self-medication with alcohol or other drugs, they did work to an extent, but with serious side-effects on both individuals and communities. Toxic therapy does not re-establish bonds between individuals severed by war, but further excludes many from the circle of the righteous. Like the past they try to deal with, these practices again create in-groups pitched against enemies without. Either you belong to the elect who fought the good war, or you are cast out of the community as a traitor or as an enemy. The fact that these ways to deal with the past serve real psychological needs born from traumatic war experiences makes them more than just cynical propaganda devices of those in power—although they are that, too. They are all the more toxic because they go so deep: as a collective response to the

---

[5] Suggestive: Nina Tumarkin, *The Living & the Dead: The Rise & Fall of the Cult of World War II in Russia* (New York: Basic Books, 1994), which has sparked a growing literature on the war cult and memory.

[6] Per A. Rudling, "The OUN, the UPA and the Holocaust: A Study in the Manufacturing of Historical Myths," *The Carl Beck Papers in Russian & East European Studies* No. 2107 (2011); Jared McBride, "Peasants into Perpetrators: The OUN-UPA and the Ethnic Cleansing of Volhynia, 1943–1944," *Slavic Review* 75:3 (2016), 630–54.

traumas of World War II, they are embedded in both individual and group psychology.

This diagnosis—that East Europeans suffered severely in World War II and that these traumas were addressed in toxic ways which repressed complexities and projected all guilt outwards and all virtue inwards—might well help us understand the viciousness of the "history wars" occurring in the region today. Ukraine's pivot towards the OUN has been critiqued with good reason, as has Russia's embrace of the myth of the Great Patriotic War.[7] However, both serve similar therapeutic ends in countries where the memory of that war was never adequately processed.

No matter that OUN-UPA were a minority terrorizing the majority; no matter that they collaborated with the Germans early in the war before turning against them when the new occupiers turned out to be hostile to Ukrainian statehood; no matter that they killed more civilians (including Ukrainians) than German or Soviet occupiers—at least their war story offers an escape from the unpalatable memories of all-pervasive fear, helplessness and community breakdown chronicled by Wylegała. The Russian war myth, too, allows one to repress the haunting memories of violence against one's own side, terror and callous disregard for the needs of individuals, both at the front and in the hinterland.

Other examples of toxic therapy, cited by Hana Kubátová, include the German myth of the "clean Wehrmacht" and the French "Vichy syndrome."[8] However, these myths have been under sustained attack for decades now and have increasingly lost their grip on contemporary German and French societies. In many places in Central and Eastern Europe, by contrast, they have been reasserted and re-imbedded more recently as post-Soviet societies try to make sense of not just the war but also of their post-war history and their position in the present.

Toxic therapy is not harmless. While it has important functions in post-traumatic societies, those come at serious costs both for the communities who develop them and in international relations. By not addressing feelings

---

[7] For example: Andreas Umland, "Bad History Doesn't Make Friends," *Foreign Policy*, October 25, 2016 https://foreignpolicy.com/2016/10/25/bad-history-doesnt-make-friends-kiev-ukraine-stepan-bandera/; Mark Edele, "Fighting Russia's History Wars," in my *Debates on Stalinism* (Manchester: Manchester University Press, 2020), 207–34, an earlier version of which was published in *History and Memory* 29:2 (2017), 90–124.

[8] See William John Niven, *Facing the Nazi Past: United Germany and the Legacy of the Third Reich* (London: Routledge, 2001), chapter 6; Henry Rousso, *The Vichy Syndrome: History and Memory in France since 1944* (Cambridge, MA: Harvard University Press, 1991).

of guilt, shame and horror, the communities project the feelings outwards, heightening hostility towards outsiders. We can observe this everywhere in Central and Eastern Europe today: Russians see Ukrainians as fascists, while Ukrainians see the Soviet war effort as nothing but a reoccupation by an imperialist power. Poles insist on their status as victims and prosecute historians who remind them of Polish guilt. And so on. As Kubátová writes, these practices are the opposite of accepting political responsibility for the past and hence allowing for inter- and intra-group healing. Antić's discussion of the link between the unprocessed war trauma and the wars of the Yugoslav succession is particularly suggestive in this regard. Toxic war memories—"the narrative of a victimized and suppressed nation, whose wartime suffering was further exacerbated by post-war humiliation and political weakening"—played a central role in Serbian national mobilization from the 1980s and eventually in the escalation of ethnic violence between Serbs and others. Toxic therapy has toxic consequences.

WHERE TO FROM HERE?

This volume, then, defines a distinct field of research: East European trauma in the aftermath of World War II. It is somewhat presumptuous to conclude a coda to such a field-defining book with thoughts on where research should go next: in the first instance, what needs to be done is to implement the research program sketched by the contributors. This work will take some time and will produce a little library of path-breaking monographs. Nevertheless, the temptation is too strong to think about where to go next. What new research could this volume open up beyond the field it has mapped out for itself?

First, there might be one way to deepen the investigations presented here. The contributions to this volume are case studies informed by a comparative perspective. Comparative history, of course, has recently been supplemented by what is variously called "entangled history" (*histoire croisée*), "history of transfers" (*Transfergeschichte*) or "transnational history," approaches which recently have also infiltrated histories of wars' aftermaths.[9] As Martin Crotty, Neil Diamant and I have argued elsewhere,

---

[9] For path-breaking transnational studies in the history of veterans see Julia Eichenberg, *Kämpfen für Frieden und Fürsorge: Polnische Veteranen des Ersten Weltkrieges und ihre internationalen Kontakte, 1918–1939* (Munich: Oldenbourg, 2011); and Ángel Alcalde, *War Veterans and Fascism in Interwar Europe* (Cambridge: Cambridge University Press, 2017).

however, transnational methodologies cannot replace the comparative method: whether or not a transfer of ideas, discourses, or practices took place is an empirical question; there are plenty of examples where "path dependency"—the history of a specific society—was more important than external influences.[10] Thus, the relative absence of "transfers" in this volume might simply be a reflection of historical reality. And yet, there might be moments where societies borrowed from each other. Commemorative practices and veterans' organizations are one possible field for such research. The recent trend to "legislate history" all over Central and Eastern Europe is another: legislators watch each other and imitate their solutions, sometimes with perverse results.[11] There might indeed be a history to be written on how such transfers enabled not the unification of historical memory in Central and Eastern Europe, but the pluralization of mutually exclusive historical memories dealing with a plurality of locally distinct wartime trauma.

Another profitable move would be to transfer the methods, skills and insights developed by the contributors back to World War I. The double shift this book performs—from the Western Front to the East as well as from World War I to World War II—might well have opened up the comparison to too many independent variables. It is true, as Mark Micale reminds us, that the fighting at the Western Front of World War I was stationary trench warfare affecting relatively few civilians. The same is not true, however, for the Eastern Front.[12] Not only was the war here much more often a war of movement, it also prefigured many aspects of the total warfare which, in a more extreme form, would characterize World War II. Population displacements, racial and other extreme ideologies, dreams of empire, ethnic cleansing, atrocities and brutal occupation policies were all part of the eastern war lands in World War I, as was the entanglement of conventional war with civil wars.[13]

---

[10] Martin Crotty, Neil J. Diamant and Mark Edele, *The Politics of Veteran Benefits in the Twentieth Century: A Comparative History* (Ithaca, NY: Cornell University Press, 2020).

[11] The Russian memory law was inspired, for example, by Holocaust denial legislation elsewhere.

[12] The classic military history is Norman Stone, *The Eastern Front 1914–1917* (London: Penguin, 1998 [1975]).

[13] Vejas Gabriel Liulevicius, *War Land on the Eastern Front: Culture, National Identity and German Occupation in World War I* (Cambridge: Cambridge University Press, 2000); Eric Lohr, *Nationalizing the Russian Empire: The Campaign Against Enemy Aliens During World War I* (Cambridge, MA: Harvard University Press, 2003); Peter Gatrell, *A Whole Empire*

Like World War II, but much more obviously, World War I "failed to end" when the conventional war was over; it seamlessly continued in the form of multiple civil wars which had been entangled with World War I in the East all along. This conflagration would cost many more civilian lives than military casualties—another parallel to World War II in this part of the world.[14]

Historians are only beginning to explore how East European societies dealt with the multiple traumas left behind by these years of dislocation and suffering. In the largest successor state of the Romanov Empire— Bolshevik Russia and eventually the Soviet Union—the psychological damage of the experience of war and civil war was worked through in landmarks of Soviet literature of the 1920s, such as Isaac Babel's *Red Cavalry* (1927) and Mikhail Sholokhov's *And Quiet Flows the Don* (1928–32), remarkably honest depictions of the brutality of war and civil war.[15] But scholars have also attempted to gauge the wider impact of the brutality of war and civil war on the new state and its cadres—an institutionalization not only of the techniques but arguably also of the traumas of mass violence.[16] The other successor states (Finland, Estonia, Latvia, Lithuania and Poland), and in fact Central and Eastern Europe more generally, faced similar, but in their details different experiences of war-cum-civil war and state building during this conflagration and its aftermath. Exploring the ways in which they dealt with the multiple traumas of this

Walking: Refugees in Russia During World War I (Bloomington: Indiana University Press, 2005); Joshua A. Sanborn, *Imperial Apocalypse: The Great War and the Destruction of the Russian Empire* (Oxford: Oxford University Press, 2014); Dietrich Beyrau, "Brutalization Revisited: The Case of Russia," *Journal of Contemporary History* 50:1 (2015), 15–37.

[14] Jonathan D. Smele, *The "Russian" Civil Wars, 1916–1926: Ten Years That Shook the World* (Oxford: Oxford University Press, 2015); Robert Gerwarth, *The Vanquished: Why the First World War Failed to End, 1917–1923* (London: Allan Lane, 2016); Laura Engelstein, *Russia in Flames: War, Revolution, Civil War 1914–1921* (Oxford: Oxford University Press, 2018).

[15] For more on this issue see Karen Petrone, *The Great War in Russian Memory* (Bloomington: Indiana University Press, 2011).

[16] Roger Pethybridge, "The Impact of War," in his *The Social Prelude to Stalinism* (London: Macmillan, 1974), 73–131; Sheila Fitzpatrick, "The Civil War as a Formative Experience," in *Bolshevik Culture: Experience and Order in the Russian Revolution*, ed. by Abbott Gleason, Peter Kenez and Richard Stites (Bloomington: Indiana University Press, 1985); idem, "The Legacy of the Civil War," in *Party, State, and Society in the Russian Civil War: Explorations in Social History*, ed. by William Rosenberg, Diane P. Koenker and Ronald G. Suny (Bloomington: Indiana University Press, 1989), 385–98; and Peter Holquist, *Making War, Forging Revolution: Russia's Continuum of Crisis, 1914–1921* (Cambridge, MA: Harvard University Press, 2002).

period, and the reasons many of them failed to do so adequately, could well inspire a companion volume on World War I.[17]

Such a history could be expanded further to investigate in a comparative, and ideally a global, context both the toxic and non-toxic ways in which societies have dealt with the psychological wounds of war in the twentieth century. As has been pointed out in the parallel discussion about "brutalization," Central and Eastern Europe was in many ways an extreme—and an extremely toxic—form of World War I's aftermaths. While the war "failed to end" here, it did so nearly everywhere else. Most combatants returned to civilian life and integrated well into post-war society; politics was not brutalized in most contexts.[18]

The reasons for more or less successful returns to peace and civility are complex, but it might be worth thinking anew about the differences in which society-wide "therapy" in the form of war remembrance and war cults, veterans' benefits schemes, aid to victims of war and population-wide welfare provision (and their respective absences) enabled some societies to leave more of the war behind and to accommodate this traumatic past in a working compromise with the present.

Although far from the only, and not always the most important, actors, historians play a crucial role in these processes. This points towards activism: to what extent, and with what means and tactics, can historians help replace the toxic therapies which have taken hold of societies in Central and Eastern Europe with more constructive approaches that allow not only healing but also prevent a slide into confrontation with other post-trauma societies? I must say that, given what is happening nearly everywhere today, I do not harbour great optimism. But that historians should try to make their voices heard is indisputable. This volume makes an important contribution to this quest.

Acknowledgment Work on this chapter was funded in part by Australian Research Council Discovery Project DP200101777 "Aftermaths of War."

---

[17] On Finland: Pertti Haapala and Marko Tikka, "Revolution, Civil War, and Terror in Finland in 1918," in *War in Peace: Paramilitary Violence in Europe after the Great War*, ed. by Robert Gerwarth and John Horne (Oxford: Oxford University Press, 2013), 72–84; on Ukraine: George O. Liber, *Total Wars and the Making of Modern Ukraine, 1914–1954* (Toronto: University of Toronto Press, 2016). For the political context in Poland, Czechoslovakia, Hungary, Romania, Bulgaria, Yugoslavia, and Albania, see Sabrine P. Ramet, ed., *Interwar East Central Europe, 1918–1941: The Failure of Democracy-building, the Fate of Minorities* (Abingdon: Routledge, 2020).

[18] Mark Edele and Robert Gerwarth, eds, "The Limits of Demobilisation," special issue of *Journal of Contemporary History* 50:1 (2015).

INDEX[1]

A

Alcohol, 70, 76, 101, 135, 308–310, 312, 317, 326

Alexander, Jeffrey, 36, 50, 50n49, 147, 153, 173, 174, 274

Autobiography, 234, 237, 245, 249–250n53, 253, 255, 258, 260n88, 261, 265, 309

Avoidance strategies, 210, 212, 213, 218, 220–222

B

Bloodlands (Snyder), 35

Brutality, 134, 156, 192, 256, 330

C

Cannon, Walter, 12

Central and Eastern Europe, vi, 4, 5, 13, 22, 34, 35, 37, 42–44, 48, 50–52, 50n48, 93, 122, 123, 154, 162, 165, 175, 176, 178, 299, 321–331

Child psychology, 151, 160, 163, 175, 176

Children, 8, 9, 13, 18, 24, 30, 38, 39, 45–47, 63, 64, 76, 110, 124–126, 128, 130, 131, 133, 135, 136, 139–142, 149–176, 178, 189, 191, 204, 218, 254, 260, 282, 283, 285, 291, 292, 294, 309, 311

psychologists, 149–151, 151n5, 152n10, 157, 161, 173, 175, 176

Civilian, 7–9, 12, 30, 33, 35, 37–42, 46, 50, 56, 63, 64, 79, 82, 103, 110, 116, 119–124, 128, 129, 134, 142, 177, 179, 185, 188, 196, 198–200, 202, 203, 205, 245, 256, 268, 269, 322, 324, 325, 327, 329–331

[1] Note: Page numbers followed by 'n' refer to notes.

© The Author(s), under exclusive license to Springer Nature Switzerland AG 2022
V. Kivimäki, P. Leese (eds.), *Trauma, Experience and Narrative in Europe after World War II*, Palgrave Studies in the History of Experience, https://doi.org/10.1007/978-3-030-84663-3

Combat fatigue, 11
Commemoration, 5, 6, 9, 14, 25, 26,
    201, 205, 210, 326
  involuntary, 9, 26
Comparative methodology, 329
Concussion, 59, 67, 69, 71, 73, 78,
    80, 81, 84, 85

D
Death
  proximity to, 122, 123, 130
  reactions to, 130, 173
Disability, 69, 83
Displaced children, 9, 144
Dreams, 18, 77, 92, 96, 97, 97n22,
    102–109, 111–113, 117, 135,
    181, 188, 197, 247, 256, 278,
    311, 325, 329

E
Eastern Galicia, 119–148, 211, 325
Eco-anxiety, 276
Education, 4, 19, 48, 65, 80, 152,
    156–161, 175, 185–187, 245,
    254, 309, 316
Ego-documents, 150, 212
Emotional communities, 6
Emotions, 6, 7, 14–19, 48, 112, 115,
    141, 144, 146, 167, 191, 210,
    212, 218, 221, 222, 226, 234,
    248, 251, 255, 256, 261, 283
Environment
  change, 270, 272, 275, 276, 286,
    288–293, 295, 296
  health and wellbeing, 276, 277,
    279, 288–291
Ethnic cleansing, 42, 119–149,
    211, 329
Experience, v–vii, 3–26, 32, 34–45,
    48, 55, 57, 58, 60–62, 64, 65,
    68, 70–72, 74, 75, 77, 78, 81,

83, 85–87, 91–93, 96–98,
    100–103, 105–117, 121, 123,
    132–136, 141, 146, 150, 151,
    153n14, 155, 157, 158, 161,
    163, 164, 166–169, 166n73,
    172, 174, 175, 178–181,
    179n3, 189, 191, 196,
    199–203, 205, 208, 210, 211,
    220–222, 226, 227–228n74,
    231, 234, 235, 238, 239,
    243–254, 245n39, 257, 259,
    264–266, 270, 272, 274–276,
    278–282, 288, 289, 292,
    295–297, 301, 316, 317,
    322–326, 330
  traumatic, vi, vii, 18, 19, 29, 58, 62,
    64, 75, 76, 80–82, 87, 94, 97,
    100, 101, 104, 106, 107, 109,
    111–117, 141, 142, 146, 150,
    165, 186, 196, 211, 261, 276,
    281, 296, 299, 315

F
Fatigue, 11, 70, 76, 180, 249
  pilots, 70
Fiction
  "Columbuses: Born 1920"
    (*Kolumbowie: Rocznik* 1920),
    234, 235, 261
  "The Stones for the Rampart"
    (*Kamienie na szaniec*, 1943),
    234, 235, 241
  The Unknown Soldier (Linna, 1954),
    109, 111n61
Film
  "Eyes in the Dark" (Silmät
    hämärässä, 1952), 110,
    111, 113n68
  "Heroes" (Delije, 1968), 186, 187,
    194, 195n34, 198
  Lazar (1984), 201
  "Moment" (Tren, 1978), 199

"Our Children" (Undzere Kinder, 1948), 164, 164n63
"The Shop on Main Street" (Obchod na korze, 1965), 207, 211, 213, 222, 224, 230, 231
Yugoslav "Black Wave," 182, 190, 198, 326
Flashbacks, 89–117, 198, 325
Fulbrook, Mary, 219

G
Guilt, 4, 48, 113, 147, 157, 165, 174, 201, 207–231, 327, 328

H
Historiography, 10, 50, 56, 59, 60, 142, 202, 219
History of emotions, 6
Holocaust, 15, 20, 27, 42, 45, 93, 120–123, 126, 128, 139, 140, 142, 164, 164n63, 169n81, 207–209, 211–214, 217–220, 222, 224, 225, 227–231
Human rights, 4, 42
Hydropower, 270, 286, 288, 289, 292, 296

I
Indigenous peoples, 13, 20

L
Lapland War (1944–45), 269, 280–282, 286, 290, 297

M
Masculinity, 29, 59, 74, 80
Memory
  flashback, 97, 106

generations, 24
Holocaust, 15, 213
1989, 8
traumatic, 4–10, 12–18, 21, 23–25, 31, 51, 63, 64, 77, 90, 92, 94–103, 106, 108, 174, 181, 187, 201–204, 262, 296
violence, 142
Mental disorders/breakdown, 63, 74, 78, 90, 92, 94, 95, 95n17, 98, 134, 252
Merridale, Catherine, 57, 60, 61, 177, 178, 324
Methodology, vi, 19, 22, 23, 329
Military psychiatry, 35, 55–87, 97–102

N
Narrative
  environmental, 267–297
  storytelling, 16, 18
  strategies, 172, 253

O
Orphans, 154n20, 159, 162, 164n65, 167, 168, 171, 175

P
"Partisan Neurosis," 22, 183, 184, 186, 187, 189
Patient files, 96, 96n19, 99–102
Perpetrator/perpetrators, 3, 4, 9, 33, 49, 114, 121–123, 132, 139, 140, 143, 144, 146, 156, 157, 198–204, 211, 218, 224, 249
Place attachment, 272, 277–279, 289, 296, 297
Politics of War Trauma, 23, 46n37

Posttraumatic stress disorder (PTSD), 12, 15, 20, 30, 34, 44, 45, 48, 49, 61, 89–93, 98, 102, 106, 114, 116, 116n78, 261, 273, 323, 325

Psychiatrists/psychiatry, 12, 31, 35, 36, 45, 47, 55–87, 90–92, 94, 95, 95n17, 97–103, 105, 114n71, 152, 160, 179–181, 183–187, 212, 259, 313

Public discourse, v, 8, 43, 59, 93, 169, 175, 186, 201, 235, 236, 243–246, 261

R

Recognition, 6, 8, 9, 12, 13, 15, 23–26, 80, 95, 95n17, 184, 187, 306

Recovery and reconciliation, 24

Red Army, 55–57, 59–61, 65, 66, 74, 80, 94, 103, 104, 121, 150–151, 169, 181, 300, 305, 306

Reminiscences, 14, 33, 77, 96, 97, 103, 107–109, 111–113, 250, 282

Resilience, 15, 16, 21, 22, 33, 56, 66, 71, 78, 84, 178, 326

Resistance, 8, 33, 39, 44, 180, 193–195, 199, 209–211, 213, 215, 216, 218, 222, 228–230, 234–236, 238–247, 251, 253–256, 259, 262, 263, 300, 305–307, 326

Responsibility, 95, 155–158, 183, 199–201, 203, 207–231, 257, 275, 276, 328

Revolution, 188–198, 200

S

Shell shock, 27–32, 34, 36, 38, 40, 41, 41n28, 41n29, 44, 46, 47, 50, 51, 60, 68, 78, 81, 111, 115n72, 177, 180

Shock, v, 11, 12, 33, 34, 48, 57, 67, 101, 115, 130, 217, 256, 259, 269, 290

Silence
public, 143
relative, 58

Slovakia, vi, 32, 126, 143, 207–231
National Uprising (1944), 209, 213, 215, 225

Socialism, 66, 200, 305

Soundscape, 287, 295

Soviet occupation, 34, 46, 169, 233–234, 268, 281, 300, 303, 305, 307–310, 316, 318

Soviet Union
psychiatry, 62, 63, 66, 68, 74, 86
society, 57, 63, 86, 87

Suicide
Durkheim's theory, 303, 305
heroic, 303, 306, 307
political, 303, 313
rates, 18, 299–318

Symptoms, 6, 12, 20, 28–30, 34, 46, 57, 64, 67, 72, 81, 90–93, 95–102, 106–109, 113, 114, 116, 134, 162n56, 185, 221, 260n86, 273, 325, 326
psychosomatic, 101, 146

T

Testimony, 23, 137, 212, 215, 225, 227, 309
Jewish, 121, 227

Trauma
bystander, 119–148
collective, 18, 58, 119, 136–141, 146, 147, 173, 203, 259, 274, 325, 326
communal, 136–141, 147, 211, 221, 230, 231, 325
cultural, v, 18, 50, 115, 147, 157, 259, 273–275, 296

environmental, 267
generations, 6
historical, v–vii, 20, 21, 30, 32, 52,
    91, 299, 301, 303–308,
    317, 318
individual, 58, 119, 259, 274
national, 201–205
perpetrator, 49, 113, 233–266
psychological, 19, 27, 30, 40, 48,
    50, 56, 57, 59–61, 64, 85, 86,
    130–135, 140, 142, 144, 146,
    147, 154, 177–179, 179n3,
    197, 273
second generation, 217
social, 50
toxic, 327

V
Veterans, 9, 12, 18, 20, 29–31, 46,
    50, 55–57, 59–63, 74, 75, 77–83,
    85–87, 95, 96, 103–105, 107,
    108n55, 109, 111, 116, 175,
    177, 196, 233–266, 324, 328n9,
    329, 331
"Vichy syndrome," 219, 327
Victimhood, 107, 113, 150,
    153, 157, 165, 174, 177, 178,
    204, 218
  heroic, 211, 224
"Voodoo Death," 12

W
War neurosis, 30, 34, 95, 180, 182,
    183, 185
World War One, 12, 28, 31, 36, 38,
    40, 41, 43, 51, 60, 68, 94, 223,
    322, 330, 331
  Western Front, 27, 32, 37, 329
World War Two
  deaths and casualties, 38
  Eastern Front, 32, 239
  Slovak participation, 223